ALTERNATIVE
HEALTH CARE

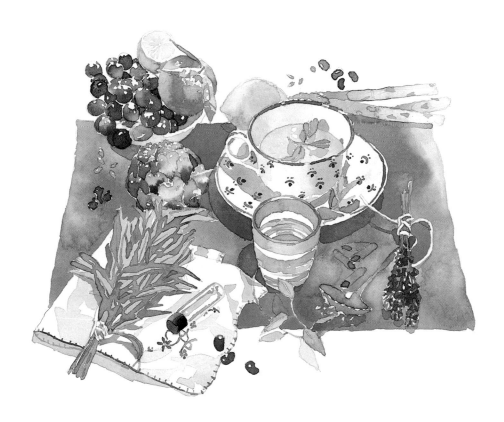

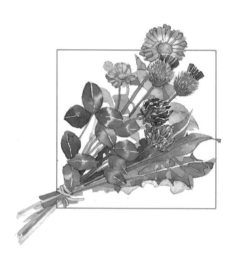

THE FAMILY GUIDE TO
ALTERNATIVE HEALTH CARE

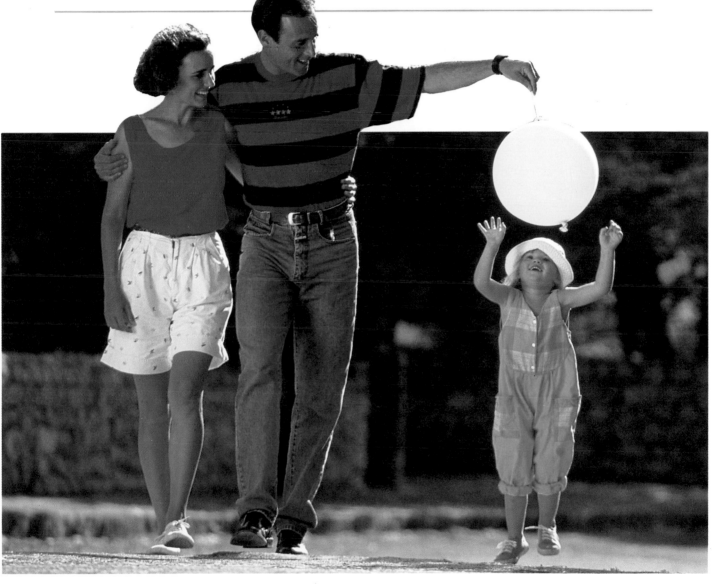

PROFESSOR PATRICK PIETRONI
FRCGP, MRCP, DCH

CLB

Colour Library Books Ltd

CLB 4097
©1995 CLB Publishing Ltd,
Woolsack Way,
Godalming,
Surrey GU7 1XW,
UK

ISBN 1-85833-484-5

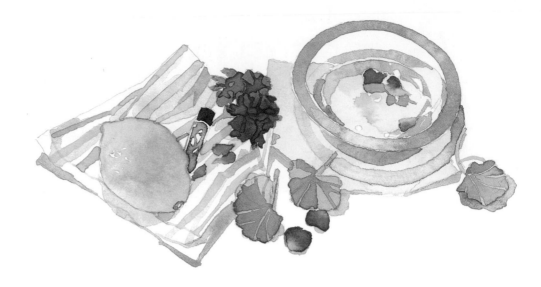

CREDITS

Editor
Philip de Ste. Croix

Designer
Jill Coote

Design concept
Roger Hyde

Colour artwork
Nicola Gregory
Lawrie Taylor

Index
Richard O'Neill

Production
Ruth Arthur
Sally Connolly
Neil Randles
Karen Staff
Jonathan Tickner

Director of production
Gerald Hughes

Typesetting
SX Composing Ltd, Essex

Colour reproduction
Advance Laser Graphic Arts, Hong Kong

Printed and bound in Hong Kong
C and C Offset Printing

AUTHOR'S ACKNOWLEDGMENTS

This book is the result of countless "clinical trials" carried out by practitioners on their patients: both groups require thanks and praise. Some of the results of these "experiments" have been collected together in separate books and their coming together in one volume is an indication of the interest in this subject and a need for an accessible *vade mecum* for the ordinary reader. I would like to acknowledge the work of others in this area from whom some of the material is obtained. I am thinking of Simon Mills, Jackie Young, Rudolph Ballentyne, George Lewith, Roger Hills, Robin Monro, and I am sure there are others whose knowledge and experience surface in different sections. Leon Chaitow, Jan de Vries and David Peters were all generous with their time and advice. The first aid section was written by Leon Chaitow. Throughout the process of assembling the material, Philip de Ste. Croix, my editor, was painstaking in his advice, support and patience. The final product is as much due to his imaginative flair as anyone's. As always, Moira Jenkins held my hand, corrected the drafts and ensured this book's emergence. A final thanks to the beauty of the French countryside where work was pleasure.

The information and recommendations in this book are not intended to substitute for the diagnosis and care of a qualified physician, nor to encourage the treatment of illness by persons not recognizably qualified.

If you are under medical care for any condition, seek the advice of your doctor before acting on any of the suggestions in the book. Do not make adjustments to any prescribed medication without the approval of your doctor. Any application of the recommendations and techniques described in this book is at the discretion and sole risk of the reader. Neither the authors nor the publisher can be held responsible for the inappropriate use of any remedy or therapy described herein.

THE AUTHOR

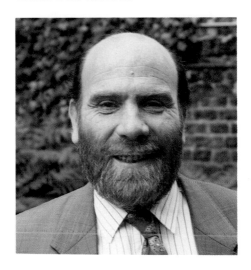

Professor Patrick Pietroni, FRCGP, MRCP, DCH, is Visiting Professor and Director of the Centre for Community Care and Primary Health at the University of Westminster in London. He is also Principal of Marylebone Health Centre, a National Health Service health centre which, as part of a research project, incorporates complementary therapies and education and self-help programmes within its curriculum of care. As a result of its research work, Marylebone Centre Trust was set up in 1988 to develop education and training programmes with the aim of encouraging similar models of health care within the NHS.

Professor Pietroni was formerly a Council Member of the Royal College of General Practitioners, a member of the Medicines Commission and was a founder member and past-Chairman of the British Holistic Medical Association, which was set up in 1983. He was also formerly Senior Lecturer in General Practice at St. Mary's Hospital Medical School in London.

Professor Pietroni has practised acupuncture and homeopathy for more than 15 years, has taught Yoga, and has lectured widely on the topic of alternative medicine. He is also a practising Jungian analyst. He is the author of *Holistic Living* (1986), *The Greening of Medicine* (1990) and was the Consultant Editor on both the *Reader's Digest Family Guide to Alternative Medicine* (1991) and the partwork *"Natural Choice"* which was published by Orbis in 1988-89.

EDITORIAL CONSULTANTS

Leon Chaitow
Leon Chaitow is a qualified naturopath, acupuncturist, osteopath and chiropractor, who has been working in the field of alternative medicine for more than 30 years. He lectures widely on the subject to academic institutions and training schools in the UK, Israel and the USA, and is a senior faculty member of the Centre for Community Care and Primary Health at the University of Westminster, London. He is currently Editor of the "International Journal of Alternative and Complementary Medicine", having previously been its consultant Editor between 1983 and 1991. He has written some 40 books on health and medical matters, and was recently a contributor to and Medical Editor of *Alternative Medicine – The Definitive Guide* (1994). Mr. Chaitow contributed the section on complementary first aid to this book.

Dr. David Peters
Dr. David Peters qualified in medicine in 1973 and is now a clinician/ researcher at the Marylebone Health Centre in London, and a senior lecturer in complementary therapy studies at the Centre for Community Care and Primary Health at the University of Westminster, London. He also holds qualifications in the disciplines of osteopathy, orthopaedic medicine, obstetrics and gynaecology, massage, acupuncture and homeopathy, and was Chairman of the British Holistic Medical Association between 1990 and 1995. He has published widely on the subject of alternative medicine and holistic health care, both in the form of papers for specialized journals and books for the general reader.

Jan de Vries
Born in Holland, Jan de Vries initially qualified as a pharmacist. A meeting with the famous Swiss naturopath, Dr. Alfred Vogel, opened his eyes to alternative methods of treating illness, and he subsequently studied homeopathy and phytotherapy with Vogel in Switzerland. Further studies mean that he is also fully qualified in the fields of naturopathy, homeopathy, osteopathy and acupuncture. In 1970 he established his first residential clinic in Troon on the Scottish coast, and he now runs seven such clinics – six in Great Britain and one in Holland. He is the author of many books on alternative medicine including 14 titles in the "By Appointment Only" series, and broadcasts regularly on national radio in the UK about complementary therapies and health.

C O N T

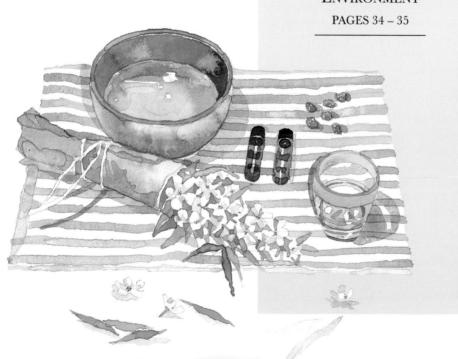

E N T S

INTRODUCTION

Health and the quest for a healthy lifestyle are among the abiding preoccupations of modern times. Increasingly, however, the general public is looking askance at orthodox medical practitioners; all too often doctors can seem remote figures, with little time to lend a sympathetic ear, and overly quick to prescribe a course of drugs to bring a consultation to a rapid conclusion. As a reaction to this, widespread and growing interest in the use of alternative medicine and complementary healing therapies is now apparent around the globe.

With this increasing interest, an understandable wish has developed for more accurate information to become available on the therapies themselves and for what purposes they can and cannot be used. At the same time, it has been important for alternative practitioners to address the requirements of professional practice. Many governments around the world have supported this developing interest in alternative therapy but have asked that these therapies should put their houses in order. This has required the establishment of proper education and training programmes for people wishing to qualify as practitioners, with regular review and accreditation procedures.

Part of the confusion arising from the term "alternative therapies" is that it is unclear what it covers and, indeed, "alternative medicine" is a very difficult term to define. Other phrases, such as complementary,

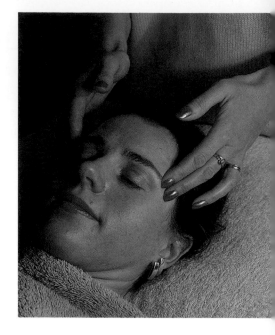

Above: *Many alternative therapies involve touch and physical closeness; healer and patient are thus in direct contact with one another.*

Below: *The high-tech nature of much orthodox medicine today can seem offputting; machines stand between physician and patient.*

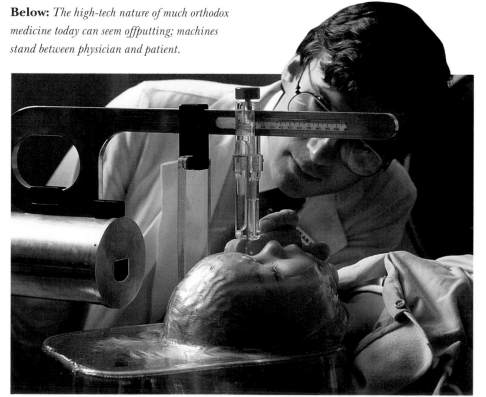

holistic, natural and fringe medicine, are often used as if they are interchangeable with the word "alternative", and under this umbrella vastly different activities and therapies are undertaken. Osteopathy and chiropractic, both requiring an extended course of full-time training as arduous as that required in orthodox medicine, are thus linked with gem therapy and kinesiology, which can be learned in a few weekend seminars. It is not surprising, therefore, that much confusion arises as to what actually constitutes alternative medicine, and whether or not the therapies described as alternative are safe and effective.

The term "complementary medicine" is preferred by many as it suggests a more co-operative and collaborative relationship with orthodox medicine. The former is seen as complementing the latter. Indeed, we are witnessing an ever increasing interest in all aspects of alternative medicine by the medical profession and patients alike. The reasons for this are many, and not least is the concern many patients have of the increasingly technical nature of modern medicine, the horrific stories of damage done by over-prescribing and the perceived coldness and aloofness of modern medical graduates. It is important to remember that every society has several approaches to health care which lie outside the professional form of medical care. Alternative medicine can be seen as a combination of folk-care and self-care, and as such is a very necessary part of the overall approach to managing sickness. It is becoming clear that the increasing cost of modern medicine will inevitably force more and more people to turn to systems of

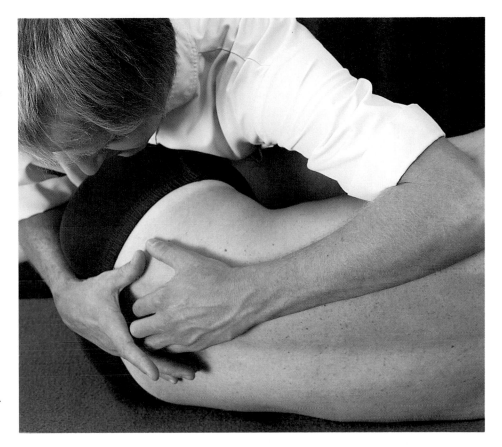

Above: *Many people first encounter an alternative practitioner when they seek relief from back pain. Here an osteopath examines a patient's spine.*

Below: *Holistic medicine ministers to the whole person – mind, body and spirit; healing has a spiritual, as well as a physical, dimension.*

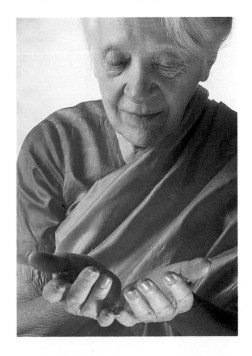

treatment which are simple, effective and a lot less expensive than conventional medical care is today.

Numerous surveys in Europe and the USA all indicate a rapid growth in the number of people using complementary therapies. The British Medical Association undertook a report on alternative therapies in 1989 and more recently 1992. Although somewhat negative in its overall findings, the first report identified certain factors which were felt to be common to a number of alternative therapies and which were acknowledged as important to the patient. These factors were:

▪ *Time* Alternative practitioners were able to offer patients more time to listen – the complaint that doctors were "too busy" was heard over and over again.

▪ *Compassion* As well as being given time, patients felt alternative practitioners were more caring and concerned. They treated the "whole person" and not just the disease.

▪ *Touch* In many of the alternative therapies, touch is used, e.g. massage, reflexology, osteopathy, acupressure (shiatsu), laying-on-of-hands. This very fundamental method of communicating healing was thought by the BMA to contrast with the high technology of modern medicine which got in the way of the doctor and patient.

▪ *Authority and charisma* As medicine had become familar, it seemed important to patients to seek out practitioners who appeared "magical". Many of the alternative therapies, with their strange words and unfamiliar practices, conveyed the atmosphere of a magical cult which was a very powerful healing force.

Many doctors and scientists, while willing to accept the increasing popularity of alternative therapies, are concerned that several of the claims made by practitioners of these therapies are unsubstantiated and difficult to prove. Partly this may be because the sorts of problems regularly seen by alternative practitioners are episodic (they relapse and recur naturally) and are non-life-threatening. Scientists are unable to find clear evidence of a *scientific* kind to prove, for instance, that acupuncture works in the case of asthma or that homeopathy helps psoriasis. They also feel that to conduct such studies would be difficult and costly.

It is this accusation of being unscientific and using unproven treatments which is the major complaint that is levelled at alternative medicine by doctors, and it must be acknowledged that alternative practitioners have, for the most part, failed to undertake the sort of studies that would reveal whether or not their therapies work. It is undoubtedly important for us to

know whether acupuncture actually is effective in the treatment of asthma, or whether patients who have psoriasis would do better with homeopathy as opposed to herbal medicine. To be able to decide which of two treatments for a similar condition is the more effective is one of the most important questions in clinical practice. Far too many treatments are undertaken where inadequate proof exists that they are effective.

Where these treatments are expensive and dangerous, it is even more important that they should be subjected to clinical trials. Because the majority of alternative medicine focuses on non-life-threatening conditions, and because most of the therapies have few, if any, side effects, very few of them have been properly studied. Fortunately, the situation is now changing and there are good scientific studies now demonstrating the effectiveness of

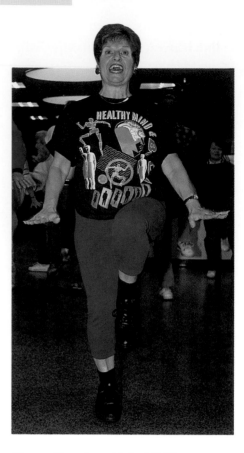

Above: *Bouncing with health? There is no doubt that, whatever your age, a sensible regime of exercise increases your sense of well-being.*

Below: *A healthy diet does not have to be boring, nor need it be difficult to prepare – nature's store of wholesome foods is abundant.*

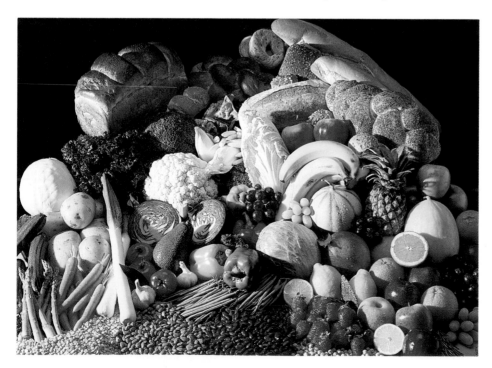

homeopathy in relieving the symptoms of hay fever, or osteopathy in the management of back pain, or acupuncture in the treatment of musculo-skeletal pain. Such studies serve both to protect the public and enhance the acceptance of these therapies by the medical community and should be encouraged by everyone concerned with health care.

Newly established research bodies have also striven to give this developing field of medicine a level of respectability and authority. Standards of education and training have been established, and regulations regarding registration and a code of conduct for practice thereafter are now in place for many of the major therapies.

Many surveys of alternative therapies suggest that the main reasons for people seeking help are related to *relief of symptoms* (mostly pain) from musculo-skeletal disorders and *relief of emotional distress* without recourse to tranquillizers. This practical guide to alternative therapies is offered to the reader with the intention that it should provide information that will enable you to make use of many alternative approaches to a wide variety of both serious and not-so-serious conditions. The emphasis is on safe, easy-to-use approaches which can be undertaken at home, together with self-help programmes to improve well-being. For serious conditions where self-help approaches are not appropriate, information is given as to how alternative remedies can be applied under the guidance of a trained therapist.

The structure of the book is quite straightforward. Part One addresses the subject of a healthy lifestyle, and shows how a fairly simple regime of healthy eating, exercise, relaxation and stress management will pay dividends in increasing your sense of well-being.

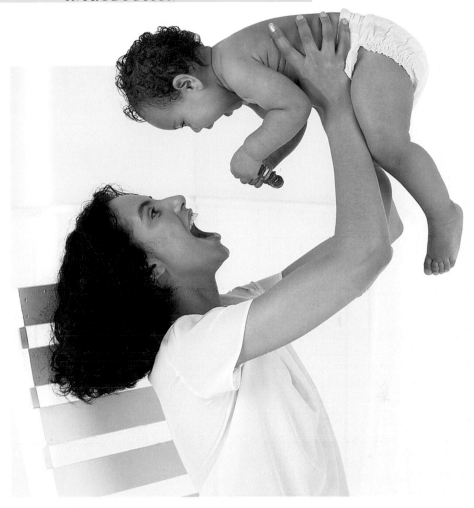

Above: *A picture full of energy and joy. A healthy family is likely to be a happy family, so learning how to deal with illness is vital.*

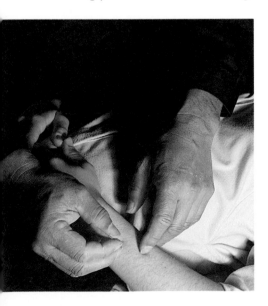

Above: *As with many alternative therapies, acupuncture has an almost magical air, as needles are inserted into invisible meridians.*

Part Two provides a guide to the major therapies that are generally encountered under the umbrella heading of "alternative medicine". Part Three is concerned with treating illness. Ailments and diseases are grouped together according to the part of the body that is afflicted, and advice is given on which alternative therapies can most appropriately be applied in each case. Part Four deals with complementary first aid and highlights the most common emergencies that you are likely to encounter for which complementary treatments have something positive to offer. The final section of the book comprises a supplementary glossary of alternative therapies, and an index.

In conclusion, I must stress that this is not a "do-it-yourself" handbook and should not be used as such. Expert opinions, both orthodox and alternative, will need to be sought on many occasions and the information given in this book is not intended to substitute for the diagnosis and care of a qualified doctor. Similarly it is important to recognize that, on occasions, treatments, either orthodox or alternative, can have limits in their effectiveness and may have side effects. The information in this practical guide will enable you to be better informed, learn some easy-to-use skills, and give you a range of self-help measures that can be of great help to both you and your family in maintaining a sense of good health and well-being.

PART ONE

A HEALTHIER LIFESTYLE

WHAT IS HEALTH?

It seems strange that with all the current emphasis on healthier living and "lifestyle" changes that there is no acceptable general definition of what "health" is. For some it is "to be able to act so as to do what you want to do, live how you want to live". For others, it is "my body functions like a well-oiled machine without having to be looked after" (quoted in *Health or Illness*, Herzlich, 1974). John Steinbeck wrote in *The Short Reign of Pippin IV*, "Pippin was healthy in so far as he knew – by that I mean his health was so good he was not aware he had it".

Scientists and researchers have also tried to define health. The World Health Organization arrived at a definition in 1946 which it still holds to – that health is the "state of complete physical, mental and social well-being".

Other researchers have equated healthiness to "robustness" or "hardiness", how much one *can do* and how one copes with the stresses of daily living. Others have linked health to *how one feels*, one's mental attitude and state of contentment. Others talk about comparative health, suggesting that standards of "healthiness" can vary from culture to culture and country to country. The term acceptable health is also used to describe "a state of perceived well-being, whether or not disease or disability is present, provided that the latter does not interfere either with the sufferer's normal life or with that of people whom he or she may

Below: *Living a healthy lifestyle does not have to be a chore. Physical exercise is an activity that the whole family can enjoy.*

affect through community living". This last definition suggests that you can be healthy even though you may have a disease, which is certainly true, although for most people health is still equated with the absence of disease. The following two examples may help to illustrate the link between disease and health:

Mr. A, aged 64, has had two heart attacks, developed heart failure and was finally given a heart transplant. Physically he feels very well, his blood pressure is now normal and the doctors cannot find any physical abnormality. However, he is still overweight, miserable and crotchety, and his wife has great difficulty in putting up with his moods. He is free from disease but not healthy.

Mrs. B, aged 52, developed breast cancer and has only three months to live. She went on a retreat and began introducing certain changes into her life (diet, meditation, walking). After two weeks she experienced a "stillness and peace" and was heard to remark "I now know what it means to be fully alive, and if it took cancer to get me to realize this, then I am glad I've got cancer." Her joy and peace transmitted itself to everyone around her and she died at the peak of her health, even though she was riddled with disease.

The definition of *disease* seems a little easier but how does it relate to the concept of *illness*. Essentially, a disease is the physical changes that occur in the organs that may or may not be detectable by a doctor, and an illness is how we, as individuals, respond to such a disease.

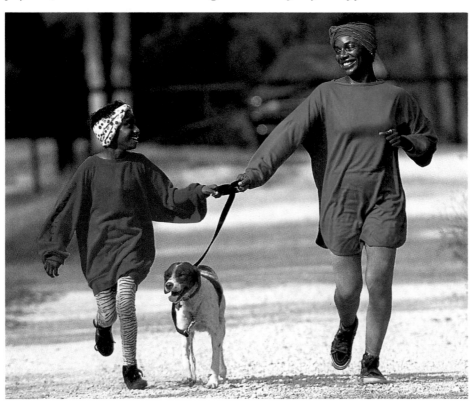

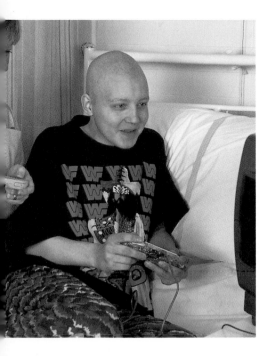

Above: *This man has a serious disease, cancer, but can still have fun. The link between health and a sense of well-being is a complex one.*

Mrs. C, aged 33, goes to her doctor for her yearly check. She is on the pill, has two children and works as a part-time secretary in an office. She feels perfectly well and is totally overwhelmed when her doctor informs her she has a small lump in her breast that will have to be removed. She does not feel *ill* but probably has a serious *disease*. On the other hand, Mr. D, aged 48, goes to his doctor because he feels unwell, he is tired, cannot sleep, has difficulty concentrating, is experiencing vague aches and pains in his body and has lost his appetite. His doctor examines him, sends him for investigations, including blood tests and X-rays, and tells him he can find no evidence of any disease. Mr. D still feels ill although no disease can be found. Then there is Mrs. E who has a severe blood disease requiring frequent blood-transfusions. She works as a supervisor in a small clothing store and other than the occasional day off, she manages very well. Following the last transfusion, she is recalled to hospital to be told she has contracted the AIDS virus through the blood. There is no sign

of any deterioration in her blood disease and she is informed that it may take years before she may develop AIDS, and that there is a good chance she will be all right. She confides to one of her work colleagues and before long everyone knows that Mrs. E is an AIDS carrier. Soon she notices that people will not sit with her in the canteen – she is asked to bring her own towel and finally the management suggests she "goes off sick". Her main problem is the way her colleagues have responded to her *disease* even though she herself does not feel *ill*. She is made to feel *sick* and is in danger of being shunned. The way we or our family and friends respond to our disease/illness constitutes the entity of sickness.

If we are labelled sick – "go and get a sick note from the doctor" – it may give us certain rights not to work, to receive benefit and to be looked after. It is therefore not surprising that people may "go off sick", feeling ill, but not having any disease. It goes without saying that this may not be a very healthy attitude.

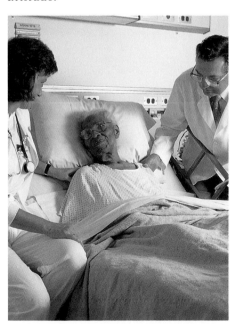

Above: *Illness can be defined as the way we respond to a physical disease. With sensitive and supportive care, even people who have serious diseases do not necessarily have to feel ill.*

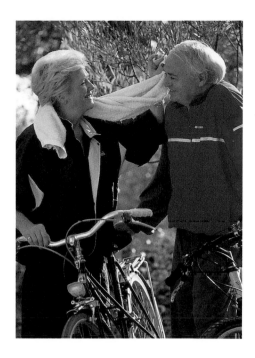

Above: *This couple look well: a combination of the absence of illness, physical fitness and emotional fulfilment creates a healthy person.*

The emergence of "holistic" approaches to health care

The great advances in medicine which began with the Renaissance have been based on sound scientific principles. These principles have required that the patient is studied as if he were a machine, or, as the 16th century philosopher Francis Bacon put it, "we must put the patient on the rack and make him reveal his secrets". This dissection of the patient has resulted in our knowing more and more about the parts (lungs, hearts, kidneys, tissues, cells, genes etc.) and has encouraged the development of specialism and specialists each limiting himself to a part of the body.

An holistic practitioner is one who tries to see the patient "as a whole" or as a very wise physician, William Osler, once put it, "It is better to know which patient has the disease than which disease the patient has". Holism, as opposed to reductionism (the study of parts), is the study of wholes. How does the liver affect the heart? How does the mind affect the body? How does what we eat affect how we feel, and how does our family or our culture affect how we act or behave? Thus an holistic approach is not necessarily about the therapy that is used but about the general approach to the patient. An acupuncturist or homeopath is not necessarily holistic, and indeed many good traditional doctors who know nothing about alternative medicine may undertake a very good "whole-person medicine".

Much misunderstanding has arisen by confusing the term holistic medicine with alternative medicine. An holistic approach involves responding to the patient as a whole, a willingness to use a wide range of treatments (orthodox as well as alternative), to focus on preventative and educational methods (dietary changes, relaxation and meditation, exercise routines etc.), and an understanding of how the healthiness and well-being of the practitioner is an important factor in how quickly the patient responds to the treatment given, i.e. each practitioner is also a healer and can make use of this factor in his approach to the patient. It is as a result of the increasing interest in holistic approaches that the focus on stress as a cause of disease has developed and the fact that many practitioners will help the client/patient to understand how he/she can cope with the stress in their lives.

Below: *Physical symptoms of stress act like a warning light on a machine. You must address the basic problem, not simply turn off the light.*

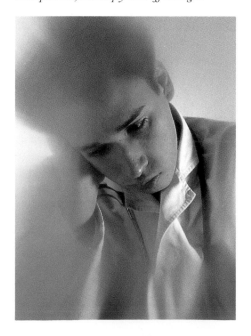

The concept of stress and lifestyle in the management of health and disease

Defining what stress is is *not* any help in understanding this difficult but most important element in our lives. Stress is *not* simply nervous tension, it is *not* just an emergency release of adrenaline, it is *not* necessarily something bad – it cannot and should not be avoided and it can result from positive events (promotion, marriage) just as from negative events (loss of a job, or a divorce). Thus stress can be seen as a very necessary part of life and something we need to learn about, rather than something we should avoid. Learning to respond to challenges in such a way that we avoid burn-out can be the ultimate goal of a successful and contented life. When we fail to respond to demands and challenges ("stressors" as they are labelled by the scientists), then we may experience symptoms and signs of the *stressed state*.

Recognizing the danger signals

Becoming aware of these danger signals is often the first step in learning how better to cope. These may be different for each person and will affect one part of the body or mind. They may also manifest themselves by a change of behaviour (such as drinking more alcohol or driving faster etc.).

Muscular system Symptoms connected with this system are the most common and they result from an increase in muscular tension. Symptoms may be felt anywhere in the body, but usually the back of the neck or lower back is the first area. Headaches are the result of increased tension of the muscles, at times accompanied by feelings of nausea or sickness. Tension in the jaw muscles leads to grinding of teeth and can produce an imbalance in alignment of the spine. Tightening of the muscles of the face leads to pain over the eyes and forehead. Any of the muscles in the body can be affected and some do not produce any obvious symptom like pain or tension. The most common groups of muscles to be so affected are the diaphragm, which is a dome-shaped

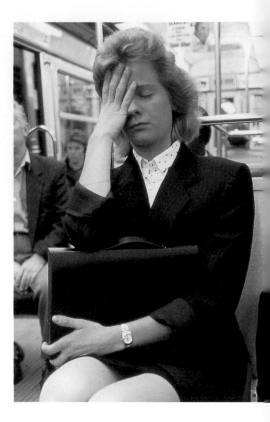

Above: *Stress is an inevitable component of modern life. How well we cope with it will determine how healthy we feel.*

muscle separating the contents of the abdomen from the chest, and the pelvic muscles deep in the lower abdomen surrounding the sexual organs.

Increased tension of the throat muscles can lead to the sensation of a lump in the throat, can affect speech, and accounts, in part, for the high-pitched and nervous laughter not uncommonly found in people under tension.

If the muscular tension is severe, then it can lead to trembling, shaking, nervous tics, or frequent blinking. If any warning sign of a stressed state is not attended to, it can produce not only short-term discomfort but long-term disability and disease. In addition to the muscles that help us move and are under our conscious control, there is a group of muscles known as involuntary muscles surrounding blood vessels and the intestines which in turn are also affected by the stressed state and produce a whole variety of warning signs, some only apparent to the doctor on examination, others causing troublesome symptoms for those individuals

affected. These include:
▪ *Raised blood pressure* because of tension in the muscles surrounding the arteries.
▪ *Migraine headaches* – the muscles surrounding the arteries of the scalp first constrict (tighten), then dilate (expand), giving rise to the throbbing one-sided headache.
▪ *Intestinal symptoms* from rumbling of the stomach to burping or increase in flatus. The "irritable bowel syndrome" which causes intermittent diarrhoea and constipation and is often associated with pain and distension of the abdomen results from a disturbance in the muscle tone surrounding the lower gut. These symptoms are also accompanied by loss of appetite.

Glandular system The stressed state may result in many disturbances of the different glands in the body, the most frequent and obvious being excessive sweating, resulting in damp palms and an unpleasant body smell. Similarly, dryness of the throat and mouth with difficulty in swallowing is a common symptom for some individuals.

Heart and lungs Rapid pulse rate, pounding of the heart, palpitations, rapid shallow breathing or overbreathing, known as hyperventilation, are common warning signs of someone in a stressed state.

Nervous system Dizziness, fainting spells and a general feeling of weakness and lethargy can develop into loss of *joie de vivre* and affect sleep. Difficulty in getting off to sleep, as well as waking up early and tired are very common warning signs. Not so well recognized but equally common is sleeping too much. Sleep which is disturbed by dreams or nightmares is frequent for those individuals who are possibly repressing some conscious thoughts during the day.

Mind General warning signs include:
▪ Inability to concentrate – not being able to focus on anything for long.
▪ General irritability or overexactingness which is often followed by periods of sadness, lethargy and depression.
▪ Floating anxiety – having a sense of mild fear or panic but not quite knowing why.
On occasions, the mind is unsettled or distressed: the only way that we can recognize this to be so is by observing our behaviour or habits. Obvious habits such as excessive smoking or drinking and increased use of tranquillizers or food bingeing are easy to identify. Other behaviours or habits that are equally destructive may include

Below: *Tension manifests itself both mentally and physically. Problems with breathing can result from being in a stressed state.*

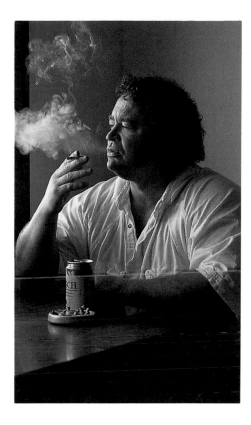

Above: *The temptation is often to try to blot out stress through agents like alcohol and tobacco. In reality, any relief they bring is illusory.*

promiscuous sexual activity or accident proneness.

It is possible to expand this list almost indefinitely, but what is more helpful is that each of us should become aware of our own warning signs. They serve to tell us that we are in the stressed state – similar to the red light on the dashboard that goes on to indicate that the car has run out of oil. Unfortunately, what tends to happen is that we ignore the red light or we divert our attention to something else. What is worse is when we visit our doctor and his approach is to prescribe a drug or treatment that only helps to "knock the red light out". These warning signs are invaluable markers and guides that let us know we are in a state of imbalance either with ourselves or our environment. By all means find something to relieve the distress or pain, but make sure it is something that helps in returning you to a state of balance and not something which affects the warning sign only. The cause underlying the warning must also be addressed.

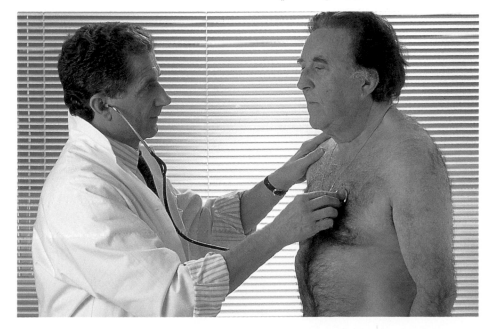

What are the causes of stress and the stressed state?

To be alive means that you have to learn to cope with stress – each event or change in your life can be seen as a stressor; a series of stressors may lead to the stressed state. So one of the first coping strategies may be to list all the stressors that are current in your life. Some changes or stressors seem to demand more from us than others. Some stressors are external, i.e. changing house or job, other stressors are internal, i.e. unhappy memories, worrying about unpaid bills etc. Use the lists provided below to calculate your various stress parameters.

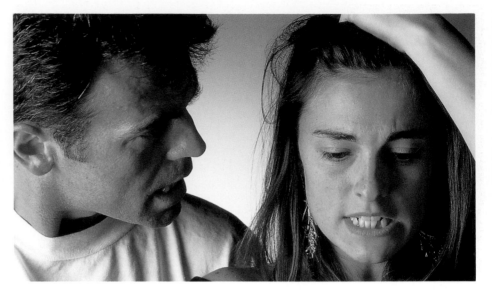

How stressed are you?

The following table lists a number of significant life events and assigns them a numerical value according to the levels of stress they engender (100 = most stressful, 0 = least stressful). Check through this list and add up all the points that you score for events that have occurred to you in the past 12 months. A score of more than 150 indi-

Above: *Disharmony in a relationship scores very high on the stress scale. When feelings get out of control, physical health can also suffer.*

cates that there is a 50 percent chance that your health will suffer in the near future, and a score of more than 300 indicates a 90 percent chance – unless you take measures to manage your response to stress more effectively.

How well do you cope with stress?

By responding to the statements in the table on the facing page you can measure how well you manage stress and whether your way of life equips you to cope satisfactorily. Select a number from one to five which matches your response to each of the statements.

Add up the total score.
More than 55
Stress is a likely risk to your health. It would be sensible to try to change your way of life to lower your stress levels.
45 to 55
Stress could be a problem for you. Try to change some aspects of your life to reduce the effects of stress.
Less than 45
You have a high resistance to stress and enjoy a healthy lifestyle.

What are your reactions to stressors?

Imagine the telephone ringing while you are busy doing an important task. How do you respond? With irritation and anger, or do you choose to ignore it and continue what you are doing, or do you accept the interruption with tolerance and equanimity. These three responses are part of everyone's repertoire of reactions to stressors.

The first, the *fight response*, is characteristic of the person who wants to control the stressor. This response is associated with competitiveness, aggression, impatience. People who

Major life event	Stress level	Major life event	Stress level
Death of spouse	100	Change in responsibilities at work	29
Divorce	73	Son or daughter leaving home	29
Marital separation	65	Trouble with in-laws	29
Jail term	63	Outstanding personal achievement	28
Death of close family member	63	Spouse begins or stops work	26
Personal injury or illness	53	Beginning or ending education	26
Marriage	50	Change in living conditions	25
Loss of job	47	Change in personal habits	24
Marital reconciliation	45	Trouble with boss	23
Retirement	45	Change in working hours or conditions	20
Change in health of family member	44	Moving house	20
Pregnancy	40	Changing schools	20
Sexual problems	39	Change in leisure pursuits	19
Gain of new family member	39	Change in church activities	19
Business readjustment	39	Change in social activities	18
Change in financial state	38	Low to medium mortgage or loan	17
Death of close friend	37	Altered sleeping habits	16
Change to different type of work	36	Change in number of family reunions	15
Change in number of arguments with spouse	35	Change in eating habits	15
		Going on holiday	13
High mortgage	31	Approaching Christmas season	12
Foreclosure of mortgage or loan	30	Minor violations of the law	11

The table is adapted from the work of two scientists at Washington University, Thomas Holmes and Richard Rahe, who identified the link between life changes and the likelihood of future illness.

How much of the time are these statements true for you?	Almost always	Usually	Some-times	Rarely	Never
1 I have a quiet time alone during the day	1	2	3	4	5
2 I enjoy seven or eight hours of sleep at least four nights a week	1	2	3	4	5
3 My religious beliefs or deeply-held personal beliefs give me strength	1	2	3	4	5
4 I exercise hard enough to work up a sweat at least twice a week	1	2	3	4	5
5 I have a group of friends and acquaintances	1	2	3	4	5
6 I discuss domestic problems with other members of the household	1	2	3	4	5
7 I have at least one friend I can confide in about personal affairs	1	2	3	4	5
8 I smoke fewer than 10 cigarettes a day	1	2	3	4	5
9 I organize my time effectively	1	2	3	4	5
10 I take fewer than five alcoholic drinks a week	1	2	3	4	5
11 My health is good	1	2	3	4	5
12 My income is adequate for my basic expenses	1	2	3	4	5
13 I am about the right weight for my build and height	1	2	3	4	5
14 I give and receive affection often	1	2	3	4	5
15 I express my feelings when irritated or anxious	1	2	3	4	5
16 I drink less than three caffeine-containing drinks (coffee, cocoa or cola) a day	1	2	3	4	5
17 I participate in regular social gatherings	1	2	3	4	5
18 I eat at least one full, well-balanced meal a day	1	2	3	4	5
19 I do something just for fun at least once a week	1	2	3	4	5
20 I have at least one relative within 50 miles (80km) of home on whom I can rely	1	2	3	4	5

This table is adapted from the work of stress psychologists Lyle H. Miller and Alma Dell Smith of the University of Boston's Medical Centre.

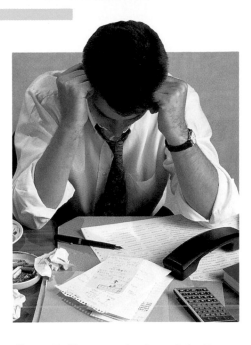

Above: *Problems at work – do you fight, flee or "go with the flow"? A balance of the three responses to stress is considered ideal.*

the world, appear dependent and timid, and are prone to depression.

The third response has been termed the *flow response*. This implies accepting the stressor without turning away from it or trying to control it. At first hand it may appear the most mature response, but if it becomes the characteristic method of responding to a stressor, the individual may appear changeable and erratic. They may be inconsistent, have little sense of their own identity and be prone to being influenced by the latest fashion or fad. Such individuals who exhibit the flow, "stay cool" response will be attracted to strong charismatic leaders and are the types who become members of religious sects and cults.

The three responses, *fight*, *flight* and *flow*, have been exaggerated slightly in this analysis to make them clearer. The successful managers of stress are those who do not overuse one or other of these responses but who are able to use each stress response appropriately as the occasion demands. It is the overuse of one stress response or the mismatching of stress response to stressor that is likely to lead to the stressed state of health. Learning to cope with stress involves a number of different strategies which can be introduced into one's daily life and help to influence the lifestyle we lead.

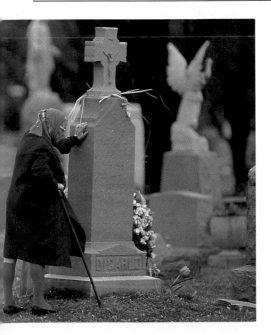

push themselves constantly and are ambitious use the fight response to manage their stressors; they have been characterized as having an "A" type personality. Some people choose a *fight* response but do not show it externally. They may appear unemotional, obsessionally "tidy" and give the impression of never being out of control.

The second stress response described involves denial or a *flight response*; the unpaid bill is buried underneath the mail, the job vacancy is not applied for – such individuals are cautious and conservative. They may feel at the mercy of

Left: *It is important that feelings like grief are expressed openly. People who exhibit a fight response to stressors can find this difficult.*

HEALTHY EATING AND HEALTHY DIETS

It is now almost impossible to avoid advice on diets, natural food, special supplements and the like if one is trying to pursue a healthier lifestyle. There seem to be as many guides and self-help books extolling one approach as there are others warning you of its dangers. Notwithstanding the enormous amount of conflicting literature on the subject, there is a consensus view which has emerged and which, if followed with the addition of some of your own personal touches, will ensure you have very few dietary problems.

Basic guidelines to a healthy diet

▪ Limit sugar intake (this means reading labels carefully); although canned foods, bottled sauces, dressings and cereals may sometimes be described as "natural", they often contain high quantities of sugar.

▪ Avoid highly processed foods with preservatives and colouring added.

▪ Eat natural wholegrain breads, cereals, pasta and rice, rather than highly processed varieties.

▪ Eat plenty of fresh fruits and vegetables, rather than those which are frozen or canned.

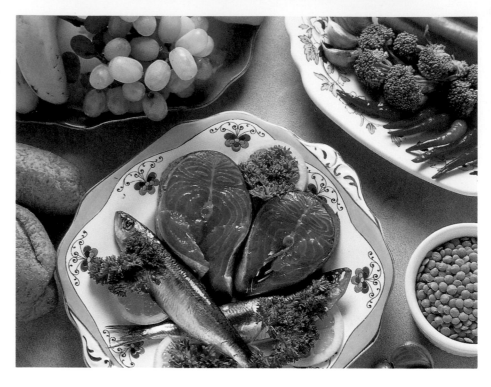

Above: *The components of a healthy diet: fish, fresh fruit and vegetables, wholemeal bread, garlic and lentils to provide extra fibre.*

Below: *Fast food is the quick way to an unhealthy body. Unfortunately, the high levels of fat in an average hot dog are not good for you.*

▪ Eat high quality protein sources (low-fat dairy products, whole grains, beans, fish, eggs, fowl) and avoid high-fat meat, high-fat cheese, red meat, and processed meats.

▪ Find suitable beverages to replace coffee, tea and fizzy canned drinks. Try a variety of juices and drink plenty of spring water.

▪ Reduce your salt intake by avoiding added salt and salty snack foods.

▪ Keep tobacco and alcohol consumption to a minimum and avoid unnecessary medication.

▪ Keep fast-food and canteen eating to a minimum.

▪ Reduce your consumption of fried foods both at home and in restaurants. Cook vegetables in a steamer rather than a saucepan.

▪ Try to eat your largest meal in the earlier part of the day to ensure the body is able to rest more at night.

▪ Give yourself time to eat slowly, peacefully, and with concentration. That way you will be aware when you have eaten enough and will be less likely to overeat. Digestion is aided by a peaceful mind and body.

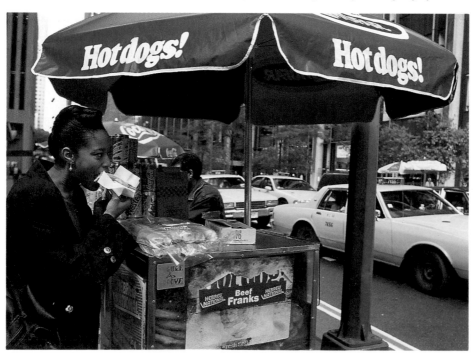

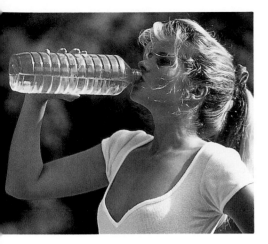

Above: *Try replacing fizzy drinks in your daily fluid intake with mineral water. It is better for your teeth, and your waistline.*

The last point is often overlooked. No matter how healthy or natural your diet is, if you eat it in a rushed and stressed state then the body's digestive processes will work against all the trouble you have taken to select and cook the food. We can now expand on some of these guidelines and add a few specific hints.

Specific hints

Carbohydrates These are the major sources of "quick energy" for the body and are converted in the body to glucose which is our basic fuel and which is stored in the liver and muscles. The major sources of carbohydrates are listed in the table. The complex forms of carbohydrate contain starch, some of which is broken down by the body to simple sugars as listed in the table, but the body can only use glucose as fuel. Over the last fifty years we have reduced the proportion of complex carbohydrates in our diet from 70 to 50 percent while our intake of simple sugars (cakes, sweets, fizzy drinks) has increased. This increase in intake of simple sugars has resulted in an increase in obesity, diabetes, atherosclerosis (narrowing of the arteries) and, on a daily basis, may cause a rapid rise and fall in blood sugar levels giving rise to mood swings, and a tendency to feel excitable and nervous, then feel down and depressed. Reducing the refined carbohydrates in your diet involves:

- Cutting down on pastries, sweets, cakes, biscuits.
- Changing from white bread to whole-wheat bread.
- Reducing added sugar to drinks and cereals.
- Avoiding processed and tinned vegetables and fruit.
- Reducing the consumption of soft drinks.
- Experimenting with other forms of sweeteners – i.e. honey, fruit, parsnips, molasses.

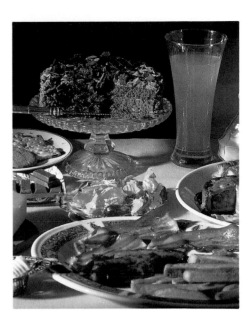

Above: *A little of what you fancy here does not do you good! The large amounts of fat, sugar and salt in these foods can lead to health problems.*

Below: *These foods offer plentiful sources of carbohydrates, which the body converts into glucose to be used as a fuel for "quick energy".*

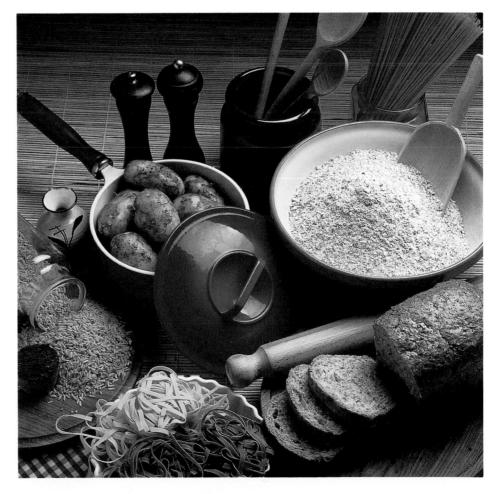

Sources of complex carbohydrates and sugars		
Complex carbohydrates	**Simple sugars**	**Glucose**
Cereals: wheat, barley, oats, corn, rye, buckwheat Rice Potatoes	Sucrose (sugar) Lactose Maltose	Fructose Galactose

Fats and cholesterol Fats are the major source of calories in our diet and like cholesterol are an essential ingredient for many of our tissues and cells. Cholesterol is made by the body from the fats we eat. It is required to make our hormones, the bile salts used to digest the food, and the hormones oestrogen and testosterone. If the level of cholesterol is increased, however, then it is deposited along the walls of the arteries (a little like the furring produced inside a kettle). This "furring" may cause the blockage of blood flow which causes heart attacks.

The advice regarding fat content in diet has often centred around whether we eat butter (animal fat – saturated) or margarine (vegetable fat – unsaturated). Whereas it is true that animal fats predispose to the formation of atherosclerosis, it is the *total content* of fat in your diet, of whatever kind, that you should reduce. If your total fat content is low, it may be quite all right to eat butter and eggs. To reduce your total content of fat does require a reduction in meat which can contain anything up to 45 percent of fat (beefsteak). Even lean meat contains 25 percent fat.

Other ways of reducing the effect of

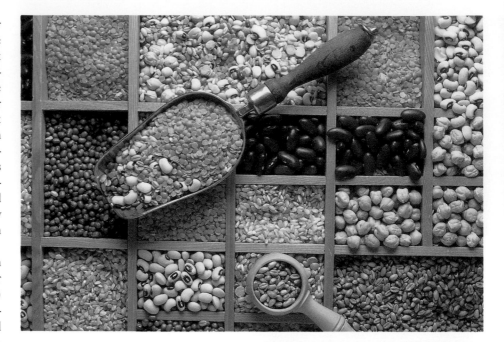

Above: *A scrumptious looking assortment of grains and pulses. By adding these to your diet, you ensure a healthy supply of proteins and fibre.*

fat in your diet is by increasing the *lecithin* content in your diet. Lecithin is one of a special category of fats called phospholipids, and is found in peas, beans, onions and garlic. It is interesting to note that many traditional high fat diets found in the Mediterranean are all combined with raw onions and garlic. The diets are thus well balanced and do not produce the fatty deposits that might lead to heart attacks, despite the high incidence of fat in the food consumed.

Manufactured vegetable oils sold as a "healthy alternative" have to pass through a complex chemical process known as hydrogenation which makes them stable at room temperatures. It is therefore advisable to choose those natural oils that are pure extracts of vegetables or grain, e.g. olive oil, corn oil, sunflower oil or safflower. Heating oils above 190°C/375°F potentiates their ability to cause atherosclerosis, which may explain the importance of reducing fried foods to a minimum.

Reducing fat content in your diet involves:
▪ Reduction in the consumption of fried foods.
▪ Changing from red meats to chicken,

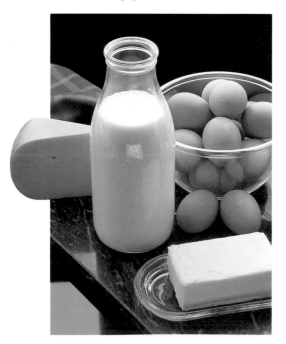

Below: *Eggs, milk and dairy produce are high in saturated fats which the body may convert into cholesterol. A high-fat diet is unadvisable.*

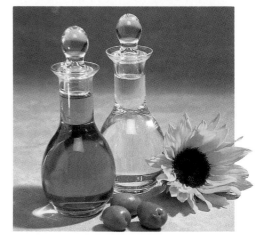

Above: *Natural oils that are extracted from products like olives or sunflower seeds are a good dietary choice. Frying food in oil, however, is still something that should be avoided.*

fish or beans as a source of protein.
▪ Increasing the intake of beans and "sprouts" as well as onions and garlic.
▪ Reducing bread-spreads of whatever variety.
▪ Changing from fatty cheese to cottage cheese.
▪ Changing from full cream milk to skimmed milk.
▪ Keeping to a maximum of three to four eggs a week.

Proteins Most people think of meat as a first-class protein and believe other sources of protein are somehow less nutritious. Another popular misconception is thinking of a meatless diet as a vegetarian diet. Proteins are the building blocks and skeleton of the body. A high protein diet is required at the time of growth (childhood, pregnancy) but we generally eat more protein than we need, and we certainly can reduce our meat-eating considerably. Some wheats contain up to 14 percent protein and the average is 7 percent. Beans are a particularly good source of protein but have become unfashionable in the West. Beans can be "de-gassed" by allowing them to soak well and changing the water at least once. *Do not cook the beans in the same water you have soaked them in, as the water will have absorbed the gases from them.*

Tips on protein consumption:
* Reduce or eliminate red meat consumption.
* Eat fish, chicken or cheese of the appropriate variety.
* Introduce a bean dish once a week.

Fibre, vegetables and fruit The reduction in the fibre content of our diet is thought to be one of the most important changes in the last fifty years leading to the development of many

Below: *A tempting harvest. Fresh fruit and vegetables supply fibre, vitamins and minerals to the body – all essential to our well-being.*

Fibre	Source
Cellulose Lignins	Vegetables
Gums Pectins Mucilage	Fruit

"Western" diseases (appendicitis, gall stones, constipation, varicose veins, haemorrhoids, large bowel cancer). Fibre derived from vegetables and fruit (see table above) is not absorbed by the body, produces "bulk" and aids in the excretion of faeces reducing the time the waste products of our diet are present in the bowel. Adding bran to the diet can be an easy way of increasing the fibre, but far better is to increase the vegetable and fruit content which will ensure an adequate supply of vitamins and minerals.

Vitamins, minerals and food additives
There is no sadder sight than to see prosperous Westerners consume dozens of extra vitamins and mineral pills each day in the misguided assumption that they are keeping to a healthy diet. Charts and tables of what each vitamin or mineral can do for you are displayed in almost every health book and pharmacy. Additional supplementation is not necessary if you ensure you

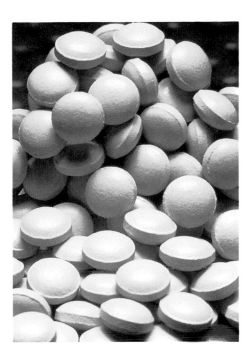

Above: *Although the body needs vitamins, the custom of popping vitamin pills is misguided. Get your vitamins through a healthy diet.*

have a good basic diet with fresh fruit and vegetables. Occasionally, and in special circumstances only, are added vitamins and minerals required. Too many people pop these pills as a way of avoiding a serious involvement in their daily diet. The evidence that high doses of Vitamin C or other supplements will reduce colds or prevent cancer is still debated in the medical journals, but recent studies do show that large doses of Vitamin C may prevent the formation of polyps in the large bowel that can cause cancer.

The various food additives found in our foods include preservatives, food colouring, oxidizers, softeners, stabilizers and anti-oxidants, and they have been shown to have a cumulative toxic effect on the body. Recently, antibiotics and hormones fed to animals have found their way into the meat we eat and much concern as to their effects has rightly stimulated the development of organic farming. Since 1986, all foods have had to have information about all additives included on their packaging. It is quite a chore, however, to keep checking them. Far more sensible is to buy fresh food and to avoid tinned, processed or packaged articles.

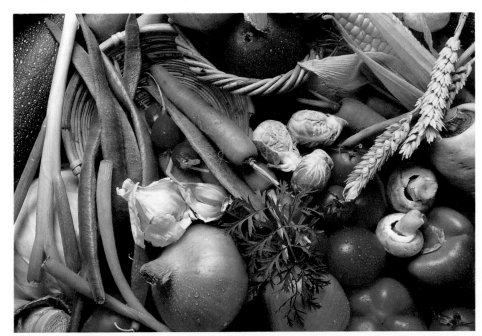

TAKING CARE OF YOUR BODY

We have seen how stress can affect our bodies and give rise not only to the painful tense muscles and headaches to which we are prone but the more serious diseased states that can shorten our life. There are several ways in which we can begin to undo the accumulated effects of stress as well as allow ourselves to become fitter and enjoy the physical aspects of our life. Such ways need not involve us in expensive or energetic pursuits and can often be done in the quietness of our own homes. The first two methods of taking care of ourselves can be seen simply as an extension of washing our faces or brushing our teeth.

Breathing exercises

Breathing is the most important and vital act we do. It happens between twelve and twenty times a minute. It is affected by what we do, think or feel and we recognize its importance in our language when we talk about "gasping for breath", "catching one's breath", "it took my breath away". Our breathing increases with

Right: *Learning how to relax and unwind in the peace of your own home is one quite simple way to start coping with stress.*

excitement, fear, sadness. On occasions, we may temporarily stop breathing altogether in anger or in breath-holding attacks seen in children having a temper tantrum. Our rate and pattern of breathing is the most sensitive indicator we have of our level of stress (rapid, uneven, shallow breaths) and relaxation (long, rhythmical, deep breaths).

Breathing occurs without our having to "think about it", but we can also consciously choose to alter the rate and pattern of our breath. This we do by using one of three groups of muscles:

■ *(Inter)-Costal Muscles*
Muscles between ribs on the chest wall – used in chest breathing for rapid entry of oxygen.

■ *Diaphragm*
The dome-shaped muscle separating the chest cavity from the abdominal contents – used in diaphragmatic breathing for relaxation.

■ *Accessory muscles of respiration*
These are situated at the top end of the rib-cage together with some muscles of the back and abdomen – used in vigorous exercise and when under great stress.

Most of us have got into the habit of using our chest muscles to breathe all the time which helps to main-

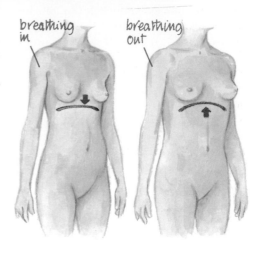

Above: *The diagram shows how the movement of the diaphragm when breathing causes the abdominal wall to move in and out. Deep, diaphragmatic breathing is a key to relaxation.*

tain the body in a state of alertness and arousal, even when we are asleep. Learning to breathe with your diaphragm and practising a ten-minute exercise daily can help restore the body into a relaxed state and requires less energy than chest breathing.

The diaphragm is a horizontal dome-shaped muscle which separates the contents of your chest (heart and lungs) from your abdomen (stomach, liver, intestines). On breathing in, the diaphragm contracts, flattens and descends, thus creating a "vacuum" in the chest, and air is sucked in. As the diaphragm descends, it pushes the abdominal contents down and the increase in pressure forces the abdominal wall (the front of your abdomen) out. On breathing out, the diaphragm relaxes and forces air out of the lungs, reducing the pressure on the abdominal contents and causing the abdominal wall to flatten.

By learning the technique of diaphragmatic breathing, you can begin to ease some of the stress out of your body. Try this simple exercise, or if you prefer, you can purchase a self-help tape or join a class to learn this routine method of relaxation practised for thousands of years by the Yogis in India.

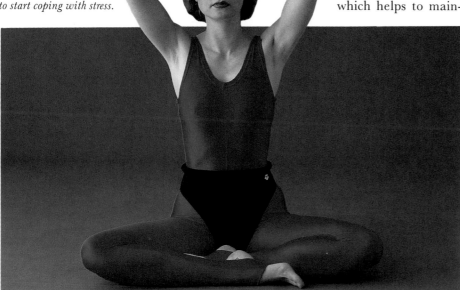

Find a quiet room where you will be undisturbed for about 10-15 minutes. Lie down on the bed or floor. Undo any tight clothing and remove your shoes. Spend a few moments settling yourself down. Close your eyes, spread your feet 30-45cm (12-18 inches) apart and check that your head, neck and spine are in a straight line. Now focus your attention on your breathing. Do not try to change your breathing for the moment. Become aware of how fast or slow you are breathing, whether you are breathing with your chest or diaphragm. Notice whether there are any gaps or pauses between your inhalation and exhalation. – *Pause* – Now put one hand on your upper chest and one hand on your abdomen just below your rib-cage. Relax your shoulders and hands. As you exhale allow the abdomen to flatten. There should be little or no movement in the chest. Allow yourself a little time to get into a regular rhythm. – *Pause* – Allow your breath to become smooth, easy and regular. – *Pause* – Now consciously slow down your exhalation and allow your inhalation to follow smoothly and easily. – *Pause* – Smooth out any gaps or pauses in your breathing. – *Pause* – If any distractions, thoughts or worries come into your mind, allow them to come, then allow them to go and bring your attention back to your breathing. – *Pause* – When you are ready to end this exercise, take a few deeper breaths in. Bring some feeling back into your fingers and toes. Open your eyes slowly and turn over on to one side before gently sitting up.

A similar sort of routine has been used in natural childbirth exercises and by heart specialists all over the world to help reduce raised bloodpressure and the effects of chronic stress. After you have become proficient at diaphragmatic breathing, check during the course of the day, while you are driving, or talking on the telephone, to see whether you have inadvertently slipped back into chest breathing.

Relaxation exercises

As well as altered and unhealthy breathing patterns, stress and tension affect the muscles of the body. Muscles get tense (contract, harden and become painful) because of an increase in nervous stimulation. Some people are not even aware their muscles are tense and it is only by increasing the tension that they can begin to relax the muscles. So the first exercise starts by getting you deliberately to increase muscle tension.

Find a quiet room where you will be undisturbed for 10-15 minutes. Remove your shoes and loosen any

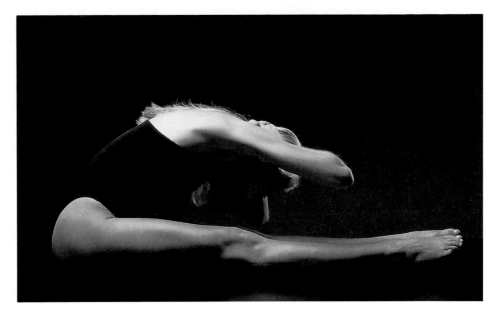

Above: *Unwanted muscular tension can lead to all sorts of unpleasant physical symptoms. Learning how to stretch and relax your muscles like this will help to ease tension out of your system.*

tight clothing. You can do this exercise sitting, but it is preferable to lie down on a bed or carpet. Close your eyes gently – make sure your head, neck and body are straight.

Start by raising your eyebrows and tensing the muscles of your forehead. Keep the tension counting to five, then relax the muscles and become aware of any difference you feel in them. Repeat once more. Now squeeze your eyes as tight as you can, forcing your eyes shut. Count to five, then release. Notice any difference. Repeat once more. Open your mouth wide, stretching the muscles of your face to the centre of the face, puckering up your lips, eyebrows and chin. Count to five – release – repeat once more. Tighten the muscles of your jaw, clenching your teeth. Count to five, release and repeat once more. Become aware of the whole of your face and any difference you feel.

Raise your shoulders to your ears, tensing the muscles of your shoulders and neck. Release and relax the muscles. Notice any difference and repeat once more. Raise your left hand and elbow off the floor/bed. Make a fist and increase the tension in your hand, forearm, upper arm. Count to five and let go, allowing the hand to fall back on

Symptoms produced by muscle tension			
Voluntary muscles	Symptoms produced by tension	Involuntary muscles	Symptoms produced by tension
Eye	Eye strain	Around arteries	High blood pressure
Back of neck	Tension headache	Around bowel	Irritable bowel syndrome (constipation/ diarrhoea)
Back	Back pain	Around stomach	Passing wind

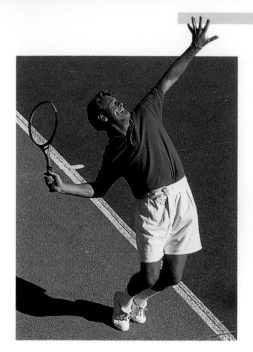

Above: *A strenuous game of competitive tennis is an enjoyable way to give your heart, lungs and muscles a thorough work-out.*

the floor/bed. Notice any difference between your left and right hand and repeat once more. Repeat the same with the right hand and arm. Now contract the muscles of the chest – notice the effect it has on your breathing. Relax. Flatten and tighten the muscles of your stomach – count to five – relax and exhale. Lift your left foot and leg off the floor by about 15cm (6in). Push your foot away from you, tensing the muscles of the foot, leg and thigh. Count to five. Let go and allow the leg to drop down on the floor. Repeat once more on the left side, then again, twice on the right.

In addition to tensing and releasing, this exercise can be repeated and a stretching element introduced into the exercises. Following this exercise, you can begin to guide yourself into a deeper state of muscular relaxation as described next.

Starting with your forehead and face, let go of any tension, relax the muscles of the face – relax the muscles of the jaw. Check that your teeth are not too tightly clenched together. Allow the tongue to lie away from the roof of the mouth. Allow your head and shoulders to fall back easily on the floor. Relax the upper arms, lower arms, hands and fingers. Let go of any tension in your chest and

abdomen. Allow your breathing to become diaphragmatic. Breath smoothly, regularly, rhythmically and without effort. – *Pause* – Relax the muscles of your feet, legs and thighs and allow your whole body to be supported by the floor and bring the focus of your attention to your breathing. – *Pause* – If any thoughts, worries or concerns come into your mind, allow them to come; then allow them to go, bringing your attention back to your breathing. – *Pause* – When you are ready to finish, bring some feeling back into your fingers and toes and take a few deeper breaths in. Open your eyes gently and sit up slowly and gradually.

Physical exercise
For most people the most enjoyable and appropriate way of keeping fit is taking some form of exercise whether it is a daily gentle walk or a weekly energetic game of squash or football. Without "medicalizing" what should be an enjoyable and normal pastime, it may be helpful and at times important to check out how fit you are and what sort of exercise routine suits you best. These can be subdivided into the following groups:

Before choosing an exercise routine, check how fit you are:

How active are you?
How often do you take physical exercise (including keep fit classes and sport) that makes you out of breath?
a Four times or more a week
b Two to three times a week
c Once a week
d Less than once a week

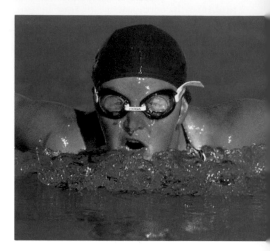

Above: *Swimming is an ideal way to maintain your level of fitness because the buoyancy of the water means that you are not imposing undue stresses and strains on your bones as you do it.*

Exercise	Comments
Very intensive Team or competitive sports. Provide opportunities for very active but intermittent bouts of exercise. Pulse and respiratory rates very rapid at times, e.g. squash, tennis, football, athletics.	▪ Need to be fit first ▪ Win or lose element may be important ▪ Can be dangerous
Moderate/rhythmical Sustained continuous exercise, maintaining a regular and increased pulse and respiratory rate. These can be team or competitive but are usually pursued individually, e.g. swimming, jogging, cycling, walking and/or walking groups, aerobics.	▪ Can be pursued at home, requires little equipment ▪ You can go at your own pace ▪ Can be taught in class and group
Static anaerobic Less intensive with little or no increase in pulse and respiratory rate. Some may involve a degree of stretching and bending which may be difficult for infirm or elderly, e.g. Yoga, gymnastics, Canadian Air Force exercise, weight-lifting, simple stretching exercises.	▪ Yoga is very popular both in class and at home. It instils balance/posture as well as being an exercise ▪ Can be practised at home, inexpensive pursuits
Breathing exercises Many more special exercises using different ways of breathing, emphasizing inhalation and exhalation techniques.	▪ Excellent for elderly and infirm ▪ Used in treatment of specific illnesses, e.g. asthma

How far do you walk each day?
a More than 5km (3 miles)
b Up to 5km (3 miles)
c Less than 1.6km (1 mile)
d Less than 800m (½ mile)

How do you travel to work, the shops?
a All the way by foot/cycle
b Part of the way by foot/cycle
c Occasionally by foot/cycle
d All the way by public transport or car

When there is a choice, do you?
a Take the stairs – up and down – always
b Take the stairs unless you have something to carry
c Occasionally take the stairs
d Take the lift/escalator unless it is broken

At weekends do you?
a Spend several hours gardening/decorating/DIY/doing some sport
b Usually only sit down for meals and in the evening
c Take a few short walks
d Spend most of the time sitting reading/watching TV

Do you think nothing of?
a Doing the household chores after a day's work
b Rushing out to the shops again if you have forgotten something
c Getting other people to run your errands even if you have time.
d Paying for a telephone call when you could make a personal visit

Add up your score, allowing
4 points for every (**a**) answer
3 points for every (**b**) answer
2 points for every (**c**) answer
1 point for every (**d**) answer

20+
You are naturally very active and probably fit.
15-20
You are active and have a healthy attitude toward fitness.
10-15
You are only mildly active and would benefit from more exercise.
Under 10
You are lazy and need to rethink your attitude towards activity. Try to reorganize your day to allow some time devoted to exercise.

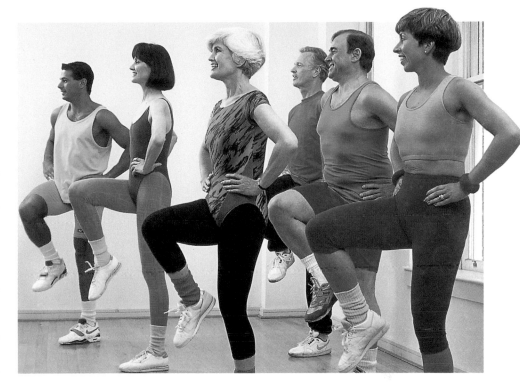

Above: *You do not have to be a supermodel to participate in aerobics. The support of a group is often an excellent motivating factor.*

What can you do?
How long does it take you to:

1 Walk 5km (3 miles) on level ground
1hr 15min (or more)	*1pt*
50min to 1hr 10min	*2pt*
45min (or less)	*3pt*

2 Swim 1,000m (1,100yds)
50min (or more)	*1pt*
35min to 45min	*2pt*
20min (or less)	*3pt*

3 Run 1.6km (1 mile) on level ground
15min (or more)	*1pt*
9-14min	*2pt*
8min (or less)	*3pt*

Scores
3-4
If you have covered these distances, you have made a start. Now keep it up until the test feels easy.
5-6
You are moderately fit. If you want to improve, increase the distance and speed up gradually.
7-9
You have reached a good level of fitness and are ready to start a more vigorous fitness programme.

Simple exercise routines you can practise at home

These routines are valuable, both for relaxation and as a preparation for more vigorous exercise.

Body awareness – *time 15 minutes*
Sway

Wear comfortable loose clothing. Remove shoes and socks. Stand with your feet apart. Close your eyes and take a few moments to settle your breath. Begin to sway slowly, first to the left and then to the right, moving at the ankles. As you sway to the left, breathe in, as you sway to the right, breathe out. Repeat six times.

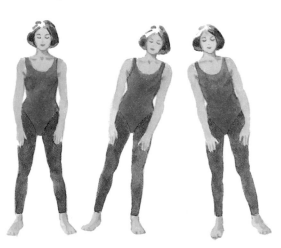

Allow your body to come to the centre position and pause. Now begin to sway backwards and forwards. As you sway backwards, breathe in. As you sway forwards, breathe out. Repeat six times, then allow your body to come to the central position and pause.

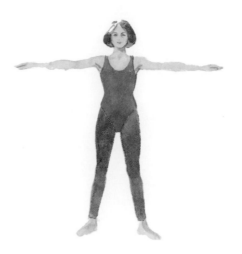

Eye rolls

Open your eyes. Focus your eyes on the top right hand corner of the room and then slowly rotate them through 360° (clockwise) keeping your head straight. Repeat three times. Close your eyes and observe any sensations around them. Repeat again, rotating your eyes in an anti-clockwise manner. Close your eyes. Pause.

Head rolls

Let your head fall down to your chest with your chin tucked in. Slowly rotate your head to the left, bringing your ear as close to your left shoulder as you can. Take your head back and round over the right shoulder and finally bring your chin round to the front. Repeat three times – with your eyes closed – breathing in as you take your head back and breathing out as you bring your head forward. Repeat in the opposite direction three times.

Shoulder circles

Raise your arms sideways parallel to the floor. With your fingers outstretched, begin to make small circles with your hands, rotating your arms at the shoulder joint. Gradually increase the circles, then decrease them. Repeat three times in one direction and three times in another, bringing the arms to rest by your side between times.

Side stretch

With your eyes closed, place your hands on the sides of your legs. Bend to the left, allowing the hand to move down the leg as far as it will go. Come up slowly. Repeat three times, breathing out as you go down and breathing in as you come up. Repeat on the other side.

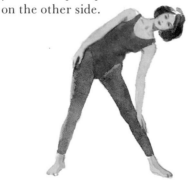

Backwards stretch

Place your hands in the small of your back supporting the back muscles. Slowly bend backwards, stretching the front muscles. Come forward slowly. Repeat three times, breathing in as you bend backwards and breathing out as you bend forwards.

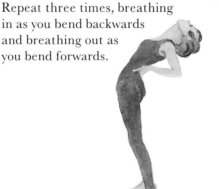

Forward stretch.

Allow your hands and arms to fall forwards. Bend at the waist and allow your head to fall towards your knees. Gently sway for a few moments. Breathe in – and then as you breathe out, allow your head to fall further towards the feet. Pause. Gradually come up, uncurling your back slowly.

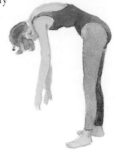

Ankle stretch

(You may need to hold on to a chair or surface for this exercise). Lift your right leg off the floor and stretch it in front of you with the foot a little off the ground. Start rotating your ankle in one direction making small circles with your foot. Repeat three times in one direction, then three times in the other. Place your foot back on the ground and repeat on the other side.

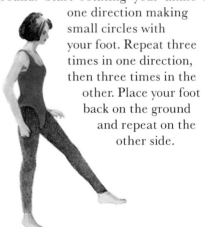

Balance

Focus your eyes on a point on the opposite side of the room. Lift your left foot off the floor and place it just above the ankle of your right leg. (You may need to hold on to a chair for balance). Balance on your right leg, taking a few slow breaths in and out. Bring your left foot back down and repeat on the other side.

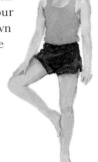

Stretching exercises *(a warm up before jogging or other more vigorous exercise)*

Hamstring stretch

Bend at the waist, clasping the backs of your calves with your hands. Hold for up to ten seconds and repeat five times.

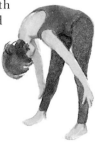

Thigh muscle stretch

Bend the left knee and stretch your right leg out as far as you can go. Balance your body over the left knee and hold for three to five seconds. Keep your right foot flat on the floor. Repeat other side.

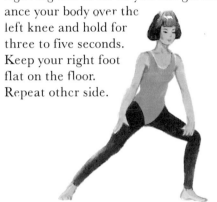

Calf stretch

Place your hands against a wall standing 50cm (18in) away. Support your body with your hands and gradually, with knees locked, bring your pelvis forward. Hold for a few seconds and repeat three to five times.

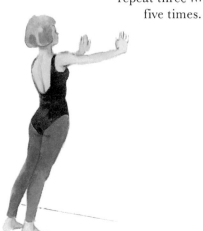

Arm circling

Lift your arms to the side and make three to five vigorous circles with both arms. Repeat in both directions.

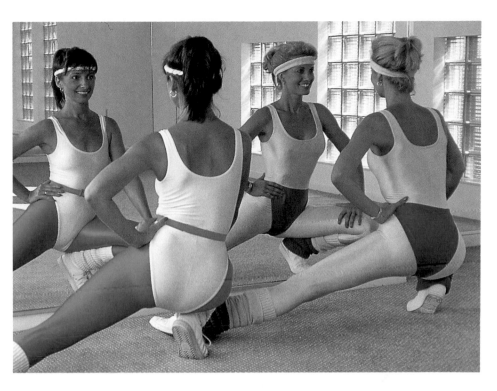

Strengthening exercises

Push-ups (shoulder and chest muscles)

a Table: Find a secure table or ledge. Stand about 60cm (2ft) away and place your outstretched arms on surface. Bend your elbows and allow your chest to come close to the surface of the table. Straighten the arms, pushing your body away. Repeat six to ten times.

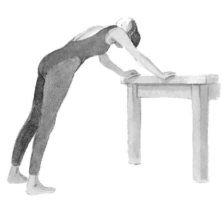

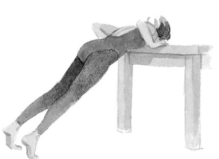

Above: *Gentle stretching is a good way to warm up for more vigorous exercise. These stretches, however, are more demanding, so be careful.*

b Floor: Lie face down on a carpet, mat or rug with your feet stretched out behind you a few centimetres apart. Place your palms on floor next to your shoulders. Push yourself up, keeping your back straight and your arms straight. Initially you may wish to keep your knees on the floor.

Sit-ups

a Chair: Find a chair with a straight back and sit with your head, neck and trunk straight. Place your feet on the floor, keeping your knees together. Raise your knees and at the same time bring your forehead down to touch your knees or as close to them as you can manage. Bring your feet back to the floor and straighten your back. Repeat six times.

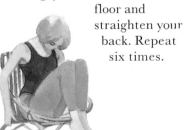

b Floor: Lie on the floor on your back, feet slightly apart. Bend your left knee and bring it towards your abdomen at the same time as bringing your forehead forward. Keep your hands either by your side or folded behind your head. Return your leg and head back to the floor. Repeat three times on the left and then on the right and finally three times with both legs at the same time.

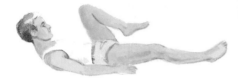

Arch-ups (back muscles)
Lie on the floor face down, hands by your side, feet together. Gradually raise one leg off the floor from the hip keeping the leg straight. Lower and repeat three times. Repeat on the other side. Repeat with both legs together.

Repeat and at the same time lift your trunk off the floor arching the back, keeping your hands by your side. Repeat three times.

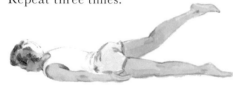

Light endurance exercises
Stair climbing / walking / jogging / running programme.
Points to remember:
▪ Enjoy your exercise.
▪ Do it with awareness.
▪ Know your strengths and limitations.
▪ Warm up before you start.
▪ Cool down after you finish.
▪ Co-ordinate your mind (thoughts and feelings) and your body (movement and speed) with your breath (regular and diaphragmatic).
▪ Ten minutes, three times a week is more beneficial than half an hour at the weekend.
▪ Be creative and develop your own routine.

Stair climbing
▪ Climb stairs rather than take a lift.

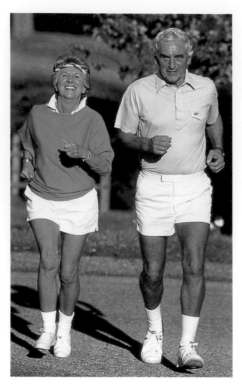

Above: *Jogging can be fun, particularly if you do it with a friend or partner. Try not to get obsessive about it, however; too much of a good thing can actually turn out to be damaging.*

▪ If you have stairs at home, spend five minutes a day climbing up and down. Start slowly and gradually increase the pace and the time spent on this exercise to 15 minutes. You can make this exercise as brisk as you like, but the important factor is co-ordinating your movement, awareness and breathing.

Walking
▪ Walk to the bus stop, railway station, or place of work. Walk to the shops and possibly arrange for any heavy shopping to be delivered. Consider joining a walking group in your area.

Jogging/walking
There is no doubt that for many adults, this activity has enhanced both their physical and mental well-being. However, it has led to many minor and, on occasion, serious health problems. If you are going to jog, jog because you want to, jog with awareness. Make sure you wear proper jogging or training shoes – not gym shoes – as running can impose quite severe stress on your feet,

knees and back. Know your limitations, learn to enjoy the long, slow jog as well as the jog with your wife/husband/friend. You may like to join a running club and for many the participation in a "fun run" or marathon can be a high point in their lives. Do not allow other people to ridicule your efforts but at the same time be clear as to why you are running.

There are many guides, programmes, routines available. Some of them are daunting and can put people off even starting. Remember it is much better to develop your own routine than to follow slavishly with a watch and pedometer someone else's. Experiment with walking slowly, "race walking", slow jogging and running. Vary your course and learn about your neighbourhood. Once a week or month, giving yourself a longer time and run/jog/walk a greater distance, allowing your exercise routine to become a "meditational" exercise for your mind as well as a physical one.

Breathing exercises
As well as undertaking physical exercises to improve general fitness levels, practising some simple breathing exercises will help both to relax you and as a quiet prelude to more vigorous activity.

Full breath (diaphragm – chest – clavicle)
Stand up straight with arms by your side. Begin by breathing in to the count of three with your diaphragm. Now continue to breathe in, expanding your chest to another count of three. Finally expand the upper part of your chest and lower neck again to the count of three. Breathe out, slowly reversing the process (clavicle – chest – diaphragm). Repeat three times.

"Bellows" breathing
This exercise should be performed with care, and if you experience any dizziness you should stop. The abdominal muscles are used to force air in and out like "bellows".
▪ Sit upright with head, neck and trunk in a straight line.
▪ Forcefully contract your abdominal

muscles, expelling air through your nostrils.

▪ Forcefully push out the abdominal muscles and breathe in deeply and quickly.

▪ Repeat this forceful inhalation and exhalation, no more than six times to begin with.

▪ Gradually increase the number as you perfect the process.

Alternate nostril breathing

This exercise helps to keep the nostrils clear and if repeated frequently will keep the body and mind in a state of balance. The breathing is diaphragmatic throughout.

▪ Sit comfortably with head, neck and trunk straight.

▪ Clear each nostril by closing first the right and then the left and exhaling moderately forcefully out of each one in turn.

▪ Close the left nostril with the left index finger.

▪ Exhale gently out of the right nostril.

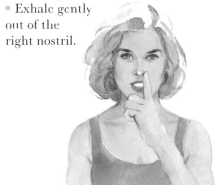

▪ Close the right nostril with the index finger.

▪ Inhale through the left nostril.

▪ Close the left nostril.

▪ Exhale gently through right nostril.

▪ Repeat the exhale/inhale sequence three times.

▪ Now change direction. Inhale through right nostril.

▪ Close right nostril.

▪ Exhale through left nostril.

▪ Close left nostril.

▪ Inhale through right nostril.

▪ Repeat this sequence three times.

There should be no pause between inhalation and exhalation. The breathing should be soundless, smooth and rhythmical.

Sex and sexuality

More has probably been written on the topic of a healthy sex life than on any other area of human life. Sex guides, how-to manuals, explicit videos, all attest to our insatiable desire for a happy and contented sex life. Most emphasis is on the mechanics and physical act of intercourse, yet for most women and, increasingly, for men "making love" as opposed to having sex is essentially an emotional and psychological activity and not just a physical act. For some lucky couples, the act of making love is an integration of body, mind and spirit where two human beings blend themselves into "one". We do not have to be athletic performers or achieve the heights of physical ecstasy: holding hands, massaging, cuddling, comforting, these are ways of making love which need not end in genital intercourse. Many people who have led promiscuous and active sex lives often acknowledge that they indulge in sex only because it allows them an opportunity to be touched and held by another human being. Their disappointment when "all that happens is sex" leads them to search for yet another partner.

What then is a healthy attitude towards sex? First, it involves knowing about your body, and understanding your sexuality. Do you make love to please your partner, because of heightened sexual desire, to express your own power, to assuage your loneliness or out of habit? Try to be as honest as you can with yourself and take the risk of expressing your needs and talking to your partner. Like all human activities, different people react in different ways. Some men and women have a heightened sexual drive and others are not so constituted. There is no "right" or "wrong" performance indicator, any more than there is a "right" or "wrong" height or colouring. Learn to accept your own pattern, allow yourself to be led or guided by your partner if you differ and above all, communicate with him or her so that you both have an opportunity to listen and learn.

The bringing together of two naked bodies in a warm and safe environment

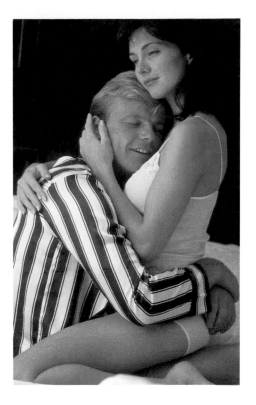

Above: *Good sex is not just about physical gymnastics; lovemaking should involve the mind, spirit and imagination also. At its best, it is one of the most enriching experiences we have.*

cannot always be easily organized, especially if children are around or if there is no privacy. Snatched or quick sex can have its own excitement but ensuring there is enough time for foreplay, with massage, music, incense, perfume and all the erotic and romantic accompaniments to lovemaking is a necessary stage for most couples to learn from one another. Do not get too concerned about a simultaneous orgasm – this is often a fantasy of filmmakers and imaginative authors. Taking it in turns to give pleasure to one another or experimenting with masturbation, especially at times of illness or pregnancy, can be a particularly intimate way of sharing. Change and experimentation is appropriate but so is regularity and habit. Actual intercourse need not be the final act on every occasion. As important is the enriching and deepening of your relationship with your partner, often aided by the sharing of your own vulnerability, as well as the exciting crescendo of full orgasm.

TAKING CARE OF YOUR MIND AND SPIRIT

For most of us, distressing thoughts, feelings, worries about the past or future are a major source of stress. We can find it difficult to switch off and even when we sleep, we may be disturbed by dreams or nightmares.

The relaxation exercises described previously will allow you to let go of muscle tension in your body and can be a good start to letting go of troubled thoughts. A more systematic way of "relaxing" the mind is through the exercise of meditation. Many of us do this naturally when we gaze into a fire or watch the ocean waves. Listening to a piece of calming music can also help, as can being "lost" in a good book. Systematic meditational practice, however, allows you to develop mastery over the process of letting go and, like the breathing and relaxation techniques, can be done at home in private and as a daily "lifestyle" routine.

Although meditation is associated with most religions and can be linked to other religious practices, it can be introduced without any spiritual connotations. Many laboratory experiments have shown that the changes in the body occurring during meditation include a slowing of the pulse rate, a lowering of the blood pressure and increased blood flow to the toes and fingers. Changes in brain-wave activity include a more rhythmical electrical pattern (alpha wave) which is found in calm, relaxed states. Blood tests carried out on people who regularly meditate show a drop in the stress hormone level and some have even managed to lower their levels of cholesterol through meditation.

Learning to meditate

It is necessary to put aside some time, say 10-20 minutes early in the morning or before you go to sleep at night. Find a quiet place in your home, preferably one where you will not be disturbed. It is helpful to keep the same place for meditation as this reinforces the habit. It also gives that place in your home a

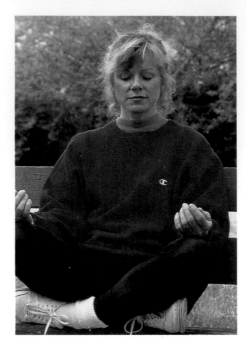

Above: *During meditation the pulse slows, blood pressure drops, the brain relaxes, stress hormones subside. No wonder you feel good!*

special significance. The next step is to find an appropriate chair. Meditation is best practised sitting up. Of course you can meditate lying down on your bed, but there is a greater likelihood of your falling asleep. Meditation is not sleeping – you should be alert and awake. However, there is nothing to stop you practising meditation to help you to go off to sleep. Choose a chair which is comfortable and which has a straight back. It is important not to slouch, although there is no reason why you should not support your back with a cushion or pillow. Keep your head, neck and body erect. If your feet do not reach the floor comfortably, put a small cushion underneath them. If you prefer to sit on the floor, find the most comfortable position for yourself and try to tilt your pelvis by placing a small cushion under your seat.

Close your eyes and place your hands just above your knees. Focus your attention on your breathing. Gradually deepen your breathing, with your diaphragm, allowing the inhala-

tion to follow the exhalation. Spend a few minutes focusing on your breath. Take your attention to your forehead – relax the muscles of your forehead – relax the muscles of your eyes – relax the muscles of your face. Check that your jaw is not too tightly closed and that your tongue is lying smooth and easily in your mouth. Relax your shoulders – relax your hands and fingers – relax your chest and abdomen – relax your thighs, knees, ankles and feet. Bring your attention back to your breathing – *Pause* – allow the breath to become smooth and even.

Now, as you breathe in, place the word "so" on your breath, silently, without moving your lips. As you breathe out, place the word "hum" on your out-breath, silently, without moving your lips. Continue to breathe smoothly and evenly, repeating the sounds "so" and "hum" on your inhalation and exhalation. If any thoughts, worries or distractions come into your mind, allow them to come and then allow them to go, bringing your attention back to your breathing and the sounds "so" and "hum".

Continue for another five to ten minutes, repeating the sounds internally in unison with your breath. When you are about to stop, bring some feeling back into your fingers and toes. Take a few deeper breaths in and out and gently open your eyes.

Tips to deepen your meditation

- Do not eat or drink for up to half-an-hour before.
- Meditate in a group.
- Buy a meditation tape.
- Practise a breathing exercise.
- Avoid stimulant foods and alcohol.

Remember, the purpose of most methods of meditation is to free the mind from the cramp of conscious control and allow it to operate in neutral gear. For most beginners, this can be a difficult notion to grasp, for if we want to do something successfully, our way is to try harder. Trying hard to meditate is not likely to help you meditate. It is important to learn how to "let go" or surrender to the deeper and quieter part of yourself.

Another way of exploring that quieter part of yourself is through visualization. Visualization is a way of using the "mind's eye" to obtain information about yourself or your situation. It can also be used to produce physical changes within the body and help you to relax. Allowing yourself to hold on to an image of peacefulness can often help to bring about that state more effectively than willing yourself to be peaceful. Visualization, or the use of imagery, has developed into a major clinical tool for many mental as well as physical disorders. Consciously constructed images (called either active imagination, guided fantasies or directed day-dreaming) have been used to treat patients with asthma, heart attacks and cancer. You can use visualization to aid your ability to work with your breathing, relaxation and meditation. On other occasions you can use this technique to reduce pain or explore creatively a problem or difficulty you are currently experiencing.

Visualization with breathing
Lie down on the floor or bed and follow the instructions for diaphragmatic

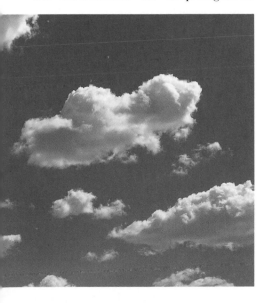

Above: *Conjuring up a restful mental image such as this is a positive help when you practise visualization. It lets your mind float free.*

breathing (pp 22-23). When your breathing is quiet and rhythmical, imagine a circle in front of your eyes. As you breathe in, imagine you are drawing half a circle with your breath. As you breathe out, imagine your breath completing the circle. Repeat this a few times, trying to make the circle as smooth and round as you can. After a few minutes allow this image to go and imagine you are breathing in from the tips of your toes to the top of your skull and as you breathe out, you breathe out from the top of your skull to the tips of your toes. Try and imagine the breath actually travelling all the way up and down the spine.

Visualization and relaxation
Once you have achieved a state of progressive relaxation as described earlier, allow a picture of a favourite, restful place to develop in front of your closed eyes. It might be a mountainside, or by the sea, or a special room. Allow whatever image occurs to form and develop the picture slowly by filling in the various objects or items associated with it. Look at each object in turn and heighten the colours associated with the object. Now fill the atmosphere a little more with the sounds and smells associated with this place. If your attention wanders, gently bring it back to the image and allow the picture to reform. After five to ten minutes, gradually let go of the image and bring your attention slowly back to your body and then slowly back to the room you are in.

Visualization for pain relief
It is usually necessary to have acquired some expertise for this process to be effective in severe pain. First, use your breath to reduce the tension surrounding the painful part. Close your eyes, focus on your breathing as described previously, slow your breathing down, then imagine that you are breathing in and out through the painful part joint, tooth, head. As you breathe into the part, imagine a warm glow being carried into the part by your breath, and as you breathe out, imagine the pain and tension being carried away by the breath. An additional image that

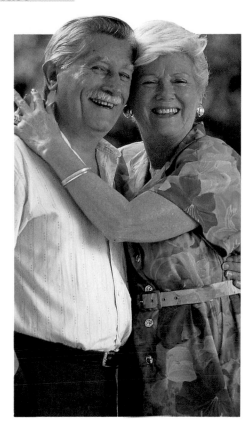

Above: *This couple's body language says "happiness and affection". Feelings, both good and bad, must be expressed, not bottled up.*

helps some people is to imagine a dial which they can turn up or down – turning the dial one way decreases the pain, and turning the dial the other increases the pain.

Working with feelings
Our feelings are often the most individual part of ourselves, and usually the most difficult to manage. Feelings are a subtle mixture of both a mental and physical experience. Observable physical changes occur when someone is overwhelmed with a feeling, such as anger, sadness, joy. We look at people's faces or posture and are able to detect how they are feeling. We get some guidance at school about our bodies and minds but very rarely are we given any advice as to how to manage our feelings. More often than not we are told in many different ways "not to show our feelings". Even to talk about managing feelings seems inappropriate. Yet there are occasions when we need to moderate our feelings or when the physical experience is so distress-

ing that it is necessary to find ways of reducing the discomfort.

Not all feelings are negative, and the joy, happiness and sheer ecstasy enjoyed in pursuing pleasurable pursuits are as important as the sadness, misery and unhappiness that are part of most people's human experience. Feelings are neither "bad" nor "good", they are there, to be experienced. Nevertheless a long-held feeling or resentment or guilt or anger may well produce a chronic mental attitude of physical difficulty. Norman Cousins, in his book *Anatomy of an Illness*, describes how a positive feeling of happiness and laughter can moderate illness and reverse its symptoms.

Exercise for recapturing a feeling

Write about a feeling of which you would like to find out more. Try and remember when you last felt angry or frightened. Notice what physical sensations occur in your body. Where do you tense – does your face change – is your breathing different? Now notice what thoughts arise as you remember that feeling. You may choose to accentuate the feeling and the physical changes to increase your awareness for a minute.

Below: *It is easy to let negative feelings overwhelm you with a sense of helplessness; but you can learn to break the vicious circle.*

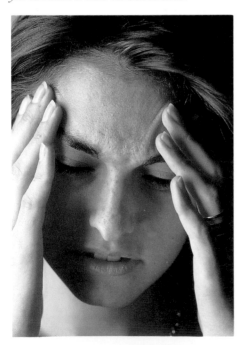

This exercise will help make you more familiar with the way your body and mind responds to feeling.

Exercise for understanding your feelings

Complete the following sentences:
- I feel angry when
- I feel that my anger is
- When others express their anger towards me I feel
- I feel that the anger of others is

Examine the sentences you have completed and ask a close friend to comment on them. Is your difficulty related to the expression of feeling, or to being on the receiving end of other people's emotions? You can then "practise" with a friend to try and learn what can be seen as a "social skill".

Exercise for shifting thoughts to help with feelings

Feelings almost invariably either follow a thought or are preceded by a thought. Thinking your way into a depression or a state of fear is not uncommon, and it is therefore possible to reverse the process and think yourself out of a distressing feeling. All too often the individual is caught up by the physical nature of the feeling and is unable to think. The previous exercise will help as it may reveal the irrational nature of the thoughts. It is necessary on occasions to use the breathing exercises to provide you with an emotional "breathing space" so that you can allow thoughts to develop and be resolved.

Often our feelings operate on a two-point scale: either we have none or the emotion is so intense that it is overwhelming. While in a calm and balanced state, it can be helpful to let the alternate emotional responses that could be more appropriate in the problem situation with which you are faced, emerge. Much of *assertiveness* training is concerned with separating inappropriate aggression (rage, fury) from assertive statements ("Please do not do that again"). Panic or severe anxiety about a piece of work can be altered to manageable concern. Guilt at having caused someone pain can be modified to regret and apology.

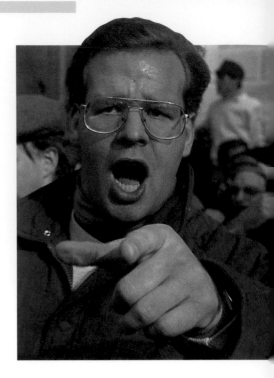

Above: *On occasions anger is a justifiable reaction; however, when it is inappropriate to its cause, it becomes damaging.*

Exercise for letting go of your feelings

Much of psychotherapy, and the church confessional for that matter, is concerned with giving people the space to "get something off their chest". Most of us have had experiences where the emotional impact of an experience has not been sufficiently well dealt with. It might be that we repressed a feeling (anger at losing a job, sadness at the break-up of a marriage) or that our feelings were not accepted as valid by our family or friends. Repressed and unexpressed emotions cause havoc with our mental life and subsequent relationships. Arriving home after a frustrating day at work, feeling resentful, irritable and angry, is a recipe for disaster on the home front. Discharging such a feeling is as important as being aware of the need to cry and sob and weep when something distressing has occurred (a bereavement or a disappointment).

Anger and frustration can often be helped by physical effort – running or jogging, or hitting a ball hard with a tennis racquet, or punching a mattress or pillow. Shouting at the top of your voice in your car as you drive home, or in a park, may appear odd and unusual, but it is much better than shouting at your wife, husband or children. Letting go of tears is more difficult and it may require the help of a friend, counsellor or sympathetic doctor. Tears contain a raised level of the stress hormone cortisol and they are the natural way of relieving the body and mind of stress. As you cry, your body is "unloading" the stress hormone.

Working with irrational thoughts

Statements such as "it's all in the mind", "it's mind over matter", "the power of positive thinking" illustrate the belief that we can train our minds to think in a particular way which will then produce changes both in our feelings and in our attitudes and relationships. There is no doubt that this sort of activity is possible, but the danger is that if it is pursued to its extreme, the idea that sadness or regret or dislike or even hate is only a negative emotion or thought develops. An holistic approach involves accepting both positive and negative aspects of ourselves and not necessarily denying or repressing the negative. With that word of caution, positive thinking can be of great help to

Below: *We all have to cope with bereavement. Allowing yourself to mourn is just as important for your health as eating the right foods.*

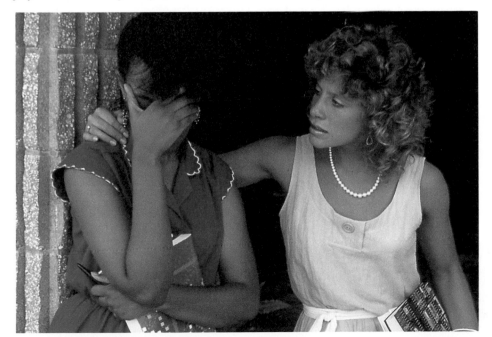

people who habitually put themselves down or feel worthless and hopeless. Giving yourself a few phrases to repeat in a difficult or stressful situation can help you to cope with that situation, e.g.
Preparation
  "There's nothing to worry about"
  "I'm going to be all right"
  "It's easier once you get started"
Confronting
  "Take it step by step"
  "I can only do my best"
  "I can get help if I need it"
Coping with fear
  "Relax *now*"
  "Breathe deeply"
  "There is an end to it"
Reinforcing success
  "I did it"
  "Next time I won't worry so much"
  "I am able to relax away anxiety"

Coping with death and bereavement

Healthy living must, at some stage, address the subject of death. The Tibetans believed that it was not possible to judge the value of a person's life until one had witnessed his manner of dying. Our culture is more geared towards denying death and retarding the aging process. Our health service could really be described as a "death prevention" service. Doctors and nurses consider themselves to have failed if a patient dies. We have developed an impressive array of procedures, chemical agents, life-support machines, transplant surgery, the aim of which is to prolong life and prevent death. The human feelings surrounding death are banished with admonitions against showing emotions. In many cases, what people are frightened of is not death itself but the process of dying. This is not surprising, given that we avoid this topic and are unwilling to discuss it openly for fear of being morbid or nihilistic. Yet the truth, and probably the only truth we can be certain of, is that we shall all die.

Recently some pioneers have attempted to bring the subject of death out into the open for honest discussion. Elizabeth Kübler-Ross interviewed many patients who were at the last stages of their lives and described four stages that many terminally ill people go through:

■ *Denial* People do not hear, or wish to hear, their prognosis. They put on a brave face and both relatives and the doctors avoid the subject of death.

■ *Anger* The "why me?" question is followed by "somebody is to blame": the diagnosis was missed or the treatment was incorrect, or "if only I had stopped smoking" etc.

■ *Bargaining* An attempt is made to "change my lifestyle", take the tablets, eat lentils or meditate regularly. We are willing to undertake heroic surgery – anything to avoid accepting that our death is imminent.

■ *Acceptance* For those who manage to "work through" their depression, the acceptance of the inevitable brings with it a sense of release, joy and spontaneous awe, which can be of major benefit to both the patient and his family.

This stage of "expect and accept" is not an easy one to arrive at but has a spiritual and religious quality which enriches everyone. It is interesting to observe that the stages described by Kübler-Ross are often experienced by those relatives who are left behind and who mourn the loss of someone they love. They are the normal pattern of human response and as such as necessary for healthy living as a dietary programme or exercise routine.

TAKING CARE OF YOUR ENVIRONMENT

These days it is not just enough to look after oneself without spending equal time looking after the environment. The effect of the environment on individual health is now so well-established that to concentrate on one and ignore the other is to do only half a job. Some of the damage done to the environment can be a direct result of our own individual actions, but the major pollution occurs from the side effects of a consumer-driven industrial society. Now that the threat of nuclear war has receded, the focus has been directed towards the pollution of the air, sea and earth through many of our manufacturing processes. Organizations such as Friends of the Earth and Greenpeace campaign to ensure that we do not lose sight of the problem and the various Green parties in Europe and America have also played their part so that now all major industrialized countries have a Minister of the Environment and participate in international agreements regarding damage to the ozone layer.

Below: *This barren landscape shows what happens if you do not care for your environment; factory pollution and emissions of noxious gases cause acid rain which kills trees.*

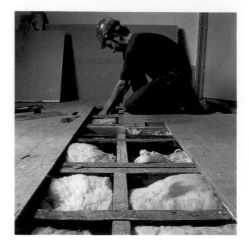

Above: *Home loft insulation is a simple way by which your domestic energy consumption can be quite significantly reduced.*

The dumping of waste in the sea is also much better controlled.

It is quite understandable that individuals, when presented with a global picture, can shrug their shoulders at the enormity of the problem and feel that personal sacrifices are pointless. The most that it seems any individual can do is to donate to a favourite charity and leave the problem to governments. This is a defeatist attitude; individuals can make a difference by changing in small ways without dramatically affecting their lifestyle. Below are some suggested "changes" that if undertaken collectively will reduce the damage done by us to the environment and, incidentally, improve the "individual environment" around and within you.

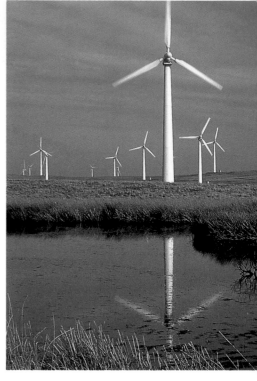

Above: *"Green energy"* – concern about the atmospheric pollution caused by burning fossil fuels has led to the development of wind farms.

▪ Eat less protein
Reduce your meat intake, or change your source of protein. The source of protein (meat/fish/beans/rice) determines the patterns of our agricultural industry. The production of meat requires ten units of energy to provide one unit of energy for the consumer, whereas rice provides 40 units of energy for the consumer for every one unit of energy required to produce it.

▪ Look out for additives on consumable purchases
Insisting that our apples look like apples means that producers wax them to give them an appealing appearance.

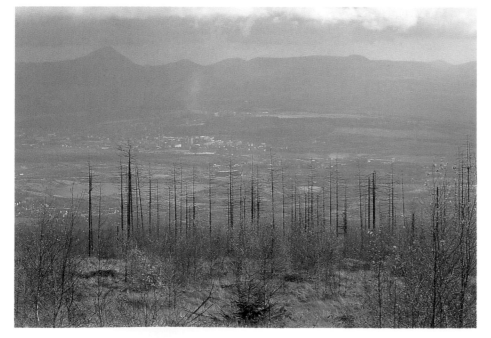

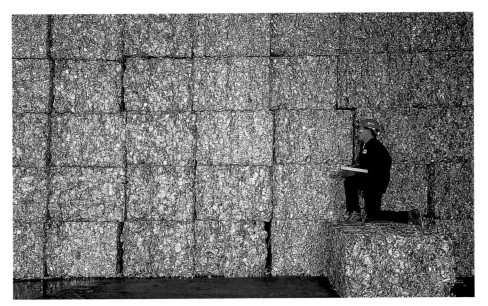

Above: Eloquent testimony both to Western consumerism and the benefits of recycling; the aluminium in these cans can be recovered.

Expecting the "right" colouring for food requires the use of artificial colouring. We eat the equivalent of 16 tablets of aspirin in food additives a day and over half of them are purely for cosmetic reasons.

▪ Use unleaded petrol

Over 25,000 tonnes of lead are released every year into the atmosphere through car exhaust fumes. By switching to unleaded fuel, you can help to reduce this figure.

Below: Destruction of the Amazonian rain forest in Ecuador. If you care about this, join an environmental group to campaign against it.

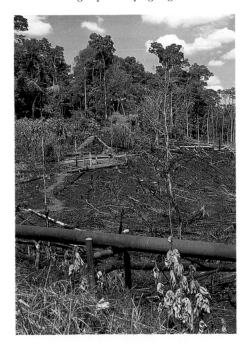

▪ Reduce your purchase of aerosols

The CFC used as propellant liquid in aerosols has caused major "holes" in the ozone layer around the Earth that protects the skin from the powerful ultra-violet light from the Sun that causes skin cancer. The use of CFCs has to be curbed.

▪ Walk to the shops and take your own carrier bag with you

Twenty-nine million acres (11.7 million hectares) of forest are destroyed annually. The average European uses 120kg (265lb) of paper and board a year – the equivalent figure for an Indian is 2kg (4.4lb) The loss of so much forest has led to an increase in carbon dioxide in the atmosphere which in turn leads to global warming. Global warming may bring about a potentially disastrous change in the world's climate.

▪ Insulate your home where possible

Hang a curtain behind your front door in the cold weather, for instance, and switch off any unnecessary lights or electrical appliances. Energy consumption has trebled since 1945 and the average person in the prosperous Northern hemisphere uses 15 times more energy than someone in the Southern hemisphere. It is not altogether clear how long our present sources of energy are likely to last, but

as Kenneth Boulding has said "Anyone who believes exponential growth can go on forever in a finite world is either a madman or an economist!"

▪ Repair and mend when you can

The life of an electrical appliance is on average five to seven years, mainly because of built-in obsolescence. Between 1900-1950, it was 20 years. A teddy bear in the early part of the century lasted for life – now it is changed every three years.

▪ Recycle where possible

Sort out your cans, papers and bottles and take them to your local recycling sites. On average in the West, we each use the equivalent of 1,000 soft drink cans a year. Throwing this quantity of waste away is undesirable.

▪ Do not smoke in public places – if possible, stop altogether

This is the simplest way to clean up your "personal environment".

▪ Join one local and one national environmental group

This will help to raise your consciousness on both a local and national level. The support of a group will also reinforce your own personal resolution. It is all too easy to overlook the problems and turn a blind eye.

Below: Tram systems are regaining popularity at the moment. It makes sense environmentally to use public transport whenever possible.

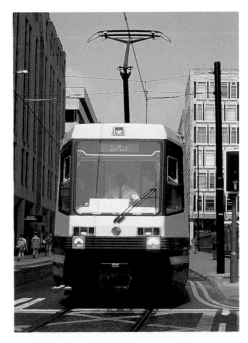

PART TWO

ALTERNATIVE AND COMPLEMENTARY THERAPIES

As mentioned in the introduction, the term "alternative medicine" covers a vast range of activities, the only thing they have in common being that they are not taught at a Western medical school. It is important to recognize that some of these activities have long traditions that predate modern medicine while others are relatively new. The following categorization will help the reader to understand the scope and range of these different approaches.

Group 1: Complete systems of healing

There are systems of healing which have had a theoretical base as to the causation of disease. They have a diagnostic, investigative and therapeutic understanding which share some similarities with orthodox medicine. Some of these systems have been around for many thousands of years, others are relatively new. The major categories that are available widely around the world are:

- Homeopathy
- Acupuncture or traditional Chinese medicine

- Osteopathy and chiropractic
- Herbal medicine
- Naturopathy
- Ayurvedic medicine
- Yoga

Most of these systems of healing have an educational framework, publish ethical guidelines and attempt to regulate their practitioners in the same way as any orthodox medical council might regulate doctors. They consider themselves, by and large, to be competent enough to deal with most of the problems that come their way, although most practitioners tend to suggest that many acute and life-threatening problems are better dealt with by orthodox medicine.

Group 2: Diagnostic methods

These are ways of determining the presence or absence of disease using methods not normally associated with traditional medicine, e.g.

- Iridology – as a test for hidden disease

Below: *The healing touch. One of the attractions of alternative therapies like chiropractic is that patient and healer are in physical contact.*

- Kinesiology – as a test for allergies
- Hair analysis – as a test for nutritional defects
- Kirlian photography/aura diagnosis – as a test for levels of well-being
- Biofeedback

Group 3: Therapeutic methods

These treatments again are not found in traditional medicine, and the list is very long. Most practitioners of these therapies do not claim any diagnostic skill, but they do claim that their treatments can and do work. It is probably within this group that the term complementary is most suitable. The treatments "complement" or "supplement" what is already on offer. This group includes:

- Aromatherapy
- Bach flower remedies
- Biochemic tissue salts
- Massage, or therapeutic touch
- Reflexology
- Hydrotherapy
- Hypnotherapy
- Spiritual healing

Group 4: Self-help measures

This group includes the package of self-help measures where patients are encouraged to undertake certain practices and exercises that will either diminish their symptoms, improve their health or maintain their well-being. These self-help measures include:

- Alexander Technique
- Autogenic training
- Bates eye exercises
- Bioenergetics
- Aerobics and other exercise routines
- T'ai-chi Ch'uan
- Breathing and relaxation techniques
- Meditation
- Visualization
- Fasting or dieting

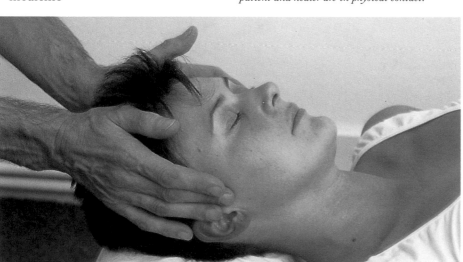

COMPLETE SYSTEMS OF HEALING

HOMEOPATHY

Homeopathy is a "system of therapeutics" or treatments which use very minute amounts of natural products to aid the patient's natural process of recovery. It has achieved wide acceptance in the UK because of the much publicized link with the Royal Family and because it is one of the few alternative therapies that is available on the National Health Service.

Homeopathy as an approach to treatment was established by a German physician, Dr. Samuel Hahnemann, who published the first basic text book in 1810. The principles involved in homeopathic prescribing were known to previous physicians and had been used in Ayurvedic medicine (the natural medicine of India) for many centuries before Hahnemann. It was he, however, who spent most of his life establishing the modern foundation of homeopathy. The basic principles include the notion encapsulated in the Latin phrase "*Similia similibus curentur*" – "Like cures like".

Hahnemann observed that many treatments used to treat disease actually caused the symptoms produced by the disease itself. His initial discovery was with quinine which was – and is still – used for the treatment of malaria. Quinine will produce the high temperatures, sweats and rigors which characterize a malarial attack. Hahnemann wondered whether this principle of "Like cures like" could be used for treating other diseases. He set about systematically testing over 4,000 substances, a process known as "provings", by taking them in high doses himself and noting all the symptoms they produced. He then gave these substances in dilute form to patients with symptoms of diseases and noted that they improved, e.g. *Nux vomica* (obtained from the poison nut tree) will in large doses produce vomiting, abdominal cramps and diarrhoea. If given to patients suffering with these symp-

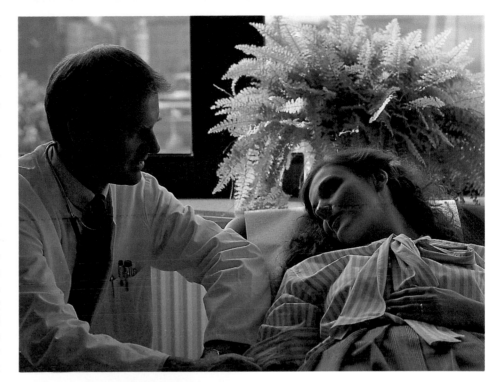

Above: *Homeopathic diagnosis is "holistic": a patient's personality and individual symptoms, or "peculiars", form part of the assessment.*

The manufacture of homeopathic remedies

After initial provings, the animal, mineral or plant extract is preserved in an alcohol solution and the active ingredient is extracted. This forms the "mother tincture". This tincture is then systematically diluted to produce the various homeopathic strengths. Each time the solution is diluted it is "potentized" by shaking in a process known as succussion. It is believed by homeopaths that this process affects the molecular structure of the liquid (water or alcohol) in such a way that the "footprints" of the active ingredient are imprinted on each molecule, so that in extreme dilutions, even though no active ingredient is present, the "energetic memory" of the remedy is transferred to the molecular structure of the dilutant. A tenfold dilution is expressed by the symbol x, a hundredfold dilution by the symbol c, and a thousandfold dilution by the symbol m.

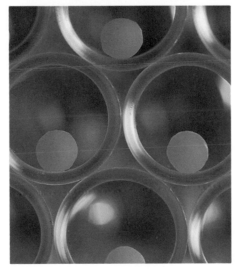

Above: *Homeopathy's founder, Samuel Hahnemann, believed that the more a remedy was diluted, the more powerful its effect would be.*

toms, *Nux vomica* is a very effective remedy. Hahnemann's second discovery, which is the most controversial of homeopathic principles, is that the more dilute the remedy, the more powerful its effect is. Thus he established a method of manufacturing remedies which is still in use today.

Thus *Nux vomica* 6x is an extract of the active substance diluted to 10^6 or 1/1,000,000 of its original strength. Homeopathic remedies are available over the counter to the public at the small dilutions of 6x while homeopaths prescribe 1m dilutions believing them to be the most powerful remedies. Science indicates that above 10^{23} dilutions no molecule exists of the original substance, and the scientific community does not accept the claims made by homeopaths that these remedies can have any effect other than as a placebo. It is this second principle of homeopaths that understandably prevents scientists from accepting homeopathy as a valid approach to treatment.

Hahnemann's third principle was that taking a case history in homeopathy involves an "holistic" approach, i.e. the patient's totality of symptoms as well as his personality should form part of the assessment before a remedy is prescribed. This leads to patients with identical diseases, e.g. asthma or the common cold, being offered completely different remedies because their personalities are different, or what are known as the "peculiars" (specific individual symptoms) vary. Homeopaths look for "peculiars", e.g. the catarrh is worse on the left side than the right, the pain is worse in the morning than at night, the skin changes colour when the room temperature changes, as very significant pointers to the remedies required. Thus a proper homeopathic case history may take as long as one or two hours to assemble.

The final principle of homeopathic medicine is the "law of direction". This law maintains that severe disease improves by symptoms moving from inside the body outwards, i.e. as asthma improves, the patient may develop eczema (a skin condition). Homeopaths believe they can treat most of the diseases to which we are subject although they accept that life-threatening conditions should be assessed by a medically qualified doctor.

Where science has studied homeopathy, it has come up with a series of not very convincing trials, and an honest onlooker would come to the conclu-sion that the jury is still out as to the effectiveness of homeopathy in treating disease. Such trials as have been conducted do not provide enough evidence to satisfy the sceptics that homeopathy is not a placebo. Laboratory experiments and the treatment of animals by homeopathy have all indicated that some changes occur and that, for instance, the prevention of recurrent abortions in pigs is successful with homeopathic remedies. These studies are felt by supporters of homeopathy to overcome the suspicion that homeopathy is "only a placebo" as animals are not thought to respond to placebos. The debate is now centring around the "transfer of energy" question and, paradoxically, high-tech medicine through Nuclear Magnetic Resonance Imaging (which uses a scanning machine that is able to produce detailed pictures of the behaviour of molecules and atoms) may help to demonstrate how vibrated dilutions of homeopathic remedies have different energy patterns from unvibrated ones, a central principle involved in the manufacture of homeopathic remedies.

Below: *The concept of Chi or energy is central to traditional Chinese medicine. The Chinese believe that Chi flows through the body in 14 channels or meridians that follow the paths indicated.*

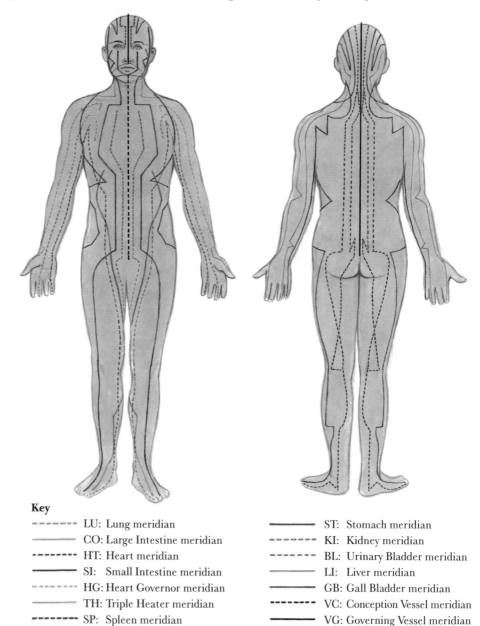

Key

------- LU: Lung meridian	——— ST: Stomach meridian
——— CO: Large Intestine meridian	------- KI: Kidney meridian
- - - - HT: Heart meridian	------- BL: Urinary Bladder meridian
——— SI: Small Intestine meridian	——— LI: Liver meridian
------- HG: Heart Governor meridian	——— GB: Gall Bladder meridian
——— TH: Triple Heater meridian	------- VC: Conception Vessel meridian
------- SP: Spleen meridian	——— VG: Governing Vessel meridian

ACUPUNTURE AND TRADITIONAL CHINESE MEDICINE

Acupunture or "treatment with needles" is the name given by a Dutch physician to traditional Chinese medicine which he first introduced to the West in 1688. The placing of needles in the skin is only one aspect of a rich and detailed system of healing that has been used for over 4,000 years and which was collected and described in the classic textbook, *The Yellow Emperor's Classic of Internal Medicine* (the *Nei Ching*) written some time between 770-476 BC, surely one of the first great books of medicine. In this book is described the basis of Chinese medicine which involves the use of herbs, diet, exercise, moxibustion (heat treatment), as well as acupuncture. The Chinese understanding of the way the body, mind and spirit works is radically different from what is understood and studied by Western doctors but its detailed description is as intricate and complex as any of the biochemical or genetic theories of causation found in Western medicine.

The Chinese understood the functioning of the human being, as well as the Universe, as following the laws of Yin and Yang. These terms refer to the nature of energy or Chi (Qi) that was thought to pervade all things. Yin energy (feminine) is said to be "soft", "dark", "cold" and "wet" while Yang energy (masculine) is said to be "hard", "bright", "hot" and "dry". In a healthy person, Yin and Yang energies flow throughout the body and are in constant flux, ever-changing to produce a balance and harmony. This energy, or Chi, is said to flow through twelve main channels or meridians and two accessory channels. These channels do not follow any anatomical pathway recognized by Western science.

A Chinese doctor will assess an individual's health and make a diagnosis by measuring the nature and flow of energy using a number of techniques, but primarily following the classic mode of pulse and tongue diagnosis. If the flow of Chi is disordered in some

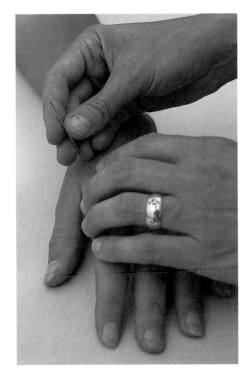

Above: *An acupuncturist is seen inserting a needle in a point on the Large Intestine meridian to stimulate and balance the flow of Chi.*

way, either blocked or deficient, then a disease ensues which may produce symptoms in an organ that may be situated some distance from the blockage. All along the 14 meridians

through which Chi flows, there are points (acupuncture points) where the Chi can be stimulated and the flow corrected. So a Chinese practitioner, after making his assessment, will place needles along selected points in order to correct any imbalances in the flow of energy he has detected.

Chinese practitioners believe that there are three major reasons why the flow of Chi is disturbed – abnormalities in the diet, emotional disturbances and the effect of climatic conditions (cold or hot weather). So in addition to the placing of needles, the patient will be prescribed a diet and told to avoid certain foods and be given instructions on exercises, ways of sleeping and postures to adopt – all thought to influence the flow of Chi. Counselling and psychological advice all form part of traditional Chinese medicine as excessive emotion is thought to be one of the causative factors of disease. The classic text describes how "joy and shock injure the heart, anger injures the liver, worry and over-concentration, the spleen" and so on.

Below: *Tongue examination is a classic diagnostic technique in Chinese medicine. The tongue is thought to mirror the state of the body.*

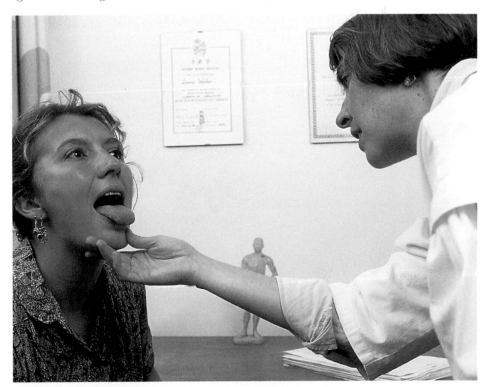

Methods of diagnosis and treatment

Pulse and tongue diagnosis In Chinese medicine, there are thought to be twelve different pulses, six points on each wrist each connected to different organ systems in the body. The Chinese practitioner will feel not just for the quality of the beat but its strength and regularity, as well as its speed and rhythm. The tongue will reveal much information as to the nature and depth of the problem. Many experienced practitioners find that tongue diagnosis is affected by the ingestion of Western drugs that can make an accurate diagnosis difficult.

The placing of needles The needles used are fine, sound, stainless steel, sterilized instruments which may vary in length. In most instances a needle is inserted a few millimetres into the chosen acupuncture point (in some special cases, the needle is inserted much deeper). It is very rare for the patient to feel the needle being inserted and, at most, it is experienced as a slight prick. Pain does not occur and when the needle is withdrawn bleeding is very rare.

Below: *Complementary medicine goes high-tech. Electro-acupuncture uses probes which deliver a low frequency electric current to acupuncture points along the body's meridians.*

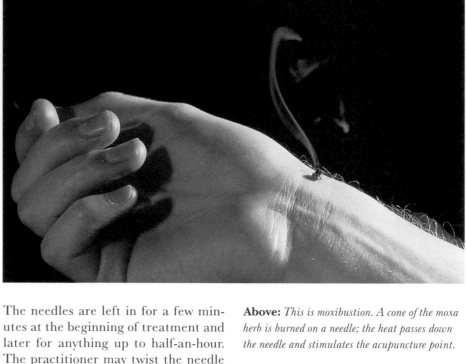

The needles are left in for a few minutes at the beginning of treatment and later for anything up to half-an-hour. The practitioner may twist the needle in the skin to stimulate the acupuncture point or he may use moxibustion and more recently electro-acupuncture (see below).

Moxibustion Moxa is a herb (common mugwort) which is processed as a stick of woolly loose material which is placed on the top of the acupuncture needle and lit, so as to warm the needle and thus further stimulate the point.

Above: *This is moxibustion. A cone of the moxa herb is burned on a needle; the heat passes down the needle and stimulates the acupuncture point.*

Electro-acupuncture More recently, various electrical machines have been constructed which both help to identify acupuncture points and to deliver a very small current through the needle to aid point stimulation.

What conditions does it treat?

In China, and many other countries in the East, traditional Chinese medicine is the normal folk medicine used to treat almost any condition. In the West, acupuncture (the placing of needles) has been developed almost as a separate treatment in itself and many practitioners, especially doctors who have received additional training, do not follow the guidelines of traditional Chinese medicine. This placing of needles or Western acupuncture is used primarily for pain relief in childbirth. One of the consequences of receiving acupuncture treatment is a general relaxation and feeling of drowsiness and for this reason it is often used in stress-related disorders where there is a lot of muscle tension and anxiety. Acupuncture has also been found to be helpful in treating addictive disorders – such as giving up of cigarette smoking and the use of drugs. Many classically trained Chinese practitioners find this

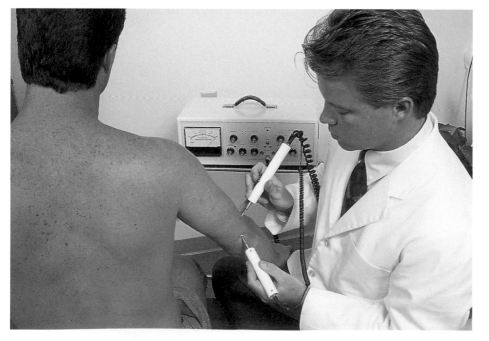

piecemeal use of acupuncture unacceptable and will practise the whole range of Chinese treatments, accepting patients who present with both simple complaints, e.g. diarrhoea and chest infections, as well as with more serious conditions, such as high blood pressure and asthma.

Scientific views

Acupuncture has been one of the most studied of alternative therapies and there is a wealth of scientific evidence supporting some of the claims made by its proponents. The effects of acupuncture – primarily pain relief – are thought to be transmitted either by the release of the body's own pain-killers (chemical substances called endorphins) or the involvement of what has been described as the "gate theory of pain". Acupuncture is thought to stimulate nerve endings which "shut the gate" on those nerve fibres that send pain messages to the brain. Studies comparing random needling to acupuncture show quite clearly that the accurate placing of needles in appropriate acupuncture points relieves pain more systematically than needles placed in the body at random. Other studies show the benefit of acupuncture in such conditions as migraine, irritable bowel syndrome and asthma.

OSTEOPATHY AND CHIROPRACTIC

Both these forms of alternative medicine grew out of the dissatisfaction of their founders with the approaches of traditional doctors to the problems that patients presented. They felt that the impotence of modern medicine to treat adequately musculo-skeletal disorders required a new approach. Initially both Andrew Taylor Still, who founded osteopathy in the mid-1870s, and David Daniel Palmer, the founder of chiropractic at the end of the 19th century, felt that their mode of treatment and their understanding of disease could be applied not just to problems of the body's skeletal system (bones, muscles, joints, ligaments) but to general conditions and internal diseases (asthma,

gastric ulcers etc.). Most modern osteopaths and chiropractors, however, now limit themselves to treating problems that are the result of damage or malalignment of the bones and joints in the body. These problems – especially affecting the spinal column – are almost of epidemic proportion, and no osteopath is without work.

The main difference between the two disciplines is in the method of manipulation used. Osteopaths tend to mobilize joints and use soft-tissue techniques more often than chiropractors, the latter using less leverage and more direct quick manipulations than the former. In the UK, osteopaths became established as a profession when John Littlejohn, a pupil of Andrew Still, established the British School of

Osteopathy in 1917. Chiropractors are few and far between in the UK, although they are fully established in the United States, which has over six separate medical schools and over 20,000 registered practitioners.

In all public surveys on the use of alternative medicine, the most often quoted reason for seeking help is for pain relief from the spine or other joints in the body. Although the differences between osteopathy and chiropractic are now largely historical, both groups have been influenced by their founders and believe that the malalignment or displacement of a vertebra or large joint can produce alterations to the working of the body which are not limited to the medical aspects. Osteopaths believe that pressure on

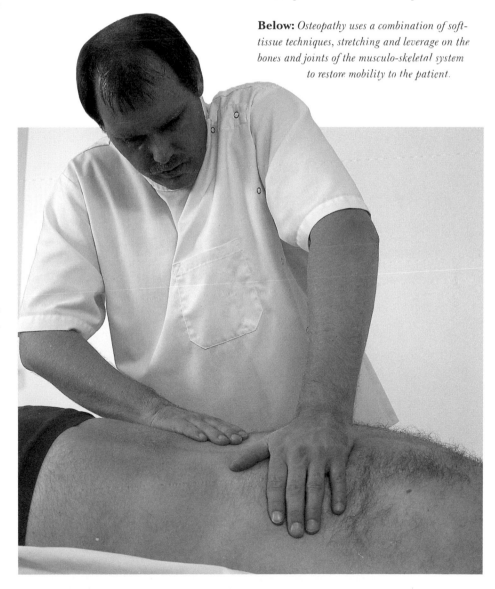

Below: *Osteopathy uses a combination of soft-tissue techniques, stretching and leverage on the bones and joints of the musculo-skeletal system to restore mobility to the patient.*

nerves around misplaced vertebrae can cause disturbances in internal organs and that secretions from the endocrine (hormone) glands can be improved by osteopathic manipulation. Similarly, chiropractors emphasize the importance of lymph drainage and believe treatments will improve circulation.

Many doctors, while not necessarily accepting these views now recognize that manipulation, whether carried out by an osteopath or chiropractor, does have a place in the treatment of many musculo-skeletal disorders. The success of these therapies is evidenced by their popularity and there are thousands of anecdotal stories that attest to remarkable recoveries. This popular success has not been translated into clear scientific trials partly because the problems presented to osteopaths can be difficult to measure and, more often than not, the abnormality the patient has is only noticeable by the osteopath

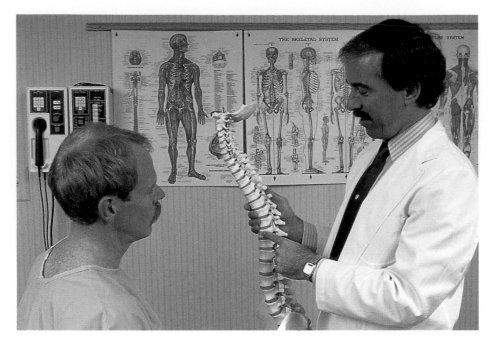

Above: *A chiropractor explains how manual adjustment of the vertebrae can release pressure on spinal nerves, and so relieve pain.*

during his examination (tight muscles, restricted movement etc.). Nevertheless several studies have now shown how osteopaths and chiropractors can reduce the painful symptoms, improve mobility and decrease the patient's time off sick, and when one considers the immense annual cost of back pain in the industrialized West caused by time off work, it seems clear that further studies need to be undertaken to ensure manipulative therapies are more widely available.

Below: *A practitioner of cranial osteopathy gently palpates the parietal bones of the skull to correct minor displacements.*

Cranial osteopathy
The term is a little misleading because the approach and techniques of this form of therapy are very different from standard osteopathy. The cranial osteopath believes that malalignment of the skull, vertebral column and pelvic area affect the flow of cerebrospinal fluid which bathes the brain and parts of the nervous system. By a system of palpating, the cranial osteopath will then help to restore the flow of cerebro-spinal fluid to its normal state. This form of osteopathy requires specialized training and is not included in the formal education of most traditional osteopaths. Nevertheless some successes have been recounted using this technique and although most doctors would dismiss this approach, it still has retained a following.

HERBAL MEDICINE

In many ways, herbal medicine is the most ancient of approaches to treatment for man has always sought some external substance to take in order to relieve his pain, distress or discomfort. This could have been a poultice, a linament, a linctus, some herbal mixture or literally the "gilded pill". The folk healers and the white witches of the late Middle Ages gave way to the apothecaries of the 17th century. The subsequent invention of the gelatin capsule (which allowed a drug to pass through the stomach to be absorbed in the gut) by French pharmacists in 1834 heralded the beginning of the modern drug industry, and the gradual disappearance of herbal medicine as a separate form of treatment. It is interesting to recall that both Thomas Beecham and Jesse Boot, who helped to establish the modern pharmaceutical industry, were herbal practitioners. The controversy surrounding the modern use of herbs rests around a number of factors.

Firstly, it has been claimed throughout the centuries that the whole plant needs to be used to make an herbal medicine and the modern wish to extract the active ingredient, purify it and standardize it does not do justice to the holistic nature of herbal medicine. Examples are given where by taking

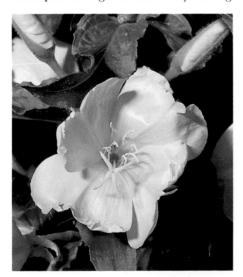

Above: *An evening primrose flower. The oil extracted from the seeds of this plant is used to treat conditions like eczema and PMT.*

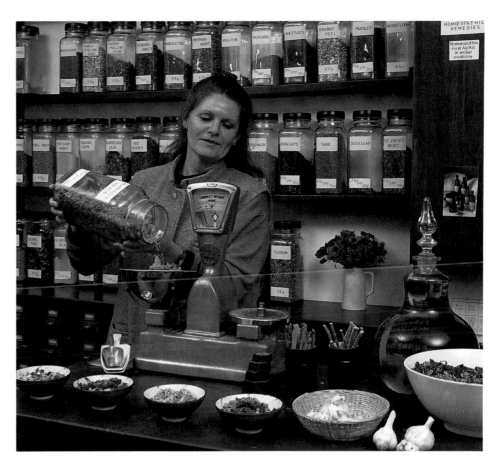

Above: *Herbalism is an ancient art, but a degree of caution is needed if you practise self-medication. Plants can harm as well as heal you.*

the whole plant, the side effects of consuming just the active ingredient are avoided as the plant contains other ingredients which protect the patient from such side effects.

Secondly, many modern herbal practitioners do not like to prescribe herbs simply for symptomatic relief, i.e. garlic is useful for infections, chamomile helps with the appetite. They believe that the true nature of herbal medicine is as an holistic approach to healthy living. They see the symptoms of disease as indicating an imbalance and their assessment of the patient will take into account emotional, environmental and lifestyle factors, e.g. diet. The simple removal of symptoms by the use of herbs is, in their view, not what herbal medicine is about. Like homeopathy, they may prescribe completely different herbal mixtures depending on the "whole patient presentation" rather than on the symptom

picture. However, it is clear from the way the public responds to herbal medicines that this view is a minority one, and to a great extent herbal medicine is a matter of self-medication, usually for minor self-limiting conditions.

The third controversial point is the claim made by many who prescribe herbal products that they are safe and do not have the side effects and dangers associated with modern drug treatment. Unfortunately, this is not true and there have been several tragic and fatal consequences as a result of this misguided view. Many of our modern drugs are indeed derived from plants and were initially discovered by herbal practitioners, for instance foxglove and digoxin used in heart disorders, and evening primrose oil, now used in a variety of conditions including eczema, pre-menstrual syndrome and multiple sclerosis. As such, both the herbal variety and the modern drug preparations contain active chemicals which can be dangerous and caution always needs to be practised if self-medication is undertaken.

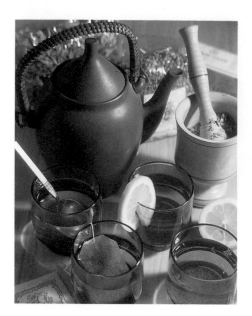

Above: *A tisane or infusion is made by steeping the flowers and leaves of herbs in hot water for around ten minutes, much as tea is made.*

Types of herbal preparation

Herbal preparations can come in many forms. The tisane common in France is made by infusing a small quantity of herbs for about 10 minutes in hot water in a teapot very much in the way that tea is made. The mixture should be strained out and can be drunk hot or cold. Tinctures are made by macerating the plant in a solution of alcohol and water (25 percent alcohol to 75 percent water), filtering the mixture and taking the resultant medicine by mouth. The alcohol acts as a preservative and a tincture can last for well over a year. Lotions, gargles, creams, ointments, poultices and inhalations are other ways in which herbal medicines can be taken. Usually the herbalist will prepare these products for you. Professional medical herbalists can be hard to find as few practitioners undertake the established and registered courses. In the UK herbs are often prescribed by the Hakims found in many Asian communities, and some Chinese herbalists have large practices, again usually servicing their own communities where herbal medicines are the normal approach to treatment. Retail herbalists operating from health-food shops or specialized outlets, although not possessing a formal qualification, possess wide experience and knowledge in the use of herbs for symptomatic relief.

Many other alternative practitioners have developed their own understanding and knowledge of the use of herbs and will incorporate this approach into their general management of disease. Herbal medicine in the West as a profession nearly succumbed to a total decline following the thalidomide drug scandal when it was required by law that all herbal products should be subject to proper analysis and testing.

NATUROPATHY

Also known as "Nature Cure" (i.e. helping the body to cure itself), this type of therapy has been practised in some form or another since time immemorial. Bathing a sprain or fasting when unwell is a form of naturopathy. It has had its famous proponents throughout the ages from the ancient Greek physician Hippocrates, one of whose principal axioms was "First do no harm", to modern orthodox physicians. As a systematic approach to healing, it was first developed by a 19th century German therapist, Vincent Preissnitz. More recently in the 1890s, an American, Benedict Lust, successfully treated by these methods under the care of an Austrian priest called Sebastian Kneipp, established a school of training in the United States and called it naturopathy. Sixty years ago Harry Benedict, an American healer, in his book *Everybody's Guide to Nature Cure* propounded the basic tenets of naturopathy and established the five approaches to treatment – fasting, the therapeutic use of diets, hydrotherapy, exercising and psychological counselling. Other approaches may include massage and osteopathy. Naturopaths believe that many illnesses arise as a result of an unhealthy lifestyle and poor posture, and that restoring the body to a natural state by natural means will allow the body to recover.

What can naturopaths treat?

Although not specifically concerned with serious diseases, naturopaths concentrate on the whole person and want to encourage healthy approaches to living. Nevertheless, many of the psychosomatic illnesses, such as migraine, asthma, and irritable bowel disorder, will respond to a naturopathic approach. Some long-standing and degenerative conditions – arthritis and

Below: *Mud, glorious mud! Naturopathy involves a combination of advice on diet and fasting, and therapies such as massage, exercise, Yoga, osteopathy and hydrotherapy like this.*

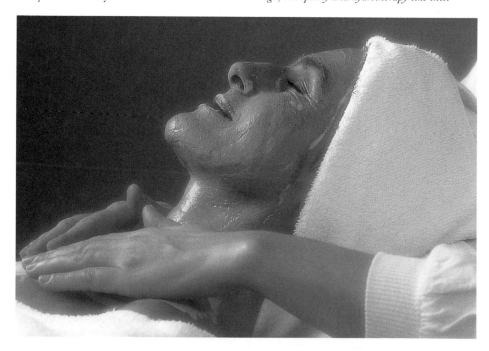

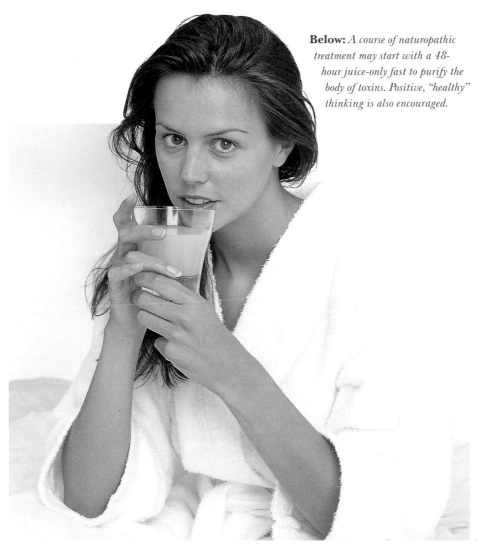

Below: *A course of naturopathic treatment may start with a 48-hour juice-only fast to purify the body of toxins. Positive, "healthy" thinking is also encouraged.*

AYURVEDIC MEDICINE AND YOGA

These are systems of health care primarily practised in India and the Far East but which have become increasingly popular in the West as their benefits become known and studied.

Ayurveda

Ayurveda is derived from two Sanskrit words, Ayur, meaning "life", and Veda, meaning "study of" or "knowledge". It is a combined system of health promotion, disease prevention and treatment. Ayurvedic physicians believe disease can arise because of *physical causes*, e.g. infections and tissue degeneration, *mental causes*, e.g. depression or prolonged anger, *accidental causes*, e.g. blows, cuts or stings and *natural causes*, e.g. old age, wrong dietary approaches.

Like most Eastern approaches to health, the basis of Ayurvedic medicine is one of achieving a balance between natural universal forces. The three basic forces (or tridoshas) are *Vata* (like the wind) – this force controls movement and the nervous system; *Pitta* (like the Sun) is the source of energy and it controls biochemical and diges-

high blood pressure, for instance – can also improve with hydrotherapy and the diets advised by naturopaths.

How do naturopaths work?

Most will have received a four-year training with examination. Some naturopaths also practise osteopathy and will want to examine the spine, and the alignment of the vertebrae. Many naturopaths, especially in Germany and France, practise in a spa or health farm where a combination of treatments is more easily available. It is important to check with your doctor to make sure you can undergo treatment in a health farm, and it is now possible to obtain reimbursement from some insurance companies who recognize the long-term value of naturopathic methods. Naturopaths will emphasize the importance of self-help and positive thinking. They believe that the

patient must be an active participant if the treatment is to work. This may start with a full fast or juice-only fast lasting 24-48 hours to "detoxify" the body. You should not try a full fast for longer unless you are receiving medical supervision. Supervision is necessary during this process as occasionally there is an intensification of the symptoms which is viewed by naturopaths as a normal occurrence. Enemas and colonic irrigation are occasionally used as well in order to detoxify the system. Other treatment may involve changing your diet, instruction in relaxation and breathing exercises, and some form of hydrotherapy.

Many orthodox doctors accept the principles on which naturopathy is based but do not agree with reducing medication or avoiding medical treatment if a treatable condition is involved.

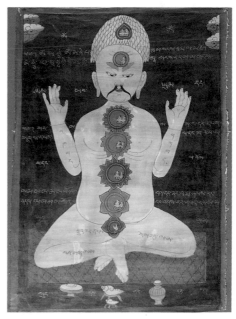

Above: *The seven energy centres, or chakras, of Hindu philosophy. Ayurvedic medicine considers energy balance as essential for good health.*

Below: *This woman has adopted the Yoga asana called the pigeon. Yoga aims to unify mind, body and spirit, and to bring peace through inner awareness.*

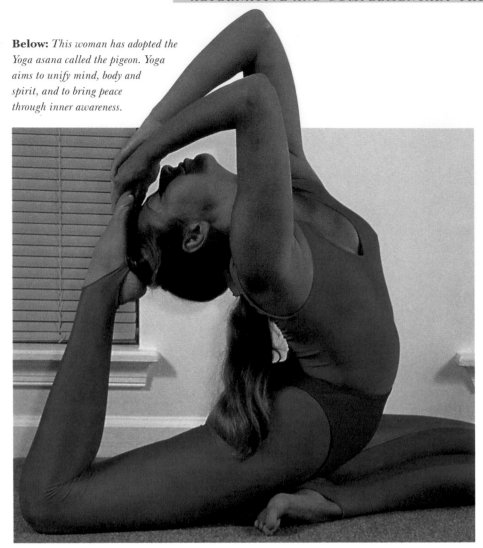

minutes to complete but which provides an excellent daily routine. Other postures (such as the Corpse) have been taken up by the Natural Childbirth Movement and have formed the basis for deep relaxation and pain control in labour. In advanced Yoga, methods of breathing with the postures become very important and many scientific studies have demonstrated benefits in diseases as diverse as high blood pressure, asthma and multiple sclerosis. For the most part, Yoga is practised as a pleasant and helpful exercise routine in classes with an expert teacher. It is generally safe to learn the simple Yoga postures from a book, but attending a class is certainly very helpful and, indeed, necessary when attempting the more advanced postures. The aspects of Yoga involving meditation and contemplation have also become extremely popular in the West for helping with anxiety, panic attacks and stress disorders.

Below: *Yoga is best learned through the guidance of a teacher. Beginners should not attempt postures like this without supervision.*

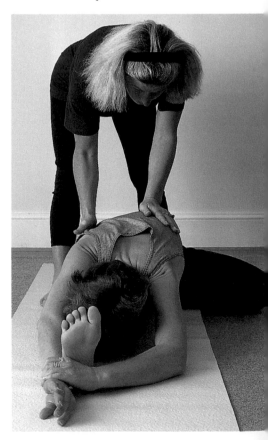

tive processes; and *Kapha*, likened to the Moon, controls cell growth and tissue development. Physicians will take a history and examine the patient but will pay special attention to diet, the tongue, breathing and sleeping patterns, and emotional and mental state.

Many of the therapies used in Ayurvedic medicine have now been incorporated in much of naturopathy and will include fasting, special diets, medicinal herbs, and homeopathic remedies. Advice is given regarding exercise, patterns of breathing and relaxation; meditation is often used as well as practical interventions such as massage and enemas. With the growth of immigration from the sub-continent of India to Europe, several physicians serve their local European communities. Centres for Ayurvedic medicine can also be found in several of the big cities in the United States of America.

Their influence on Western medicine has been much greater than that implies, however, as Western-trained doctors have turned to their holistic model of health care and combined it with the more orthodox methods of drug prescribing and surgery.

Yoga

Yoga, meaning "yoke" or "union" in Sanskrit, was introduced to the West in the late 19th century and has been popularized for its simple but very intricate system of health promotion and disease prevention. The purpose of Yoga is to bring about union between body, mind and spirit. In its entirety it has eight separate stages of spiritual, mental and physical training, of which the asanas (the physical postures) are only one. Many such postures are grouped in a sequence, e.g. the Sun salute which can take less than five

DIAGNOSTIC METHODS

When we are ill, most of us want to know what is the matter. We would like to have a name given to our particular set of symptoms. For doctors, making a diagnosis or naming the illness is seen as the first necessary step before commencing treatment. It is true that many of the problems seen in general medical practice are never properly diagnosed even though treatment may be commenced. Alternative practitioners also think a diagnosis is important but, like the famous American physician William Osler, they believe it is more important to know which person has the disease than which disease the person has. Accordingly they will concentrate on finding about the "whole person" as well as undertaking certain physical examinations not used in traditional medicine.

Taking a history
This will include the sorts of questions most clinicians would ask – How long have you had the symptoms? Where does it hurt? What makes it better? What makes it worse?, and so on. In addition, most homeopaths will ask about what are known as mentals and peculiarities. This will mean that they will be interested to find out your mood state, your likes and dislikes as well as whether the pain or symptom is only on the left side or right side, or lasts for only one hour etc. This helps to create the pattern that will allow them to choose an appropriate remedy.

Chinese practitioners (acupuncturists) will pay especial attention to diet as will naturopaths. You may be asked to keep a diet diary for one week and this can prove to be a very revealing exercise. It is something you may want to do at home. Write down everything you eat and drink for one whole week and then ask an expert to analyse it for you. If at the same time you note your mood and energy level during the course of the day, this may help to identify any particular responses you may

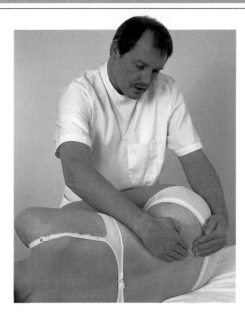

Above: *Like any reputable holistic healer, an osteopath will want to build up an accurate picture of his patient's whole physical nature.*

have to specific items in the diet. Chinese medicine pays special attention to the effect of the weather on your symptoms, and you may be asked questions regarding your body temperature – do you feel hot or cold, do you like hot or cold drinks etc.? Osteopaths will want to hear about any accidents or injuries you may have had and may want to know something about your chairs, bed

and car, as this will help them build up a picture of your posture, throughout the day.

Physical examination
Alternative practitioners do not always use the same examination methods as doctors do but they will generally take the blood pressure and examine the skin and nails. Pulse diagnosis forms a very important part of Chinese medicine because it allows the practitioner to determine the flow of Chi or energy in the major meridians or channels. There are twelve different pulses the practitioner feels for and this may take a little while to accomplish. The practitioner will feel with three fingers along the radial artery on the side of the wrist. There are twenty-eight different qualities to each pulse (choppy, rapid, stringy, etc.) so a very complex and intricate picture will often be developed. Sometimes you may be asked to return at a different time of day as the pulse is thought to be affected by changes in weather and time. Following the examination of the

Below: *Chinese pulse diagnosis is more complex than its Western counterpart. The practitioner will feel for twelve different pulses.*

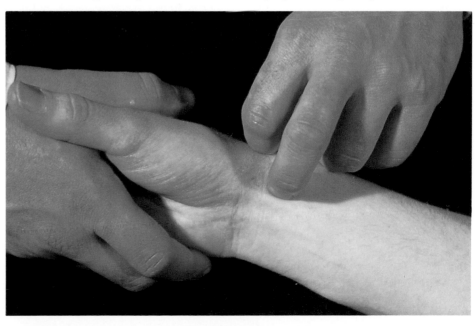

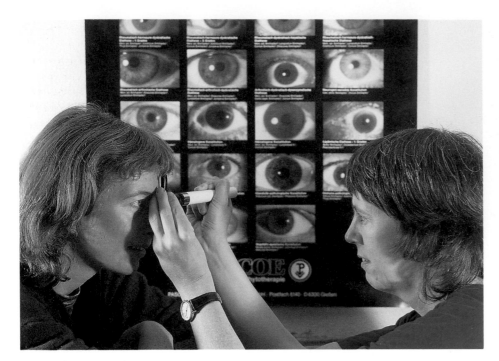

pulse, the practitioner will go on to examine the tongue which again can reveal not only the general state of the body and mind, but may give specific clues as to imbalances, vitamin deficiencies and allergic responses to food you have eaten. Whether the tongue is moist or dry, whether it is coated, what colour the coating is, whether there are any teeth marks or indentations on the tongue, these are all thought to be important signs in Chinese medicine.

Osteopaths will be interested in your spinal column, whether it is properly aligned, how much movement there is and how "springy" the joints are. Most alternative practitioners will also pay attention to your pattern of breathing and how that is or is not co-ordinated with your movements, speech and posture. A fixed chest-breathing pattern will be seen as requiring a particular intervention to help you free up the way you breathe.

Once the initial examination is complete, like doctors, alternative practitioners will want to undertake further tests to enable them to develop a more accurate picture of your problem. There are a number of specifically diagnostic disciplines within the canon of alternative medicine, and we shall now look at the most important of them.

Above: *Beauty may be in the eye of the beholder, but iridologists believe that they can identify illnesses in various parts of the body by minutely examining the eyes of a patient.*

IRIDOLOGY

Iridology is the ability to detect illnesses in parts of the body (liver, kidney, spleen) by examining the iris or coloured portion of the eye. This technique was first developed in the 19th century by a Hungarian doctor, Ignatz von Peczely, who had noticed a discoloration in the iris of an owl which had a broken leg. He went on to study this phenomenon in more detail and published his results. These were largely ignored until an American physician, Dr. Bernard Jensen, picked up on his research in the 1950s and established the modern map of the iris.

The iris is divided into several portions, like slices of cake, and each slice is said to represent parts of the body. Examination of the iris may be made with a torch and magnifying glass but special cameras now exist that will take accurate close-up pictures which are processed into slides and projected on a screen. Special training centres exist both in the USA and Europe where practitioners are taught how to chart accurately the various discolorations

and patterns of the iris. Orthodox doctors have found the claims made for iridology incredible and various tests and trials have been undertaken to check whether those claims are accurate. In a well-controlled study, it was found that the accuracy of iridology was no more than could be predicted by chance, and most conventional doctors dismiss this method as both unscientific, unsound and inaccurate.

KINESIOLOGY

Kinesiology is a form of "muscle testing" which is said to be able to detect imbalances in the body, food allergies, and disturbances in energy flow which may indicate actual disease or the precursor of disease. As a diagnostic method it was developed by American osteopaths early in the 1930s and subsequently popularized by George Goodheart in the 1960s. The theory underlying kinesiology is drawn from Chinese medicine in that it is believed that subtle change to energy flow in the body occurs when an individual is in contact with a substance to which he or she is allergic. This can also take place if there is a mental "allergy" or distressing emotion or memory associated with a

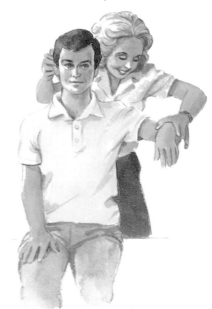

Above: *By testing the relative strength of muscular resistance to pressure, kinesiologists believe that they can identify allergies.*

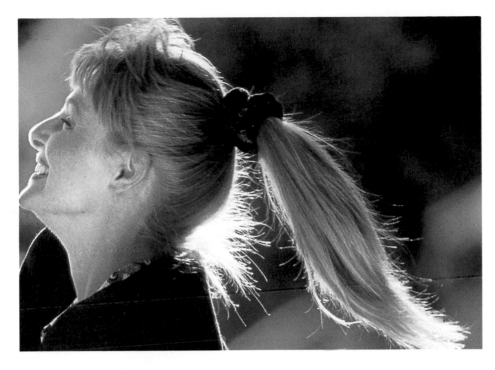

Above: *Hair analysts claim that laboratory tests on a lock of hair can reveal mineral imbalances in the body. Orthodox doctors dispute this.*

particular person. The test itself is deceptively simple and involves two people and can be tried at home:

Kinesiology allergy test

1 Stand or sit facing your partner.
2 Stretch out your left or right arm so it is parallel to the floor.
3 The tester then tries to lower your arm by gently pressing on your wrist.
4 You resist the downward pressure.
5 Place the food you wish to test either in your other hand or in your mouth.
6 Repeat steps 3 and 4 while at the same time the tester places the first two fingers of his other hand just behind your ear to complete the circuit.
7 If you are able to resist the downward pressure, then all is well.
8 If your arm feels less strong and is unable to resist the pressure, it is thought you are allergic to the piece of food or other substance you are testing.

Kinesiology has not been shown to have any scientific validity and, like iridology, is not accepted by most doctors as an accurate diagnostic test.

HAIR ANALYSIS

This is another simple and attractive method of determining the state of health of the body, especially in terms of measuring the mineral, vitamin and dietary deficiencies. Hair is made from a protein, keratin, which as it grows "traps" and mirrors the minerals, e.g. sulphur, mercury, aluminium, that are present in tiny quantities in the blood. By laboratory analysis of the mineral content of a lock of hair, it is possible to detect the levels and imbalances present in the body. Following a hair

analysis, a practitioner may suggest a dietary regime which can include a fasting programme or the prescription of a mineral supplement if deficiencies are detected. Again, unfortunately, this simple test has not proved in trials to be reliable or accurate enough to convince orthodox scientists, and most responsible practitioners no longer place as much reliance on its findings as once they did.

KIRLIAN PHOTOGRAPHY

One of the major differences between alternative and orthodox medicine is the belief by many who practise alternative medicine that the body possesses an energy flow system, much like the blood circulating in the arteries, or the peripheral nervous system. Kirlian photography is thought to be able to detect this energy flow that exists as a very thin layer encircling the body (a bit like the aura or halo seen in paintings of saints and mystics). The technique was discovered by accident by a Russian husband and wife team of radiologists (Semyon and Valentina Kirlian). By passing a high voltage, high-frequency electric charge through a very sensitive photographic plate and placing first a hand on the

Below: *Hands-on diagnosis? Here a Kirlian photograph is taken of a woman's hand which is held on a discharge plate over reactive paper.*

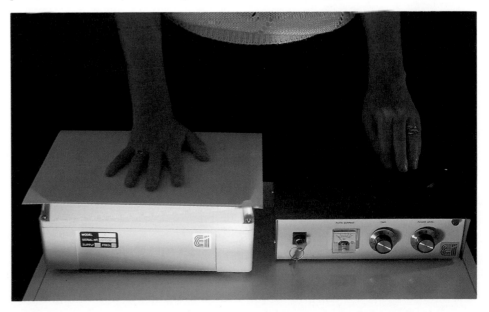

plate, then plant material, the Kirlians were able to demonstrate, once the photographs were developed, pictures of what appeared to be "electrical emissions" surrounding the substance photographed.

By experiments initially with themselves, the Kirlians thought they could detect changes in the photographs that occurred before one of them developed a cold, thus reinforcing what many Chinese practitioners believe, that physical disease results from a prior disturbance of energy flow. Kirlian photography had great appeal for some years and research laboratories existed in America, England and Europe. Unfortunately, the early enthusiasm for this test rapidly diminished when it was discovered that many of the so-called "electrical emissions" could be affected by "artefacts", e.g. the relative pressure of the hand on the plate, the temperature of the hand and its distance from the photographic plate. Although it is still available as a diagnostic method in some research centres, very few alternative practitioners now make use of it, partly because of its expense and partly because it proved not to be particularly reliable.

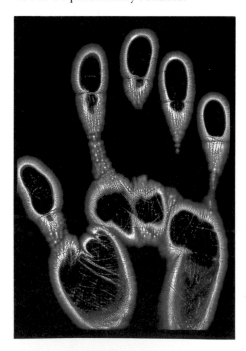

Above: *A Kirlian photograph of a hand. The image is not created by a light source, but instead is the result of an electrical interaction.*

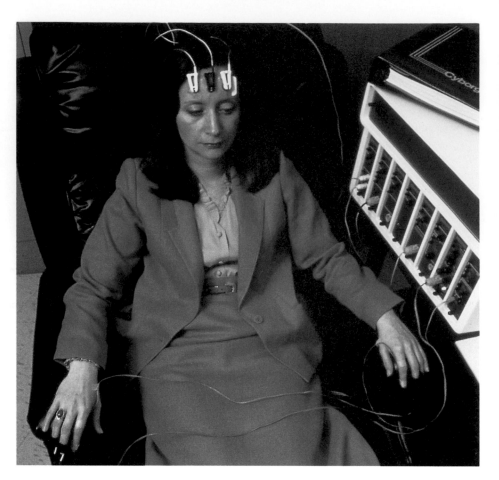

Above: *This woman is attached, via electrodes on her skin, to a biofeedback machine which allows her to monitor physiological changes in her body by reacting to visual or aural messages.*

BIOFEEDBACK

Although not specifically used as a diagnostic test this is, however, one of the most reliable and accepted methods of detecting changes in the body that has been developed in alternative medicine. It is now used in several orthodox centres, both as a research tool and as a treatment method. Like the lie detector, biofeedback provides information on the body's systems – pulse-rate, sweating pattern, temperature and muscle tension. These are obtained by attaching electrodes to the patient's skin which are connected to a machine that can register changes in skin temperature, muscle tension or brain wave activity. These measurements are transferred to a visual dial (you can see your temperature rising or falling) or to an auditory system (the frequency of the clicks will tell you how tense the particular muscle being tested is). By giving someone direct and immediate "feedback" concerning the state of their body systems, it is then possible to teach them how to reduce muscle tension or raise body temperature or reduce the blood pressure or induce a sense of mental relaxation.

Conditions that can be detected by biofeedback include:
▪ High blood pressure by measurement of blood pressure.
▪ Migraine by measurement of skin temperature.
▪ Muscle tension by measurement of muscle tone.
▪ Anxiety by measurement of brain-waves.

These conditions can be altered and improved by self-help exercises such as breathing, relaxation and simple meditational techniques. The effectiveness of biofeedback as a diagnostic tool is beyond doubt and some of the machinery involved is simple enough to be used at home.

THERAPEUTIC METHODS

AROMATHERAPY

This is principally the use of essential oils during massage. They can, however, be used in the bath, taken in inhalation, dabbed on pulse points, used as compresses and occasionally, but only under proper direction, ingested. Oils are the extracts of plants which are obtained from the tiny glands in the petals, leaves, stems and bark of the plant. They are extracted by being heated and then concentrated and purified. The use of essential oils is an ancient art that dates back to the time of the Egyptians and Persians, but it was rediscovered and established in its modern form by a French chemist, René Gattefossé, who noticed on an occasion when he accidentally plunged his hand after receiving a burn into a bowl of water containing lavender essence, that it healed very quickly. Aromatherapy is mostly used in combination with massage by adding 15-30 drops of the required essential oil to 60ml (2 fl. oz.) of massage oil and then shaking the mixture. It is now possible

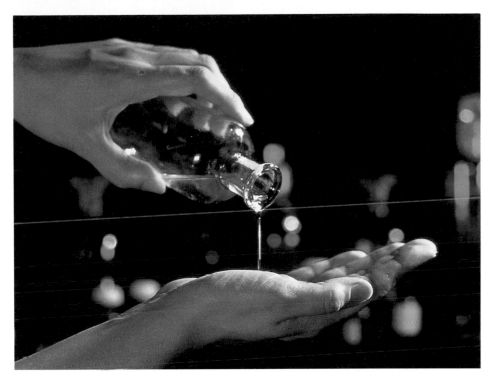

Below: *You can almost see tension being eased out of this woman's shoulders. Massage with essential oils induces a deep feeling of well-being.*

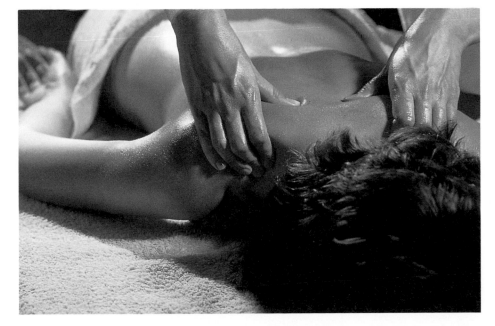

to purchase these massage oils already prepared.

The science of aromatherapy is not particularly precise and very little, if any, research has been undertaken to evaluate the claims made for the different uses to which oils are put. Most, if not all aromatherapy is safe, except during pregnancy when it is important to

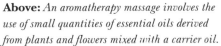

Above: *An aromatherapy massage involves the use of small quantities of essential oils derived from plants and flowers mixed with a carrier oil.*

avoid certain oils that can be absorbed through the skin and can prove toxic to the baby. Some oils should also be avoided by people who suffer from epilepsy. In either case, seek the advice of a qualified aromatherapist.

Aromatherapy is safe to use at home. In the bath, add six to eight drops of essential oil and stay in the bath for at least 15 minutes. As an inhalation, pour ten drops on a paper towel or handkerchief and inhale – sometimes it can be helpful to do this at night, placing the handkerchief on your pillow so that you inhale while asleep. Oils can also be used in a steam inhaler, but guidance is required from a qualified aromatherapist. Hand and foot baths can also be used by gently rubbing warm water (ten drops of oil in a bowl of water) over the legs, feet and hands. You should not use the concentrated oils directly on your skin unless under the supervision of a qualified practitioner.

BACH FLOWER REMEDIES

These are infusions of various flowers in water preserved in alcohol, which are supplied in small bottles with a dispensing dropper. They are taken directly in the mouth (two or three drops on the tongue) or diluted in water and drunk. They are named after an English physician, Dr. Edward Bach, who discovered their use in the 1930s after some 20 years of research into human nature, and the relationship between the personality and mental outlook and its effect on chronic disease. The remedies are produced at the Dr. E. Bach Centre, Mount Vernon, Wallingford in the United Kingdom, this being the house in which Edward Bach lived and worked.

Bach believed that the body had inherent power to heal itself but that a

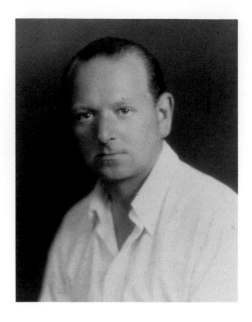

Above: *Dr. Edward Bach, who gave up a flourishing medical practice to devote himself to discovering the healing properties of plants.*

long-standing worry or fear hindered the recovery of health and slowed convalescence. The remedies therefore do not address physical complaints directly, but rather aim to improve the sufferer's state of mind. Once mental peace has been restored, Bach maintained that the life force would flow freely again allowing the body to regain health. In the course of his research, he developed great sensitivity to plants, and eventually identified 38 flowers to counter all the negative states of mind that we commonly experience. These are described in the accompanying table.

The remedies have become popular throughout Europe and the United States where centres exist with trained therapists to advise on their detailed use. Self-help books are also available and these, together with the table, can be used as a simple guide for their use

Bach Flower Remedies

This table, issued by The Bach Centre and reprinted with their permission, lists the flower remedies and the negative states of mind that each can counter.

Flower Remedy	State of mind	Flower Remedy	State of mind
1 Agrimony	Those who hide worries behind a brave face.	22 Oak	Normally strong/courageous, but no longer able to struggle bravely against illness and/or adversity.
2 Aspen	Apprehension for no known reason.		
3 Beech	Critical and intolerant of others.	23 Olive	Fatigued – drained of energy.
4 Centaury	Weak willed; exploited or imposed upon.	24 Pine	Guilt complex – blames self even for mistakes of others. Always apologising.
5 Cerato	Those who doubt their own judgement, seek confirmation of others.		
6 Cherry plum	Uncontrolled, irrational thoughts.	25 Red chestnut	Obsessed by care and concern for others.
7 Chestnut bud	Refuses to learn by experience – continually repeats same mistakes.	26 Rock rose	Suddenly alarmed, scared, panicky.
		27 Rock water	Rigid minded, self denying.
8 Chicory	Over possessive – (self-centred) – clinging and over-protective especially of loved ones.	28 Scleranthus	Uncertainty/indecision/vacillation. Fluctuating moods.
9 Clematis	Inattentive, dreamy, absent-minded, mental escapism.	29 Star of Bethlehem	For all the effects of serious news, or fright following an accident, etc.
10 Crab apple	The "Cleanser". Self disgust/detestation. Ashamed of ailments.	30 Sweet chestnut	Utter dejection, bleak outlook.
		31 Vervain	Over-enthusiasm – fanatical beliefs.
11 Elm	Overwhelmed by inadequacy and responsibility.	32 Vine	Dominating/inflexible/tyrannical/autocratic/arrogant. Usually good leaders.
12 Gentian	Despondency.		
13 Gorse	Pessimism, defeatism, "what's the use!".	33 Walnut	Assists in adjustment to transition or change, e.g. puberty, menopause, divorce, new surroundings.
14 Heather	Talkative, (obsessed with own troubles and experiences).		
15 Holly	Hatred, envy, jealousy, suspicion.	34 Water violet	Proud, reserved, enjoys being alone.
16 Honeysuckle	Living in the past – nostalgic. Home-sickness.	35 White chestnut	Persistent unwanted thoughts. Preoccupation with some worry or episode. Mental arguments.
17 Hornbeam	"Monday morning" feeling – procrastination.		
18 Impatiens	Impatience, irritability.	36 Wild oat	Helps determine one's intended path in life.
19 Larch	Lack of self-confidence, feels inferior. Fears failure.	37 Wild rose	Resignation, apathy.
		38 Willow	Resentment, embitterment, "poor old me!".
20 Mimulus	Fear of *known* things. Shyness, timidity.	39 Rescue Remedy	A combination of cherry plum, clematis, impatiens, rock rose, star of Bethlehem. All-purpose emergency composite for effects of anguish, examinations, going to the dentist, etc. Comforting, calming and reassuring to those distressed by startling experiences.
21 Mustard	"Dark cloud" that descends, making one saddened and low for no known reason.		

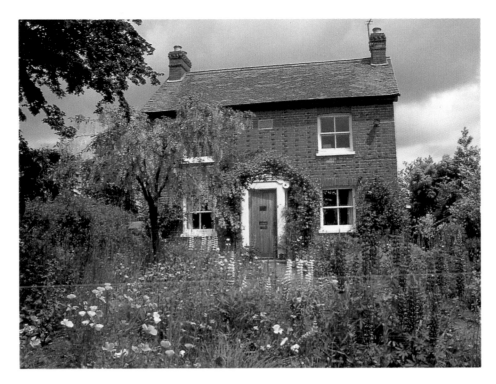

Below: *The Bach Centre in Mount Vernon. Bach lived here and worked in the surrounding fields identifying his healing plants.*

your symptoms and consult a trained practitioner if in any doubt. The tissue salts are added to a lactose-containing tablet (so these are *not* to be taken by anyone suffering from lactose or milk intolerance). The tablets can be taken quite frequently – every half-hour – if there is an acute condition or every two hours if the condition is long-lasting. There is no medical evidence as to their efficacy but they are harmless.

Wilhelm Schuessler's 12 original tissue salts
Calcium fluoride (*Calc. fluor.*)
Calcium phosphate (*Calc. phos.*)
Calcium sulphate (*Calc. sulph.*)
Iron phosphate (*Ferr. phos.*)
Magnesium phosphate (*Mag. phos.*)
Potassium chloride (*Kali mur.*)
Potassium phosphate (*Kali phos.*)
Potassium sulphate (*Kali sulph.*)
Silicon dioxide (*Silica*)
Sodium chloride (*Nat. mur.*)
Sodium phosphate (*Nat. phos.*)
Sodium sulphate (*Nat. sulph.*)

at home. Bach also combined five of these remedies together (cherry plum, clematis, impatiens, rock rose and star of Bethlehem) into a "Rescue Remedy" which he advised should be used at times of great shock or stress.

These simple remedies have been used successfully by individuals, as well as medical and complementary health professionals, for the relief of a variety of emotional problems. However, few, if any, scientific studies have been undertaken to validate whether the good results achieved in relation to the treatment of physical disorders, as reported by some practitioners, can be substantiated.

TISSUE SALTS

Also known as Biochemic Tissue Salts, they were developed in the late 19th century by a German homeopathic physician, Dr. Wilhelm Schuessler, in conjunction with homeopathic remedies. They are extracted from plants and herbs and are used to correct mineral imbalances which are thought to exist in the body – they help to restore

the appropriate balance. They are available from homeopathic chemists and because they are dilute and non-toxic, they can be a good self-help approach to many minor aches and pains. The 12 salts originally listed by Schuessler are shown in the table. It is helpful to keep an accurate record of

Below: *Tissue salts are available in tablet form from suppliers of homeopathic remedies. They are used to correct mineral imbalances in the body.*

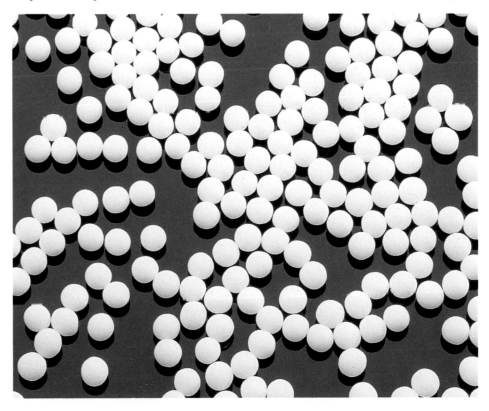

MASSAGE

Massage is one of the oldest healing interventions. In 3000 B.C. there are records of it being used for soothing purposes. The ancient Greek physician Hippocrates (c.460-c.377 B.C.) himself wrote: "The way to health is to have a scented bath and an oiled massage each day". Until the 19th century, references to massage commonly occurred in medical text books, but with the advent of drug therapy, it lost its appeal and it is only recently that it has regained a respectability within the medical and nursing professions.

There is nothing more natural or human than the use of touch to relieve pain and distress, whether it be a hug, a consoling hand on the shoulder or a mother rubbing the injured knee of her young child. The skin is in fact the largest organ in the body. It has millions of nerve endings and touch is the first "sense" the foetus possesses. The baby's perception of its external world

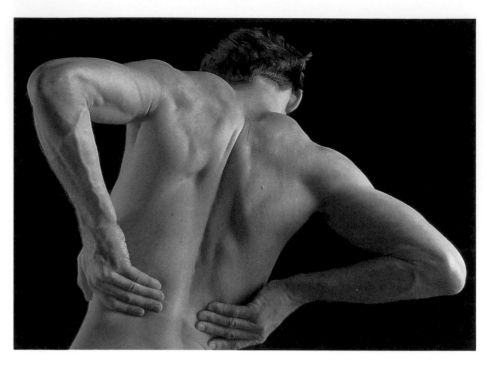

Above: *One of the most natural reactions in the world is to rub an ache or hurt. Although massage is most beneficial when peformed by an expert, self-massage like this does relieve pain.*

Below: *Long, rhythmic, gliding strokes such as this are known as effleurage. They promote blood flow and drainage of the body's lymph system.*

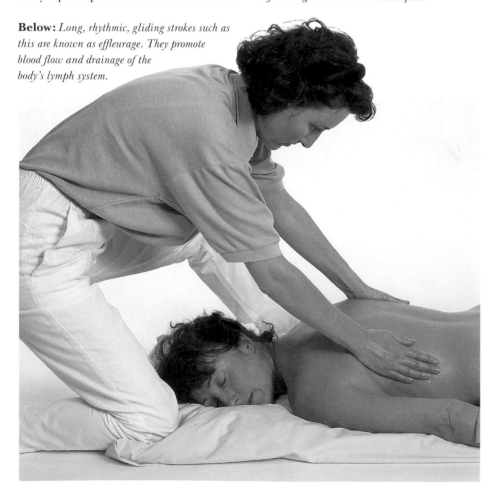

is largely arrived at through touch and its subsequent learning pattern is largely shaped by how it was or was not touched during its first few months. In animals, licking, patting and stroking are equivalent activities, and in adults, oiling our bodies, preening, head-scratching and even sunbathing are viewed as ways in which we reaffirm our need to be touched. "Deprivation dwarfism" is a well recognized condition that occurs in institutions where children, in spite of good food and medical care, fail to thrive because they are not petted and cosseted enough.

Massage can be seen as a form of "structured touch" or "therapeutic touch". It not only reaffirms our bodily sense of being human but can be used systematically to bring about a sense of relaxation and relief from muscle tension. In the care of the dying, it can be most powerfully used to help with the sense of hopelessness and despair that surrounds the death bed. Most modern Western forms of massage techniques are derived from the work of Per Henrik Ling (1776-1839), a Scandinavian practitioner who devised what is now called Swedish massage. This incorporates four basic techniques which can be learnt without great difficulty by almost everyone. These techniques include:

Percussion: short, sharp, fast, rhythmic movements, known as *tapotement* in France, delivered with the side of the closed wrist of the open hand. They are used on the buttocks, thighs, and lower back and should not cause pain.

Effleurage: slow, rhythmic, gliding strokes using the palms of the hands close together. The finger tips and "ball" of the thumb can be used for firmer pressure and deep massage can be given with the knuckles or thumbs.

Petrissage: This involves grasping and squeezing sections of the skin such as those close to the waist or stomach. The skin is treated as if it were bread dough and squeezed between fingers and thumbs. This can be slightly painful at times but it helps to improve and stimulate circulation, and to relax tense muscles.

Frottage or friction: consists of a series of small, circular movements made by one or more fingers, the heel of the hand or the pads of the thumbs. Increasing pressure will release muscle tension and improve circulation, but this technique should not be used too vigorously over injuries or bruises.

For massage to be successful and easy, a firm couch should be used and a warm room is necessary. Oils are used to avoid unnecessary friction between the skin and hands, but talcum powder can also be effective. A hand, foot or face massage can be enjoyed anywhere as undressing is not necessary.

Massage is relatively easy to learn and can be both enjoyable and health promoting. Certain precautions are, nevertheless, important: avoid open wounds, vein thrombosis and areas of extreme sensitivity. Avoid working over the spine area or the major organs of the abdomen. Seek advice before massaging someone with cancer, or anyone who is pregnant. Always seek your "patient's" approval before embarking on any deep massage. Wear comfortable clothes yourself and do not continue to massage if either your client or yourself become tired. Learn the few basic strokes by attending a weekend course and then practise on family and friends. Always use a carrier oil or powder, and use the latter sparingly only.

Massage is one of the many different forms of therapeutic bodywork that has gained increasing popularity in the last ten years and specialized versions of it include aromatherapy and reflexology (q.v.). Two systematic forms of touch therapy are Shiatsu and Rolfing.

Below: *A Shiatsu therapist working on acupressure points located on the Stomach meridian. Similar self-help techniques can also be learned.*

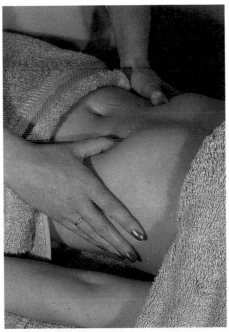

SHIATSU

This is a Japanese system of "finger-pressure" or acupressure. This form of therapy follows the Eastern understanding of life which sees Chi, or energy, as the basis of both health and disease. Shiatsu has been used for centuries in the Far East but has only recently been formulated into a systematic therapeutic model. The therapist will make a diagnosis using both tongue, eye and pulse as guides to the state of the Chi. He will then go through a series of movements pressing with his fingers, thumbs, fists, knees and feet on "pressure points" along your body that lie along the meridians. Unlike massage, it is not necessary to disrobe and each treatment session may last up to an hour. Many musculo-skeletal problems as well as allergic and functional problems (migraine, irritable bowel, digestive disorders) respond well to Shiatsu. Certain self-help techniques of acupressure also exist, and several of these are illustrated in Part Three.

Below: *A woman receiving a Shiatsu massage. The word Shiatsu is derived from two Japanese characters signifying "finger" and "pressure".*

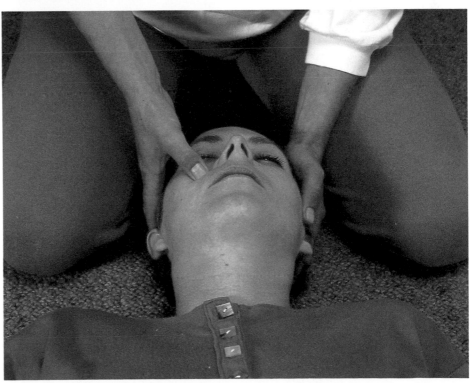

ROLFING

Rolfing is a system of manipulative movements devised by an American biologist, Ida Rolf (1896-1979), that are a modification of osteopathy, Alexander Technique and Shiatsu. Dr. Rolf believed that by realigning the body's mechanical structures (bones, ligaments, muscles and tendons – a process she called a structural integration) it was possible to restore the balance of energies and ensure the body functioned more efficaciously. Rolfing is practised by relatively few practitioners in Europe, although it is more popular in America and Israel. It has been used, like osteopathy, to treat specific bony malalignments, but, like Shiatsu, can also be used by skilled practitioners for common ailments not related to the bony skeleton (asthma, migraine, etc.).

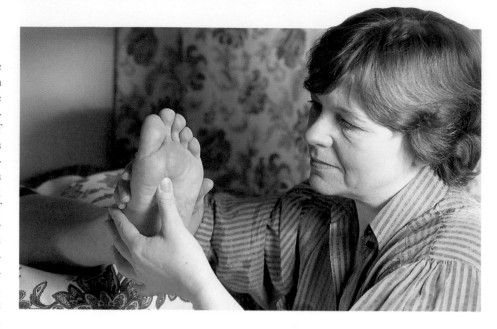

Above: *Reflexologists believe that they can treat ailments in the major organs of the body by stimulating specific reflex points on the foot.*

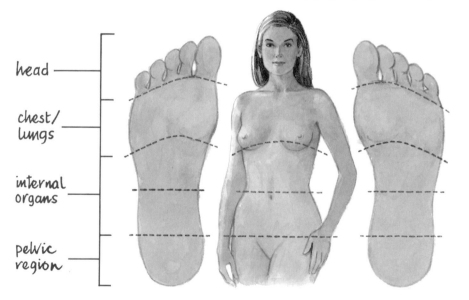

head
chest/ lungs
internal organs
pelvic region

REFLEXOLOGY

Reflexology, or zone therapy as it is sometimes called, is a form of specialized foot massage which concentrates on specific areas of the soles of the feet. These areas, or zones, are thought to be connected to the major organ systems of the body and by stimulating and kneading these specific points, therapists believe they can both detect and treat several conditions and ailments afflicting the body as a whole. Much as Chinese medicine, acupuncture and acupressure, reflexology is

Above: *The diagram shows how zones on the soles of the feet correspond with specific parts of the body. Reflexology aims to stimulate energy flows so that the body can better heal itself.*

based on the belief that an energy system connects the various areas of the body and that blocks or disturbances in this energy flow will produce disease. Reflexology as a modern treatment was developed in the early part of the 20th century by an American physician, Dr. William Fitzgerald, who divided the body into ten different zones and identified these zones on the

soles of the feet. The reflexologist applies firm pressure with the thumb on specific pressure points in the foot that are linked via the nervous system with the body's organs. Stimulation of the nerve endings in the foot is believed to cause a reflex response in the appropriate organ, helping it to return to health.

When visiting a reflexologist, you may be asked certain questions regarding the problem you may have and then the practitioner will examine the soles of your feet and possibly give them a gentle overall massage with talcum powder. Following this he or she will spend some time identifying treatment points, usually by locating those areas on the foot that are tender and painful. Reflexology with aromatic oils can safely be used as a self-help technique for minor conditions, and books specifically devoted to this therapy are now widely available.

HYDROTHERAPY

Spa treatment or "taking the waters" is probably the oldest and most natural form of therapy in everyday use, from showering and sea-bathing to sitting in a warm bath or taking the waters at a warm natural spring. Water can stimulate blood flow, relax muscles, ease pain, invigorate the system and help to cleanse and remove toxic substances. Many of the original healing centres in ancient Greece and Rome were sited specially over naturally occurring waters with special mineral content. It is the healing effect of this mineral content when used to bathe arthritic limbs or rheumatic joints that has given spas their appeal.

Hydrotherapy is the use of water for special treatments, and with modern technology the techniques may include steam baths, jacuzzi, aerated pools, fine shower sprays or sitz baths (sitting alternately in cold and hot baths). Compresses – cold and hot – can be used for painful joints, and in the special spa sites, water is also drunk for its mineral content. More recently, water baths have been used in childbirth with great effect, reducing the discomfort and distress to both mother and child. M. E. (myalgic encephalomyelitis), a particularly disabling condition for which there is little effective orthodox treatment, has responded well to daily cold baths and showers which stimulate and "kick start" the hormonal and immune systems which appear to be non-functioning in this condition. Hydrotherapy can sometimes be found in some physiotherapy units in large hospitals, but is mostly available from health farms and spas where treatment can often be paid for by medical insurance if the treatment is recommended by a doctor.

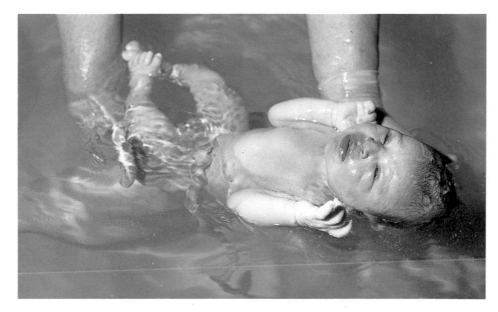

HYPNOTHERAPY

This is one of the more controversial methods of alternative treatment probably because of some misconceptions ("In a trance you might make me do what I don't want to do") and because of its use on stage as a form of popular entertainment. You should certainly not seek hypnotherapy from anyone other than a properly qualified practitioner, preferably one who has a clinical

Below: Hydrotherapy in action: a woman relaxes while her body is massaged by 50 high-pressure water jets in a mineral water bath.

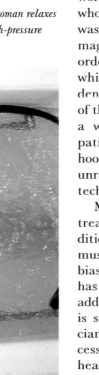

Above: *The use of water baths to ease the strain of childbirth has become increasingly popular with mothers in recent years.*

psychology training or is himself a doctor or dentist. Hypnotherapy is a form of induced sleep which was originally used to diminish pain during surgery, but which, with the development of safe anaesthetics, became redundant. In the 18th century it became something of a *cause célèbre* because of the work of Austrian Franz Anton Mesmer who used hypnosis, or mesmerism as it was called, together with the use of magnets, to treat a whole variety of disorders. Immensely fashionable for a while, Mesmer was eventually denounced as a fraud. Later, at the end of the 19th century, Sigmund Freud for a while used hypnosis to help his patients remember traumatic childhood episodes, but found the method unreliable and went on to develop the technique of psychoanalysis.

Modern hypnotherapy is helpful in treating a number of psychological conditions like anxiety states, stress and muscle tension and also specific phobias (fear of flying, or spiders) etc. It has been used to help people overcome addiction (to tobacco, food, drugs) and is still used by dentists and obstetricians to help reduce pain. It is also successful in treating migraine, general headaches, ulcers and sleeping difficulties. Most people can be hypnotized and there are several methods and techniques which are used by trained practitioners. You may be taught to hypnotize yourself and be asked to remain in this relaxed auto-hypnotic state for anything up to 20 minutes. It is usual to have a series of sessions and although some hospitals provide this free, most hypnotherapists will charge for their services. During the trance-like state, you may be given specific instructions but the popular idea that you can be forced to do something against your will is mistaken. During the trance your body will gradually relax, and several scientific studies have demonstrated beneficial changes in pulse, blood pressure and breathing patterns.

SPIRITUAL HEALING

The laying on of hands is undertaken by spiritual healers who are particularly conscious of spiritual practice and who often derive their authority from the scriptures. Notwithstanding the onset of science in modern medicine, spiritual healing is still one of the most popular of alternative therapies. The

Below: *Hypnosis has been successfully used to treat phobias, addictions and stress-related conditions. As a means to recover suppressed memories, however, it remains controversial.*

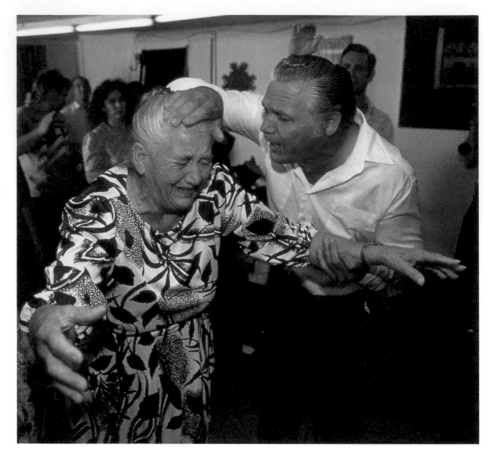

miraculous cures claimed for it, however, have never stood up to proper scientific investigation and caution about raising hopes and expectations must be expressed.

Healing as it is practised today is usually considered to be a two-way

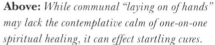

Above: *While communal "laying on of hands" may lack the contemplative calm of one-on-one spiritual healing, it can effect startling cures.*

process. The healer will ask some questions about the problem but is not trained or able to diagnose as such. He will, after calming himself down, induce a deep state of relaxation in the patient and will then focus his "energies" and endeavour to transmit this "power" to the patient through his hands which he usually places just above the client's body, possibly near his head. Patients may be asked to focus on their breathing or concentrate on a white light or warm glow. Patients report a feeling of calmness, and tingling in their limbs. The session lasts about an hour and may be repeated weekly for a while. There is little doubt that much of the beneficial response comes from the relaxation and the sense of hope that is transmitted by the healer. Nevertheless, some preliminary research studies suggest that some healers may be responding to energy flows in the body of the client.

SELF-HELP APPROACHES

ALEXANDER TECHNIQUE

This is a form of specialized sequence of exercises that are taught in classes that help to re-educate you as to the postures you adopt for sitting, standing, lying, answering the telephone, etc. It is not used generally as a remedy for any particular illness, but is a regime to increase your overall sense of well-being. The exercises were developed at around the turn of the century by an Australian actor, Frederick Matthias Alexander, who found he could cure the temporary loss of his

Below: *The Alexander Technique concentrates on correcting a person's posture so that the body's muscular system is not put under undue strain.*

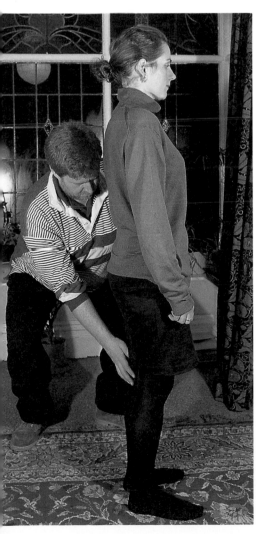

voice through changing his posture, particularly with regard to his head, neck and spine. The Alexander Technique has been further developed to help pupils co-ordinate posture, breathing and voice control and has become particularly popular among actors, dancers, singers and public speakers. It is generally taught in classes over ten to twelve hour-long sessions but once you learn the technique you can practise it at home.

As well as being a general educative system for good postural control, the system of exercises has been found to be helpful in stress-related conditions such as insomnia, tension and anxiety as well as general conditions such as raised blood pressure and asthma. More specifically it is of great help in persistent back problems, sciatica, lumbago, etc.

The scientific attitude is positive and supportive and several studies have indicated that it is a safe and appropriate treatment for many general complaints. The writer Aldous Huxley gave Alexander much publicity by supporting his work in the early 1930s and there are now training centres throughout Europe and the USA.

AUTOGENIC TRAINING

A systematic form of relaxation exercises for both body and mind, autogenic training is often referred to as Western Yoga. These simple exercises were developed in the late 1920s by a German physician, Dr. Johannes Schultz, practising in Canada, who felt that the body had an untapped capacity to cure itself (auto – self, genic – producing). Initially three simple exercises (reclining, armchair and simple sitting – names that relate to the position in which they are undertaken) are taught and these are co-ordinated with breathing and relaxation techniques. Then other exercises (warmth, heaviness, heart-beat [slowly], breathing [deep] stomach and forehead) are

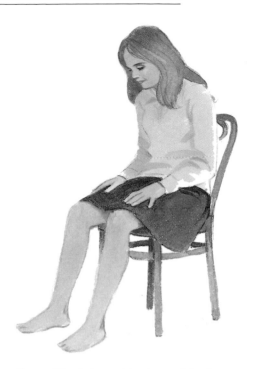

Above: *The sitting position is one of the three postures that beginners in autogenic training are taught as a means to deep relaxation.*

taught, which give the client more control of his physiological processes.

Autogenic training has been used as a stress-reduction programme as well as for treating insomnia and high blood pressure. It is also used for helping with other conditions, such as asthma, irritable bowel syndrome, migraine and chronic pain. Many people who learn the technique attest to its ability to release energy and induce a general level of calm and invigoration.

Scientific studies of the effectiveness of autogenic training exist aplenty as this has been one of the most closely researched forms of relaxation training, and orthodox doctors have no difficulty in accepting this mode of work. Training centres exist in Canada, the USA and Europe. Initially, clients are seen in groups of six to eight persons; while self-help cassettes exist for using at home. Like many self-help approaches, the success rate depends on the client maintaining the practice routine and keeping a diary, and a daily discipline is of great importance.

BATES EYE TRAINING EXERCISES

These are a series of specially designed eye exercises that help to restore the ability of the eye to focus by strengthening the muscles of the eye. Bates exercises have helped individuals avoid wearing spectacles and, practised as a daily routine, have meant that many individuals have kept good eyesight well into old age. They can be seen as an equivalent of brushing the teeth but for the eyes. They were developed by an American ophthalmologist, William Bates, in the early years of the 20th century. He developed this system while treating not only adults but young children. He argued that better development of the muscles that control each eye and its ability to focus would cure sight problems that were otherwise only treated by the prescription of glasses. He published his findings in his book *Better Eyesight Without Glasses* (1919).

The exercises are simple to learn and include palming, remembering, focusing, splashing, swinging and blinking. They can be of help to anyone who has eye problems, eye strain or suffers from headaches. Teachers are not easy to come by, but several self-help books have the exercises well illustrated and their simplicity makes it possible for all to follow. Although few scientific studies have been undertaken, no harm can come of pursuing

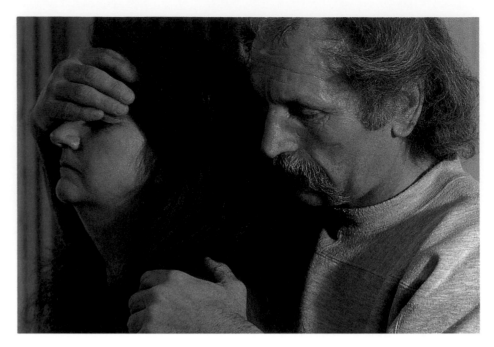

these exercises and much good has been reported of them.

BIOENERGETICS

Bioenergetics developed from the work of psychotherapists Wilhelm Reich and Alexander Lowen, and is an approach to body-mind integration using a set of exercises which concentrates on the breathing as the basis of the person's health. Like any Eastern approach to health, bioenergetic therapists believe in the life-force, Chi or Prana. The key to working with and liberating this force is proper breath control. Lowen believed the body had a memory, just as

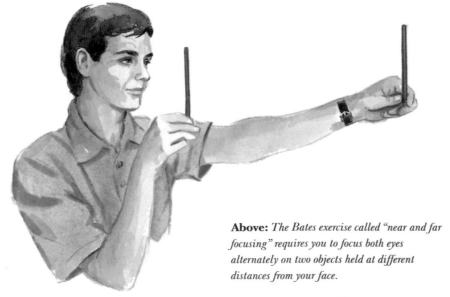

Above: *The Bates exercise called "near and far focusing" requires you to focus both eyes alternately on two objects held at different distances from your face.*

Above: *Bioenergetics recognizes a link between physical posture and mental state, and aims to "unlock" the body so that it functions properly.*

the mind did, and that we develop a "character armour" in our body, so that our posture and movements reflect our psychological and emotional state. The body literally becomes "overburdened with grief", or if we are "flushed with pride" then that would be observed in our chest muscles and blood circulation. Through a system of exercises, often done in groups, students are encouraged to make links between physical posture and psychological states, thus facilitating the body-mind link, especially through the breathing exercises.

Although not specifically developed to help with disease, bioenergetics has been found to be helpful in many of the recognized psychosomatic illnesses. It is more useful, however, as an educational and therapeutic approach to stress disorders and forms part of the humanistic growth movement, the group of therapies that stress the individual's responsibility for his or her actions which grew up in the 1960s, mostly in California, under the influence of Fritz Perls and Carl Rogers.

Attitudes in the scientific community are mostly sceptical and the theories of Wilhelm Reich, whose concepts of energy flow form the basis of bioenergetic therapy, have largely been discarded. Centres in America, the UK and Western Europe exist and it is popular among the growth movement.

AEROBICS AND CALLISTHENICS

These activities are popular and effective exercise routines that are usually geared for young, fit individuals and attract a large following, as they are often associated with music, dance and the self-promotion of attractive film stars. Unlike Yoga, aerobics aim to exercise the heart and lungs by fast repetitive movements which increase the breathing and pulse rate. It is important to check you are reasonably fit before joining a class and a period of "warming up" is a necessary prelude to prevent muscle and joint damage. Usually most classes will end with a period of relaxation. Those people suffering from blood pressure or heart problems should seek medical advice before starting on any vigorous exercise routine, and it may be safer to follow an audio or video tape at home, where it is easier for you to stop when you wish to.

Below: Joining an aerobics class is fun and very motivating, but take care that you do not push yourself too far too fast.

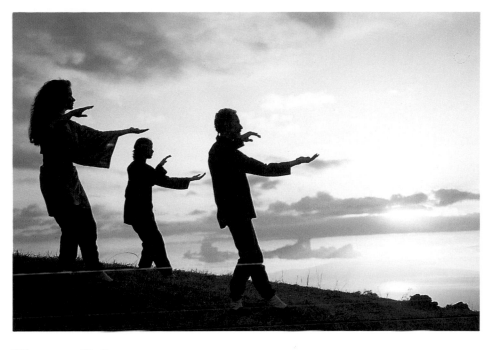

T'AI-CHI CH'UAN

Many of the Chinese forms of exercise routines are linked to the martial arts, but the development and popularity of T'ai-chi is related to the fact that it avoids a link with aggressiveness and the use of force. The word means "supreme ultimate" and, as practised in China as long ago as the 14th century, it developed into a system of simple, slow, beautiful and graceful movements of the body linked together in a dance-like formation, often prac-

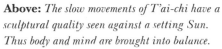

Above: *The slow movements of T'ai-chi have a sculptural quality seen against a setting Sun. Thus body and mind are brought into balance.*

tised in the open air. Although allied historically to the martial arts, it replaced aggression with slow, contemplative movements that help the practitioner focus on the integration of body and mind. T'ai-chi became instantly popular when introduced into America and Europe and can often be seen being practised in the early morning in many of the public parks.

T'ai-chi, although appearing deceptively simple, is quite difficult to learn and requires attendance at a number of weekly classes taught by an experienced teacher. Loose clothes are essential and the student is taken through each movement cycle in stages. The short form of movement consists of about 40 movements, while the long form contains over 100 movements which can take over half an hour to perform. T'ai-chi, like many of the self-help therapies from the East, is not used specifically for treating a particular condition but is held to be of value as a health promoting and life-enhancing daily routine. Nevertheless, those who use T'ai-chi feel that its effects help them to manage stress and tension particularly well, as well as diminishing any long-term muscular pains.

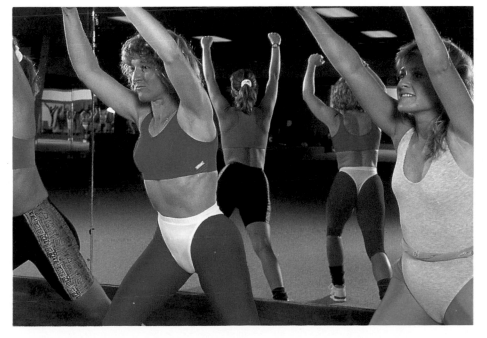

PART THREE

TREATING COMMON ILLNESSES

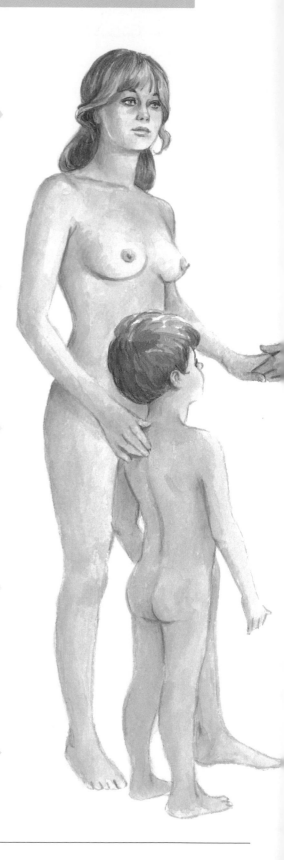

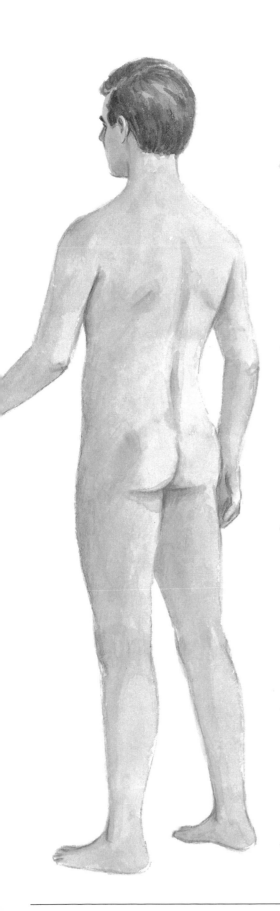

ASTHMA

Asthma is a relatively common condition affecting both children and adults, which has recently increased in its incidence. It can be both frightening, especially for parents with small children, and serious. Asthma is characterized by a narrowing of the small tubes of the lungs (bronchioles) which produces the characteristic wheeze and rapid breathing associated with this condition. Many babies, especially in the first year of life, sometimes wheeze, especially if they have a cold, but this will not necessarily develop into asthma. In fact, it is a quite common occurrence due to the narrowness of the child's bronchioles, i.e. all wheezes do not necessarily signify asthma.

CAUSES

The narrowing of the bronchioles results either from sticky phlegm and catarrh causing obstruction, or because the muscles surrounding the small tubes contract, so narrowing their diameter. Asthma can run in families, especially when it is associated with the skin condition known as eczema. It is generally accepted in Western medicine that asthma is caused by one of three different possibilities:

Infection allergy and stress anxiety Any respiratory infection that results either from viruses or bacteria can trigger off an asthmatic attack because of the increased phlegm produced. Certain infections caused by moulds or fungi will also trigger off an attack, but usually this is the result of an allergic response to the fungus.

Allergenic asthma Sometimes

Below: *Narrowing of the airways in the lungs, either through blockage or muscular spasm, characterizes asthma.*

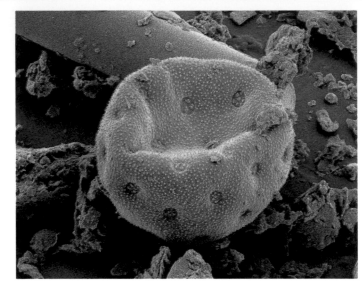

called extrinsic or atopic asthma, it usually starts in childhood and is associated with other allergies such as hay fever, allergies to pets (feather and fur), dust mites, certain foods, especially dairy products, and air pollutants.

Non-allergenic asthma or intrinsic asthma This tends to start in adults, is not necessarily

Above: *Possible causes of asthma. This is a pollen grain and specks of house dust magnified over 5,300 times.*

allergic and can be associated with emotional tension, certain forms of exercise, and is often worse at night (nocturnal asthma).

SYMPTOMS

A persistent cough without any wheeze, especially if there is no phlegm or sputum. Wheezing, which can be audible, and difficulty in breathing out, often associated with a feeling of tightness in the chest. The respiratory rate and pulse are increased, and in severe cases a drawing in of the lower ribs can be observed, especially in babies and children.

PREVENTION AND SELF-HELP

Asthma is a serious and potentially fatal condition. Medical treatment is both effective and life-saving and before consulting a complementary therapist, you should ensure that you see a medical doctor. There are, however, several things you can do to help yourself.

▪ Keep a diary recording the frequency of the attacks, when they occurred, and what possibly brought them on (infection, allergy, stress). You may obtain a Peak Flow Meter from your doctor that actually measures your lung capacity and so gives you a more accurate estimation of the severity of the asthma attack.

▪ If you are allergic, keep a record of the various items that trigger the allergic attack and avoid them. Get rid of your blankets, feather pillows or eiderdown, heavy rugs or (unfortunately) any pets. The house dust mite is a common cause of asthma and regular vacuuming of your bedroom and mattress will help.

▪ Eat plenty of fresh fruit and vegetables – avoid cheese, butter, eggs and milk. If your baby or infant has developed asthma, changing to soya milk can often be of great help. Supplement with Bifidobacteria Infantis for babies (three drops twice a day).

▪ Take regular light exercise (swimming, running). Check your posture and obtain a breathing and relaxation tape to help you breathe with a regular diaphragmatic breath.

▪ Know your limitations and avoid pollutants (tobacco smoke, heavy fog), but do not allow yourself to become an invalid. Many Olympic sportsmen and women have been asthmatics. Do not over-protect your asthmatic child, let him/her lead as normal a life as possible.

▪ Take your medication regularly if prescribed, both before and during an attack, but do not exceed the recommended use of inhalers, especially as this can be potentially fatal.

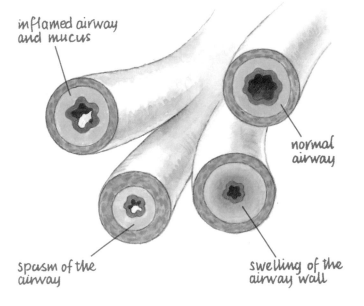

inflamed airway and mucus

normal airway

spasm of the airway

swelling of the airway wall

ACUPRESSURE

Learn the acupressure points that are helpful and if you think you are going to have an attack, try and get a massage to help you relax. There are two acupoints that are particularly useful: Lung 7, which is found two fingers' width above the wrist on the inner forearm in line with thumb. Support the wrist and apply pressure firmly with the index finger towards the thumb for up to two minutes. Secondly, there is the Asthma Relief point, found on the back of the neck, one finger's width to the side of the seventh cervical vertebra. Apply pressure with the thumbs on either side of the spine.

TRADITIONAL CHINESE MEDICINE

This is now a well-accepted approach to asthma, although it is important not to stop any orthodox medication without

Below: *Gentle manipulation of the neck vertebrae by an osteopath can help long-term asthma sufferers.*

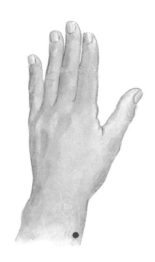

Above: *Acupoint Lung 7 is found on the inner arm, just above the wrist.*

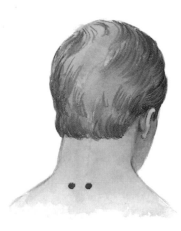

Above: *This point is specifically designated for asthma relief.*

proper supervision. Chinese practitioners view asthma as a dysfunction of either the lung or kidney Chi, and will prescribe a course of treatment which may last up to six months, initially concentrating on reducing infection and catarrh with the help of both diet and herbs. Acupuncture alone, or together

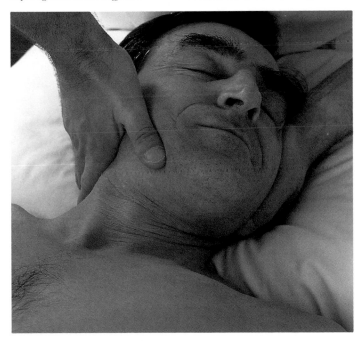

with acupressure (Shiatsu), can relieve an acute attack, especially if there is an element of tension and stress.

OSTEOPATHY AND CHIROPRACTIC

Often in people with long-term asthma, chronic muscle spasm and spinal malformations can occur, which not only cause physical pain and discomfort, but can restrict chest movement and make the asthma worse. Gentle manipulation of the neck, shoulders, vertebrae and rib-cage will loosen the restriction and help to improve movement. The use of Yoga postures or the Alexander Technique will ensure that the re-adjustment will be maintained.

HERBAL TREATMENT

Will be used by both Chinese practitioners as well as naturopaths, and specific remedies are best left to trained practitioners to prescribe. They may use any of the following herbs: euphorbia and thyme as infusions will help both to loosen phlegm and relax the tight bronchial muscles; chamomile will

act as an anti-inflammatory agent and will reduce general tension and stress; ephedra is a powerful herb which may also stimulate the heart and blood pressure, and therefore regular checks are required when it is prescribed.

HOMEOPATHY

An extensive history would be taken by a homeopath to try and identify the appropriate remedy and it is not advisable to rely on homeopathic self-medication in asthma as there is no clear evidence that it can help. Nevertheless, a homeopathic consultation can sometimes pinpoint the problem, especially in children. Remedies that have been used include *Arsenicum albicum, Natrum mur.* and *Ipecacuanha.*

OTHER THERAPIES

Hydrotherapy, massage, reflexology, aromatherapy will all help to relax the body and reduce stress. Inhalations as used to treat bronchitis will loosen the mucus.

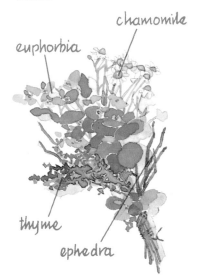

chamomile
euphorbia
thyme
ephedra

Above: *Herbs such as euphorbia, thyme, chamomile and ephedra can help, but take them under the supervision of a qualified herbalist.*

ORTHODOX TREATMENT

Because asthma is potentially fatal, it is important to obtain conventional medical advice and take the regular orthodox medications, either tablets or inhalers, that cut short or prevent attacks. In severe cases, injections (including steroids) are used. Because of the long-term side effects, it is now no longer customary to keep patients on steroids and many doctors will now recommend the use of acupuncture as a supportive measure for people with asthma.

CHRONIC CATARRH AND SINUSITIS

The lining of the nose, throat, sinus cavities and upper part of the lungs (trachea, larynx and bronchi) contains small mucous glands that secrete a watery substance (mucus) which helps to lubricate the airways and protect us from infection and pollutants that may be inhaled. If the secretions are too productive, or if they become thick and infected, the common symptoms of a runny nose, a blocked and stuffed-up feeling, together with a cough or even a temperature and facial pain can occur. The sinuses are hollowed-out cavities (four pairs) in the bones of the face which normally contain air and which are lined by mucous membranes. The mucus normally flows between the nose and the sinuses through little openings and ducts. If these become blocked, neither air nor mucus can flow and infection can set in, leading to dull pain (face, forehead or nose) together with a temperature.

CAUSES

The major causes of chronic catarrh that can lead to sinusitis are infections, allergies, air pollutants, smoking, and stuffy office buildings (which can lead to a condition known as sick building syndrome). Cold viruses and influenza are the commonest cause of episodic catarrh, but allergies, especially to pollen (hay fever) or house-dust mites, can lead to persistent nasal stuffiness. Some individuals, especially small children, can be allergic to dairy products and wheat, which will also produce an inflammation of the mucous membranes leading to the symptoms described. The persistent use of anti-histamines or nasal decongestants in hay fever or other allergies will thicken the mucus initially and may stop the symptoms, but it can lead to blockage of the tiny ducts and actually bring about a sinus infection.

SYMPTOMS

In addition to those mentioned above,
▪ A chronic discharge from the nose – yellow or green, occasionally tinged with blood.
▪ Blocked nose with loss of sense of smell or taste.
▪ Watering of the eyes with redness or swelling over the sinuses.
▪ Facial pain on stooping, bending, coughing or sneezing.
▪ Soreness in the face which occasionally may be located over the teeth.

PREVENTION AND SELF-HELP

Dietary changes
▪ Avoid mucus-producing foods – dairy products, including eggs, white flour, sugar, chocolate.

Below: *This shows the location of the sinuses around the nose. Infection in the sinuses leads to facial pain.*

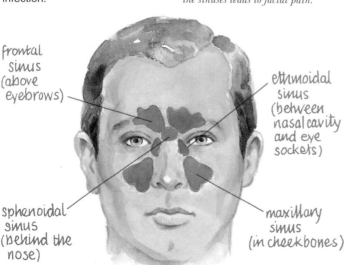

frontal sinus (above eyebrows)

ethmoidal sinus (between nasal cavity and eye sockets)

sphenoidal sinus (behind the nose)

maxillary sinus (in cheekbones)

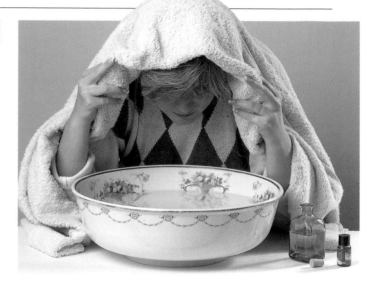

▪ Drink plenty of spring water or fresh juices.
▪ Introduce a "wholefood diet" including garlic (see section on diet, pages 18-21)

Environmental changes
▪ Remove any potential allergic products.
▪ Keep the room well ventilated.
▪ Use an ionizer if there is air conditioning in the building, together with a humidifier.

Supplementary vitamins and minerals
▪ Vitamin A and Vitamin C will help to restore the mucous membranes and prevent infection. One tablet a day.

CHILDREN: Children should only be given extra Vitamin C – half the adult dose.

▪ Zinc tablets (one daily) will sometimes be suggested by naturopaths.

CHILDREN: Take half the prescribed adult dose.

Above: *Inhaling the steam from a bowl of hot water and Friar's Balsam is an effective way to relieve sinus pain.*

Fasting
This can often be very helpful (take water or fruit juices only), but should not be prolonged for more than 48 hours unless under expert supervision. This can be done by children as well.

Inhalations
These are helpful both in an acute attack as well as a preventative measure, and can either be done with steam over a bowl of hot water containing Friar's Balsam, or directly in the form of a nasal wash (use a bowl of warm water, body temperature, together with half a teaspoon of salt – the water should be slightly salty like tears). Inhale the water through one nostril and let it run out of the mouth; repeat on the other side. Special nasal wash pots can be obtained from natural food stores to help with this technique.

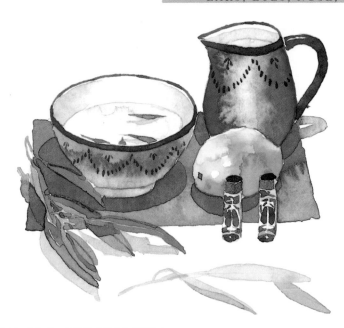

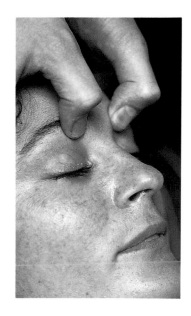

HYDROTHERAPY

Treatments such as mustard baths are traditional and very helpful: put a teaspoon of mustard in a bowl or bucket, and pour in hot water until it is deep enough to cover the feet and ankles. Make sure the water is not too hot before you immerse your feet. Saunas and steam baths are helpful in the acute phases, and a daily cold bath is a good preventative measure.

ACUPUNCTURE

This can be helpful in cases of chronic catarrh and sinusitis by reducing the production of mucus. Needles are inserted on the lung, large intestine and stomach meridians.

ACUPRESSURE

Pressure on any one of three points will reduce discomfort and feelings of stuffiness. The points to use are:
Urinary Bladder 2, found on the inner edge of the eyebrows on either side of the nose. Press gently upwards towards the skull for one minute.

Above: *Gentle pressure on the Urinary Bladder 2 acupoints is soothing.*

Urinary Bladder 10, found on the back of the neck below the hair line, two fingers' width on either side of the spine and level with the lobes of the ears. Press gently but firmly for one minute. Stomach 3, on the cheekbone directly below the middle of the eye. Press straight into the cheekbone for one minute.

AROMATHERAPY

The use of essential oils in a bath or a steam inhalation or directly as a gargle are all recommended. **Bath/inhalation** Use two drops of pure essential oils (eucalyptus, lemon or cedarwood). Add to your bath or a bowl of hot water (for inhalation). The same amount (i.e. two drops) can be added to an eggcupful of neutral carrier-oil and rubbed on the upper chest.

CHILDREN: Care must be taken if oils are used on children under 12 years of age – use half the adult dose.

Gargle One drop of the above oils in half-a-cup of water – gargle but do not swallow. The same dose can be used for children.

HOMEOPATHY

These remedies can be very helpful for sinusitis but it may require the skilled help of a homeopathic practitioner to identify the right one. The following guide may be helpful for self-medication:

Above: *Inhaling fragrant oils like eucalyptus, lemon and cedarwood can ease that "blocked-up feeling".*

Nat. mur. Catarrh is runny, like egg white.
Kali bichrom. Catarrh is stringy and yellow.
Hydrastis Continual post-nasal drip.
Graphites Chronic catarrh with irritation of the nose.
Pulsatilla Yellow nasal discharge
Hepar sulph. Face is tender and sensitive
Sambucus "Sniffly", blocked-up nose in children.
In each case take one tablet (6c potency) every two hours (six doses only), then three times daily until better.

CHILDREN: Infants and children can take the same dosage but it can be given as drops.

BIOCHEMIC TISSUE SALTS

These are also useful, *Kali sulph.* being the most commonly prescribed. Take one tablet a day; half for children.

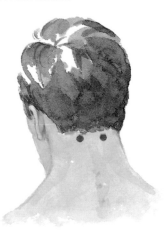

Above: *Urinary Bladder 10 is another acupoint that may help.*

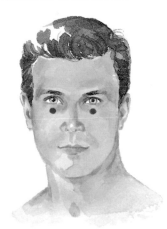

Above: *The Stomach 3 point is under the eye, on the cheekbone.*

ORTHODOX TREATMENT

Ordinary symptoms are often treated with anti-congestants or anti-histamines which can, however, cause problems in the long run. Acute infections respond well to antibiotics, but on occasions surgery or sinus wash-outs are required to clear out all the sticky mucus. Nasal sprays will also be prescribed, especially when allergies are present. None of the alternative therapies described is considered harmful, but many doctors do not believe that they are effective. However, because these conditions are so common and orthodox treatment can be harmful, it is a good idea to try an alternative approach, especially some of the preventative measures outlined.

THE COMMON COLD

The common cold is the "folk illness" of the Anglo-Saxon world and is most prevalent in Britain, but it is also frequently found throughout Europe and the USA. Although "colds" are popularly believed to occur in the winter and in damp, wet weather, there seems to be no actual link with outside temperature and their prevalance. The symptoms are well-known – sore throat, running or blocked nose, headache, slight temperature and occasional cough. Because a cold is caused by a virus, antibiotics are not only unhelpful, they may be harmful (antibiotics are only effective against bacteria). If you suffer from persistent colds, it may be that you are run down and that your immune system is not working as well as it might. If you are under constant stress, catching a cold may be your body's way of telling you to slow down or that you need a day or so of rest.

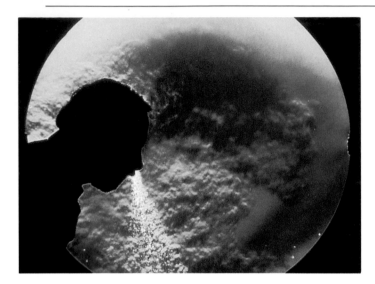

CAUSES

A cold is caused by a virus of which there are over 200 varieties and is "caught" by breathing in the tiny infected droplets that are expelled when someone coughs and sneezes. Most adults can expect to have at least two or three colds a year and as yet no magical treatment exists that will cure colds. The link with cold weather arises because we tend to remain indoors during the winter months, in crowded situations, and it is therefore easier to catch the virus which is present in the air we inhale. You can also catch the virus from an object, such as a cup of tea or a book, if the person with a cold has sneezed on it and you subsequently touch the object.

PREVENTION AND SELF-HELP

It is not always possible to prevent catching a cold, but some of the following may help in boosting your immune system

Above: *A special camera allows us to see the explosive power of a sneeze jetting mucus drops out of the nose.*

and strengthening your ability to manage the symptoms. Research has shown that we are more likely to catch a cold if we are suffering from stress. Useful preventative measures include:
■ Vitamin C: 1g (children 500mg) three times a day as tablets.
■ Acidophilus capsules: Three capsules three times a day (half this dose for children).
■ Zinc gluconate: This is one of the few substances that research has shown is effective in preventing a cold. Lozenges can be sucked or chewed. Adults and children over 27kg (60lb), one lozenge every two hours.

CHILDREN: For children weighing less than 27kg (60lb), half a lozenge every two hours.

■ Honey propolis and pollen have all been used both to treat and prevent colds. Take by mouth, one teaspoon daily.

If you have been in contact with someone who has a cold, Vitamin C, garlic supplements and zinc gluconate (25mg daily) can be effective from time to time in preventing you from catching it.

TREATMENT

However bad you feel, it is important to remember that a cold is not a serious condition and may require no treatment at all. General measures include resting, taking things easily, not eating heavy meals, keeping your room warm, stopping smoking and maintaining the humidity using a humidifier or vaporizer. Diet is important – avoid dairy products (eggs, milk, cheese) and eat fresh fruit, especially citrus fruits (oranges, grapefruit, mandarins, limes and lemons) and pineapples.

REMEDIES FOR SPECIFIC SYMPTOMS

Blocked nose Make a mixture for inhalation using a bowl of hot water with three or four drops of any of these essential oils: rosemary, eucalyptus, juniper. Allow the steam to rise and breathe it in deeply with a towel over your head. Steam on its own may be sufficient to ease congestion and a herbal pillow at night will relieve some of the stuffiness. Drinking a bowl of hot onion soup with cayenne pepper is often used to clear the sinuses, and if there is any sign of infection, a garlic clove or garlic capsules will act as a natural antibiotic.

Below: *Eating plenty of citrus fruits such as these can help the body combat the symptoms of a cold.*

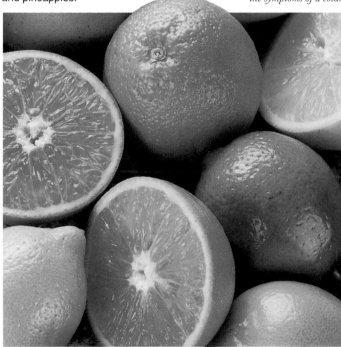

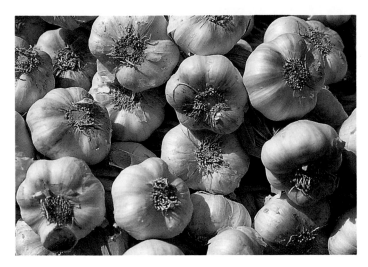

Above: *Garlic has powerful healing properties; try eating a finely sliced clove in honey if you have a cold.*

Sore throat Gargling with hot water, honey and lemon drinks is particularly helpful and the mixture can be swallowed. Thyme is another herb that is used and you can buy oil-based lozenges to suck. The traditional salt and water gargle – three or four teaspoons of salt in a tumbler of warm water – helps to remove excess mucus. You should not swallow it, however. Spit it out instead.

Headaches These are caused by swollen mucous membranes and many of the previous remedies will help to reduce the congestion and pain. Acupressure is also useful – apply a gentle pressure for five to ten seconds just above your nose on the centre of your forehead using your thumb and forefinger, and then work slowly down the nose. If there is muscle tension, then a massage or warm bath will help a great deal.

Earache Especially in young children, this problem should be seen by a doctor, but again it may only be a symptom of congestion. It is important to avoid sniffing with a cold as this may force the infected mucus into the inner ear. A warm pad placed over the ear will help. Do not use oil drops unless they are prescribed by a doctor.

elderflower

hyssop

thyme

red sage

chamomile

Above: *Red sage makes a soothing gargle, while teas of chamomile, hyssop and elderflower can also help.*

HERBAL MEDICINE

Gargle with red sage (half a teaspoon) steeped in hot water, or use the traditional salt water gargle (see remedy for Sore Throat above). Do not swallow the gargle. Honey and lemon drinks are also popular, but try finely sliced garlic (one clove) in three to four tablespoons of honey (no water). Teas or infusions with the following help

with specific symptoms: chamomile (calming, and reduces temperature), elderflower (reduces stuffiness and catarrh), hyssop (helps with coughing and infection). These can all be taken as teas and do not forget the soothing lemon-balm and rosehip. Echinacea tablets (anti-infective) are a general cold and 'flu remedy – take one four times a day (children twice a day). The traditional mustard foot bath is also helpful. Dissolve a tablespoon of dry mustard powder in a bowl of hot water. Place the feet in the bowl and pour on more warm water. Soak for ten minutes and then dry. Repeat before going to bed.

HOMEOPATHY

Homeopathic remedies are particularly helpful for the common cold and include *Belladonna* (sore throat), *Bryonia alba* (headaches), *Aconite* (sneezing), *Pulsatilla* (general remedy), *Natrum mur.* (chronic runny nose), *Euphrasia* (watery eyes). Take the remedies (as tablets) at 6x potency every three hours.

CHILDREN: The same dosage applies to children and they can be obtained in drop form (four to six drops on the tongue).

BIOCHEMIC TISSUE SALTS

Take *Ferr. phos.* (fever and sneezing, or just before the cold develops), *Nat. mur.* (for runny nose), *Kali mur.* if there is chesty congestion or cough. Take two tablets four times a day.

CHILDREN: One tablet four times a day for children under 12.

AROMATHERAPY

Many oils have been used in inhalers (see recipe below). Coughs can be helped by dropping four drops of lavender essence on a little brown sugar and swallowing the mixture.

CHILDREN: Take half the adult dose.

How to make your own inhalation mixture
One litre (1¾ pints) of boiling water
Three tablespoons of 90% alcohol
30g essence of eucalyptus
14g essence of thyme
14g essence of pine-needles
10g essence of lemon
10g essence of lavender

Below: *Two tablespoons of honey, two of glycerine, one of lemon juice and a pinch of ginger make a good gargle.*

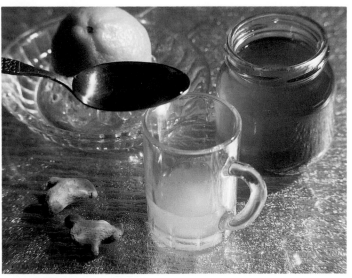

ORTHODOX TREATMENT

While none of these remedies is harmful, most doctors would suggest that they may also be unnecessary. A cold usually lasts two to three days and recovery is not shortened by such treatments, although the symptoms can be better tolerated while your body overcomes the virus.

COUGHS AND CROUP

Coughing is a reflex activity involving the diaphragm, chest wall and larynx which is often a normal protective response to a variety of different factors. It is helpful to think of coughing as resulting from three different situations. These are an increase in catarrh or saliva, excess production of sputum and irritation of the larynx. Each of these causes of coughs is examined below.

CAUSES

Increase in catarrh (common cold), or saliva (teething) The excess catarrh can collect at the back of the throat, and coughing prevents it from entering the trachea and lungs, i.e. the cough is protective and is a sign the body is responding well.

Excess production of sputum or phlegm This can occur in the lungs either from infection or chronic irritation (bronchitis). Coughing helps to "bring up" the sputum, unplugging the tubes of the lungs and thus helping to rid the body of excess fluid. Both these coughs are called "productive" because they are usually accompanied by expectorant (coughed-up phlegm) which can be clear or coloured.

Irritation of the larynx (voice-box) or throat The third type of cough arises if the larynx or throat is irritated in some way, e.g. laryngitis, croup or whooping cough. In this instance, the cough is usually dry, rasping and can be painful.

A cough in itself should rarely be suppressed unless it is clear it is caused by an irritation and is not part of the body's protective system. Other more serious conditions accompanied by coughing include pneumonia, bronchitis, heart failure, tuberculosis, lung cancer, and in young babies, a viral infection of the lungs called bronchiolitis. People with asthma can find an attack is preceded by a series of wheezy coughs often brought on by irritation (pollution) or allergy.

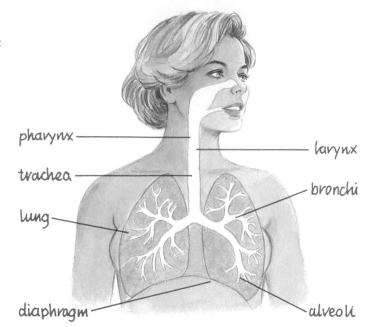

Above: Coughs can arise because of irritation of the larynx, phlegm accumulating in the lungs, or raised levels of catarrh or saliva.

In this instance, the cough occurs because of the spasm of the muscles surrounding the large air tubes (bronchi).

SYMPTOMS

Simple coughs related to colds or sinus infections usually last less than ten days. The sputum may be coloured or occasionally blood-stained. The dry, rasping cough from croup or whooping cough is often quite characteristic and is described as "barking" and "deep". Fits of coughing are often associated with allergy or asthma, and coughing with lots of phlegm occurs in chronic bronchitis. Coughs accompanied by discoloured or blood-stained sputum should be seen by a doctor, especially if there is any temperature or chest pain.

PREVENTION AND SELF-HELP

It is first important to recognize that a cough in itself is not something that should be removed or suppressed as it can be the body's own way of removing or preventing infection.

- Avoiding irritants – tobacco, smoke, pollution (wear a face mask if cycling in a city) – is important.
- Humidifying the atmosphere in a home, especially if there is central heating, will help both irritating coughs, as well as ease productive coughs. Putting a wet towel over the raidator, or allowing a steam kettle to boil in a room, or buying a humidifier will all help. Taking a hot bath or hot shower, with plenty of steam, also helps.
- Inhalations are a traditional way of soothing and helping infections or laryngitis. The simplest way is to pour some boiling water in a large bowl, place a towel over your head and breathe in the steam. A tablespoon of Friar's Balsam or menthol crystals added to the water will help to release sticky mucus and soothe the soreness in the face or throat.
- Hot drinks of honey and lemon will also help to reduce irritative coughs.

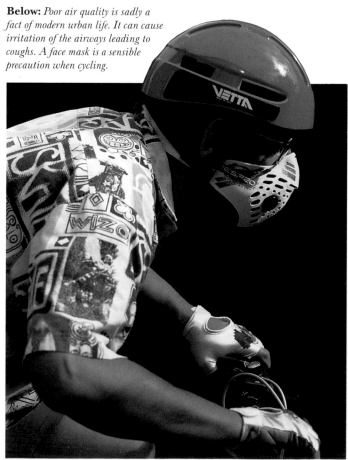

Below: Poor air quality is sadly a fact of modern urban life. It can cause irritation of the airways leading to coughs. A face mask is a sensible precaution when cycling.

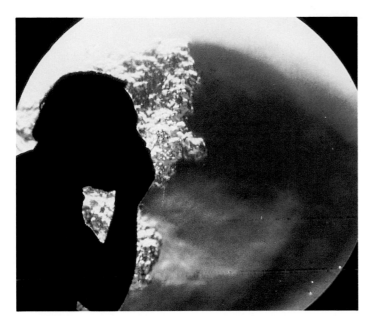

Above: *Coughs and sneezes do spread diseases. This Schlieren photograph shows how a hand has contained the jet of droplets expelled from the mouth.*

NATUROPATHY

All of the above self-help tips will be recommended, Taking two garlic tablets three times a day for one week, together with extra Vitamin C (1,000mg a day) may help prevent colds and infections. Wrapping a towel soaked in hot (but not boiling) water around the throat will ease pain.

HERBAL MEDICINE

An infusion of white horehound can be helpful. Put a few leaves in a cup of boiling water, allow them to steep for about ten minutes and take a teaspoon three times a day (half-dose for children under 12). Wild cherry bark is a remedy often used for children, and elderflower can be given when the cough is quite productive. These both can be made as teas and drunk (three cups) during the course of the day.

Herbs can also be used in inhalations (see above) or added to a hot bath (excellent for children). In this case use tinctures, two drops in a bath: hyssop and thyme for productive coughs, mullein and liquorice for a dry cough. A hot compress impregnated with three drops of tincture can be used to rub a child's or adult's chest. Add three drops to a bowl of warm/hot water, soak the towel and wring it out, and apply it to the chest wall until the towel is cool. Repeat every four hours.

BIOCHEMIC TISSUE SALTS

A combination of salts known as Combination J containing *Ferr. phos., Kali mur.* and *Nat. mur.* is often used as a general remedy for coughs. Adults shold take one tablet 6x, every two hours, up to six doses.

CHILDREN: Children under 12 should take one tablet 6x, every three hours.

AROMATHERAPY

Aromatherapists suggest using essential oils in a bowl of steaming water as an inhalation (take great care if you are using this with children). Oils suggested include eucalyptus, thyme, cypress and sandalwood. Add three drops of one of these oils and inhale for no more than ten minutes. Repeat up to three times a day.

HOMEOPATHY

Aconite: Hoarse, dry and painful.
Bryonia: Bronchitis.
Drosera: Barking, dry cough.
Hepar sulph.: Thin, yellow sputum.
Rumex: Tickling cough.
In each case, take one tablet, 6x potency, three times a day, for up to three days.

CHILDREN: Same dose as for adults.

Below: *Try making an inhalation mixture with hot water and oil of eucalyptus to soothe a cough.*

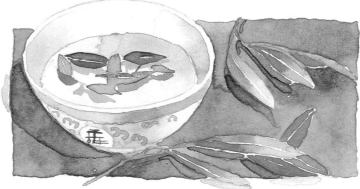

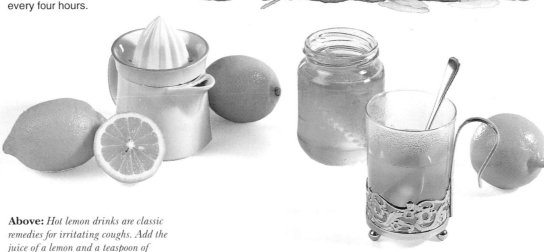

Above: *Hot lemon drinks are classic remedies for irritating coughs. Add the juice of a lemon and a teaspoon of honey to a cup of hot water, and sip.*

ORTHODOX TREATMENT

A diagnosis is usually arrived at before any treatment is prescribed. Often, if there is no sign of bacterial infection, the patient will be advised to use their own preferred remedy. Many cough lozenges and linctuses exist which both soothe and help to loosen the cough. "Drying up" linctuses are not often recommended as they may make the sputum dry. Investigations to rule out bacterial infection or cancer will be undertaken if appropriate. No cough which persists for more than ten days should be treated without seeking medical help.

BRONCHITIS

Two distinct types are recognized: acute bronchitis, which often follows a cold or influenza, is an acute inflammation of the lining of the large tubes of the lung, causing a cough, sometimes painful, with discoloured yellow or green sputum (phlegm). It can be associated with a temperature, muscle-aches and a tightness of the chest. Occasional actual pain on coughing is experienced, and wheezing can be heard. It usually lasts up to seven days but can take up to three weeks to clear. Chronic bronchitis is the result of permanent damage to the delicate lining of the tubes of the lung which causes an accumulation of phlegm or sputum resulting in a persistent productive cough which will get worse if the sputum becomes infected. This eventually leads to damage of the tiny air-sacs in the lung leading to shortness of breath and occasionally heart failure.

CAUSES

Acute bronchitis is most commonly caused by a virus or bacteria. Occasionally it may be the result of toxic fumes and polluted air (exhaust fumes) irritating the lungs.
Chronic bronchitis arises as the result of long-term irritation of lining of the lungs from smoking, coal dust (miner's disease) and other long-term damage.

PREVENTION AND SELF-HELP

Prevention requires effective elimination of the irritant (stop smoking or wear a face mask if cycling in the inner cities). Use an ionizer and humidifier in your rooms, especially the bedroom, to remove airborne particles of dust. Self-help measures include concentrating on a wholefood diet, reducing or omitting all dairy products, and creating a warm, humidified environment. All contact with smoke or pollution should be avoided and an ionizer will help improve the air breathed in. Occasionally steam baths and saunas are recommended. Additional Vitamin C (a gram a day) and garlic capsules (two a day) will help to treat and prevent secondary infection.

HERBAL TREATMENTS

Inhalation with essential oils (eucalyptus or pine) is recommended by herbal practitioners who would also prescribe some of the following. Echinacea (improves circulation), ginger (stimulates lung function), elecampane (stimulating expectorant), wild thyme (loosens phlegm). These should be taken as a tincture if prescribed by a herbalist. At home you can make an infusion or a herbal tea.

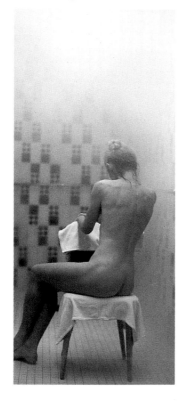

Above: *Steam treatments, such as this woman is enjoying in a health spa, can be helpful preventative measures against bronchitis.*

AROMATHERAPY

Aromatherapists would suggest some of the following oils				
Method	Eucalyptus	Hyssop	Sandal-wood	Carrier
Bath	6	2	2	Warm, half-full bath
Compress	6	2	2	In half-cup of water
Inhalant	6	2	2	In half-basin of hot water
Massage oil	15	10	5	In 60ml (2 fl. oz.) of carrier oil
Medicine	2	1	1	In honey

Amounts: These figures indicate the number of drops of essential oil that should be added to the "carrier". These figures are for adults.

CHILDREN: Under 12, use half this prescribed dosage.

HOMEOPATHY

A therapist would focus on the "total" history and would prescribe one of a number of remedies depending on the characteristics of the cough and quality of sputum. *Bryonia* is the classic remedy for bronchitis, but *Kali bich.* is also used (if sputum is loose and green). *Aconite* is often given for fever and muscle aches. You should use 6x potency and take one tablet three times a day for three days. Repeat in one week if no better.

CHILDREN: Can take the same dosage, four to six drops orally.

ACUPUNCTURE

This can be of great help, especially in chronic bronchitis to help with the shortness of breath. The needles are placed in the lung meridian and the circulation is improved by further needles affecting the blood Chi. A recent scientific study indicated that this treatment can be effective although it does not restore the lung tissue that has been damaged.

BIOCHEMIC TISSUE SALTS

Preparations that can be taken include *Ferr. phos.* 6x and *Kali mur.* 6x. They should be given frequently in the first four days, then halve the dosage for the next four. Start with two tablets every two hours for adults.

CHILDREN: One tablet every two hours.

ORTHODOX TREATMENT

For acute bronchitis a course of antibiotics, occasionally a cough expectorant (linctus), rest and a pain reliever (aspirin) would be prescribed. Chronic bronchitis may require long-term antibiotics, physiotherapy to help remove excessive sputum and inhalers to improve air-flow into the lungs.

SORE THROATS

At the back of the mouth and nose (known as the pharynx) there is a "ring" of glandular tissue – the tonsils and the adenoids. They are part of the immune system of the body and can be likened to policemen or doorkeepers which protect the body from invasion by foreign and dangerous particles (viruses, bacteria, dust particles, pollen etc). They are prone to become inflamed and infected, giving rise to painful but not serious infection (pharyngitis, tonsillitis, adenoiditis). These infections can be regarded as protective: they prevent the bacteria/viruses from invading deeper into the body. On occasions, however, the pharynx can become so infected that treatment is required either for the painful symptoms or because there is a danger of the infection spreading to the ear (otitis), or developing into an abscess (quinsy), or spreading to the blood (septicaemia). Most commonly, however, these infections are minor, last three to five days, leave no scars and require very little treatment.

CAUSES

Sore throats and "colds" are very common in childhood as children get in contact with viruses from other children – it is a way for them to develop immunity later in life. People who are run-down, have poor diets and have other illnesses, are susceptible.

PREVENTION AND SELF-HELP

Vitamin C tablets (1 gram a day, 500mg for children) have been used frequently to prevent sore throats, as has garlic (see below). An infusion of thyme (two pinches of thyme in a cup of warm water before going to bed) can be an effective preventative remedy. If you are under a lot of stress, one or two dessert spoonfuls of wheatgerm daily can be taken both by adults and children. Stopping smoking is important, both to avoid catching sore throats as well as during an attack.

HERBAL MEDICINE

Fresh lemon juice and honey in water is both soothing and helpful in reducing inflammation. It can be taken as a gargle or as a drink. Common herbal teas used include myrrh, thyme or sage (they are not particularly pleasant to drink so a teaspoon of honey can be added to sweeten the

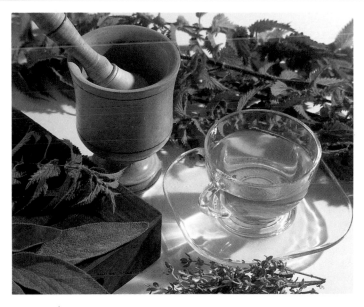

Above: *An infusion of sage, thyme and young nettles such as this often helps relieve soreness in the throat and bronchial congestion.*

taste). Garlic, like sage is a natural antibiotic and two garlic capsules daily can reduce the length of the infection. Some people are quite happy to have a fresh garlic clove shredded in half a glass of water.

CHILDREN: Find gargles difficult and may not like the taste of herbal teas, so it may be more helpful to try a homeopathic remedy in their cases (see table).

with hot water and add two teaspoons of Friar's Balsam. Inhale the steam under a towel for ten minutes. Take care with children not to spill hot water.

BIOCHEMIC TISSUE SALTS

Ferr. phos. in the initial stages (one tablet three times a day). This chemical (iron phosphate) is a constituent of red blood cells which distribute oxygen around the body. Use *Calc. phos.* for "chronic" tonsillitis and *Nat. mur.* when there is a lot of saliva. *Kali mur.* is also useful in combating respiratory disorders and sore throats.

CHILDREN: May find a tincture easier to swallow than tablets. Two to three drops three times a day.

Inhalations are helpful especially if the adenoids are affected or if the nose is blocked. Fill a bowl

HOMEOPATHY		
Homeopathic remedy	Symptom picture	Dose
Aconite	Hot, dry, sudden onset	6x, one tablet three times a day.
Apis	Redness and puffiness of throat	**CHILDREN:** May take the same dose as adults, or give as tincture, three drops three times a day if throat is very sore.
Belladonna	High temperature, red face	
Hepar sulph.	Very sore, green mucus	
Mercurius	Bad smell, slimy saliva. Sweating and thirsty.	

ORTHODOX TREATMENT

Most sore throats are caused by viruses and you may wish to gargle with soluble aspirin or suck antiseptic lozenges. If there is evidence of bacterial infection, then the policy is to give a short course of antibiotics, usually penicillin. In chronic infections, surgical removal of the tonsils is advised, although this is becoming much less frequent. If there is constant nasal obstruction, mouth breathing and snoring, then surgical removal of the adenoids may be advisable.

EARACHE AND EAR INFECTION

The ear is a complex sensory organ embedded in the skull and traditionally divided into three parts (external ear, middle ear and inner ear). The external outer ear includes the fleshy and cartilagenous part that we see on the side of the face. It contains the canal that secretes wax to keep it oily and it stops infections entering the more delicate middle ear where sounds are registered. The middle ear is embedded in the mastoid bone and contains the delicate hearing mechanism. This small "boxlike" cavity is connected to the back of the throat by a narrow tube called the eustachian tube. If the latter is blocked with mucus or inflammation, the middle ear can become infected and give rise to a very painful condition known as otitis media. Infection of the outer ear is known as otitis externa. The inner ear consists of a complex set of structures – known as the labyrinth – that are concerned with hearing and balance.

CAUSES

Earache can be caused by blockage or infection of either outer or middle ear and will lead to a pain which is dull or throbbing, together with a temperature, and if severe, discharge, which can be yellow/green, thick mucus or blood-stained. Often in children all that will be noticed is a distressed, fretful child refusing his or her feeds, and running a high temperature. It is important to differentiate between otitis externa and otitis media as treatments are different. Usually the former has no long-lasting effects, but if not properly treated otitis media can lead to chronic serious otitis which may lead to deafness. Blockage of the ear canal can arise from wax and water (swimmer's ear). Infections can arise when people try to clean their ears and in doing so damage the delicate lining. Pain also occurs when the ear is blocked because of a cold, or because of cabin pressurization when flying in an aeroplane.

SYMPTOMS

- Earache, discharge from either ear.
- Temperature and vomiting (small children)
- Uncontrollable crying and (in small babies) diarrhoea.
- Partial deafness or ringing in the ear.

PREVENTION AND SELF-HELP

Because this problem can arise so quickly, it can be difficult to prevent, but general measures encompass avoiding damage to the outer ear (i.e. do not clean the ear canal with a matchstick), and trying to prevent colds and infections (concentrate on a good wholefood diet, and take extra Vitamin C). It is important to avoid leaving the ear canal wet, especially after swimming.

CHILDREN: Children who regularly get colds and suffer from chronic catarrh should follow the measures described in those entries. Avoiding dairy products will help, as will a 24-hour fluid (water) fast.

Acute infections can be so distressful and worrying that it is usual and advisable to follow orthodox medical treatment but the following self-help measures can be helpful in relieving the symptoms:
- Ice-packs will bring immediate relief for pain when placed next to the ear.
- A small piece of cotton wool soaked in garlic (squeezed from a capsule) and inserted gently in the ear is soothing.
- A gauze plug soaked in an emulsion made from mixing a 40 percent alcoholic tincture of propolis with olive oil and inserted in the ear helps to relieve pain.

BIOCHEMIC TISSUE SALTS

Treatments here include *Ferrum phos.* for fever, pain and congestion, and *Kali sulph.* when there is a thin, watery yellow discharge. Take one tablet twice a day.

CHILDREN: Should take half the adult dose.

AROMATHERAPY

A small drop of warm olive oil dropped into the ear canal will help to relieve pain. Take care that it is not too hot, as the ear will be sensitive.

HOMEOPATHY

This can be very effective both as a first-aid remedy in the middle of the night and also in long-term problems. The following may be taken according to the symptom picture:
- *Aconite* Severe pain, irritation, due to chilling.
- *Chamomile*: High temperature, crying/restlessness, discharge.
- *Belladonna* Severe, boring pain, worse at night.
- *Mercurius* Sweating, very cold sensation, maybe a delirious child.
- *Pulsatilla* Yellow/green discharge, temperature, tearful. All these should be given at 6x potency, one tablet (or equivalent drops) every two hours, up to six times in the first instance and then repeated three times a day.

CHILDREN: Children over two years may take the same dose as adults. For children under two, use drops – administer two drops every three hours.

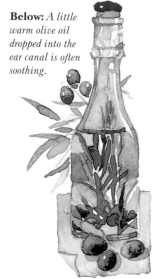

Below: *A little warm olive oil dropped into the ear canal is often soothing.*

ORTHODOX TREATMENT

Symptom relief with aspirin (which reduces pain and temperature) and tepid sponging (bathing the body with tepid water) will be advised. Antibiotics will often be prescribed, although increasingly some doctors no longer believe these to be appropriate as their use may lead to the chronic condition known as "glue ear", in which fluid accumulates in the middle ear and which causes deafness in children. It may require an operation and the insertion of grommets in the ear to relieve the sticky mucus that accumulates in this case.

EAR DISCHARGE

This is a common, unpleasant and potentially serious condition affecting children more commonly than adults, usually as a result of an upper respiratory tract infection. Two varieties are known: one is characterized by an acute discharge with yellow/green pus and is the result of an infection (acute otitis); the other, chronic otitis, is also known as serious otitis or glue ear. Other causes of ear discharge are the result of a foreign body in the ear (such as a peanut or matchstick), or may follow a blow to the head when there is an accompanying fracture leading to a bloody discharge. Occasionally soft wax may be confused with an ear discharge. Otitis externa is a skin infection of the ear canal and does not usually affect the ear drum or inner ear. Skin disease, such as eczema or psoriasis, can affect the skin lining the ear canal, also giving rise to a troublesome ear discharge.

CAUSES

These are generally as explained above, and usually as a result of a viral or bacterial (haemophilus, streptococcus) infection.

SYMPTOMS

Clear, yellow/green or blood-stained discharge, all accompanied by pain, tinnitus (ringing in the ears) and dizziness. Painful ears often result from changes in atmospheric pressure that can be experienced during flying or deep-sea diving.

PREVENTION AND SELF-HELP

Children should not be allowed to poke matchsticks in their ears and care must be taken with cotton buds if they are used to clean the ear canals. Chewing gum will ensure the Eustachian tubes connecting the middle ear to the nose are kept open, which will ensure drainage occurs from the middle ear. Babies and children can be encouraged to

Below: *If an earache is accompanied by discharge, the probable cause of the trouble is an ear infection.*

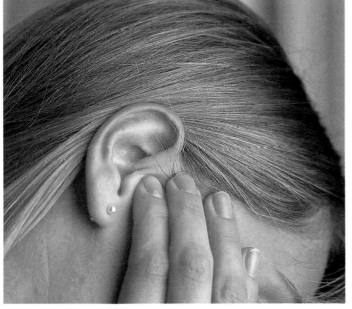

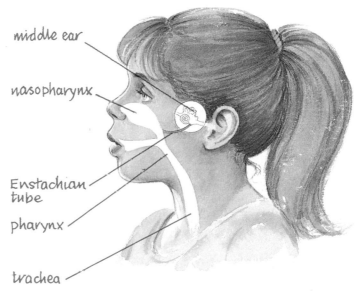

middle ear

nasopharynx

Eustachian tube

pharynx

trachea

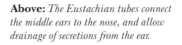

Above: *The Eustachian tubes connect the middle ears to the nose, and allow drainage of secretions from the ear.*

swallow if they are flying by using a bottle to reduce the pressure in the middle ear. Pain from ear infection can be treated with ice packs. A hot salt bag is also helpful: heat a cup full of salt gently in an oven – place the salt in a cloth bag and hold against the ear. A little warm olive oil will help ear ache, but ear discharge will need to be seen and examined by a qualified doctor to ensure there is no damage to the ear drum.

TRADITIONAL REMEDIES

These include using a warm clove of garlic placed in the ear itself (garlic contains a natural antibiotic). Homeopathic remedies to relieve pain include *Aconite* 6x, one tablet three times a day (adults and children), and *Belladonna* 6x (one tablet three times a day for three days, adults and children). If recurrent ear infections occur in children, it can be helpful to change from cow's milk to soya milk. Added Vitamin C will aid resistance to infection.

ORTHODOX TREATMENT

Ear discharge is taken seriously, especially in children, as unless properly treated it may lead to deafness and permanent loss of hearing. Careful cleaning of the ear is undertaken and antibiotics prescribed either locally (in the form of ear drops) or by mouth. Some doctors now believe that antibiotics are not helpful and may actually lead to the chronic serious otitis or glue ear. The latter condition presents as deafness accompanied by a thick, sticky discharge and for a while it will be treated with the insertion of grommets (small plastic tubes that allow the discharge to drain from the middle ear).

GINGIVITIS

The gums are medically known as the gingiva and inflammation of this structure is known as gingivitis. The gums should be healthy and pink in colour, with a stippled appearance like the skin of an orange. Gum disease and infection is the most common cause of tooth loss in adults due to loosening of the base of the tooth socket. Chronic gingivitis is a condition that is difficult to treat but easy to prevent.

CAUSES

The most common and almost only cause of gum disease is the accumulation of dental plaque around the gums. Plaque is a sticky, soft, non-calcified film of bacteria and other organic material that accumulates on the base of the tooth and spreads to the gum. If the plaque is not removed, the bacteria attack the tooth enamel and cause holes, which are then further invaded and lead to caries (cavities) and dental decay. Plaque is most common in someone eating a high starch, high sugar diet who does not take the trouble to brush his or her teeth regularly and so remove the plaque. Occasionally gingivitis will result from a more serious bacterial infection which will invade the mouth and pharynx.

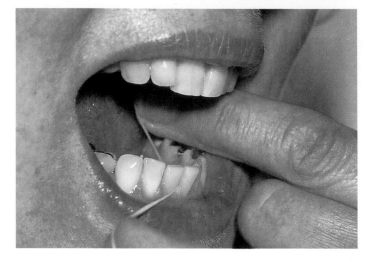

Above: *Flossing between the teeth, though boring to do, is vital to your dental health, so keep at it!*

SYMPTOMS

- Soreness of the gums.
- Bad breath (halitosis).
- Bleeding of the gums on soft brushing of the teeth.
- Dental cavities or loose teeth.

PREVENTION AND SELF-HELP

- Reduce consumption of all starchy food and foods containing sugar, including drinks.
- Brush teeth regularly, especially immediately after you have eaten a meal.
- Use special plaque-removing toothpastes obtainable from healthfood stores and most chemists.
- Regular use of dental floss (waxed string) to rub between the teeth will allow for removal of harmful plaque.
- Mouthwashes, medicated or salt, will sweeten the breath but do not actually reduce plaque.
- "Disclosing dyes" that colour the plaque red will allow you to see how successful you are in your plaque-removing efforts.
- Eat healthily – chew hard food regularly; chewing helps to stimulate saliva that destroys plaque. For instance, chew raw carrots or a stick of celery.
- Use cheese as an after-meal dessert, as it helps to restore the acid balance in the mouth.
- Visit your dentist regularly and have your teeth scaled every six months.
- Learn how to brush your teeth properly.

Below: *The action of chewing hard on raw food, such as a stick of celery or a carrot, stimulates the flow of saliva in the mouth, which in turn destroys the build-up of plaque which is the main cause of gum disease.*

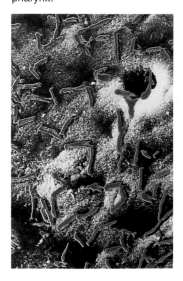

Above: *These objects are bacteria on a human tooth magnified x1,700. If plaque is not regularly removed, such bacteria attack tooth enamel and gums.*

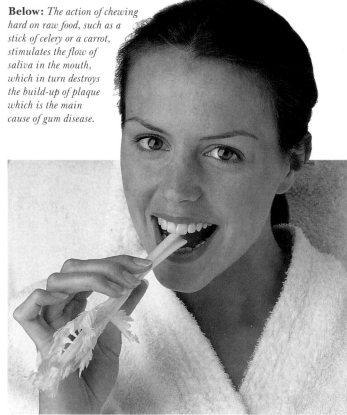

ORTHODOX TREATMENT

Most doctors will refer you to a dentist to check for gum disease or infection which may occur with heavy plaque formation. Occasionally, and especially if the gums are bleeding, an antibiotic may be prescribed (metronidazole) to reduce the presence of the bacteria that can also cause bad breath odour.

HAY FEVER

This condition, so common in the spring and summer months, is neither caused by hay nor does it result in fever. It is, in fact, an allergic reaction to pollen which is released by plants in spring and summer. It produces the characteristic symptoms of an itchy, runny nose, red, sore, watery eyes, sneezing, a prickling sensation in the mouth and a sore, itchy throat. Occasionally it will give rise to asthma.

CAUSES

Hay fever or seasonal allergic rhinitis is the result of an allergic response to pollens released into the air by grasses, trees and flowering plants. The pollen is trapped in the hairy linings of the nose and sinuses, and causes the cells in the lining of the respiratory tract to release histamine and other chemicals, which produce the symptoms described above. The common pollens include those of timothy grass, rye grass, mugwort and the beech, plane and elder trees. Symptoms can also be caused by house dust, feathers or cats' and dogs' fur. Hay fever can occur at any age, but seems to be particularly common among young adults. It does seem to run in families and some people will only experience the symptoms during the specific time of flowering. Like all allergic conditions, it can be made worse by stress and emotional tension.

SYMPTOMS

These are as described above and can be worse at particular times of day or during certain weather conditions. They vary depending on the amount of pollen present in the atmosphere and pollen counts issued by meteorologists during the summer months can be helpful in helping you to avoid contact with pollen by staying indoors at times of high pollen concentrations.

PREVENTION AND SELF-HELP

▪ Keep a diary of your symptoms and try to identify the causal pollen. It is now no longer the practice to carry out allergy testings, as this has proved not only inaccurate but dangerous.
▪ Stay indoors during high pollen times keeping doors and windows shut.
▪ Avoid smelling fresh flowers, mowing the lawn, dusty atmospheres.
▪ Wear sunglasses to reduce irritation of the eyes and apply a damp towel over face and eyes. During the allergic season, bathe your eyes regularly with cold water by using an eye bath.
▪ Nasal washes (as described in Catarrh entry, pages 66-67), will remove pollen trapped in the nose.
▪ Warm honey and lemon drinks will ease the pain of sore throats.
▪ Smear a little vaseline around the nose to trap pollen, and wear a nose and mouth mask when venturing outdoors.

Below: *This image, magnification x4,000, shows the inflamed lining of the nose caused by an allergic reaction to pollen in the air.*

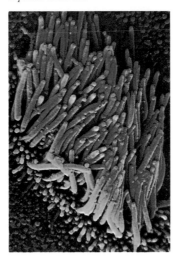

Above: *When your hay fever symptoms are bad, try inhaling a few drops of the essential oils of hyssop or fennel sprinkled on a handkerchief.*

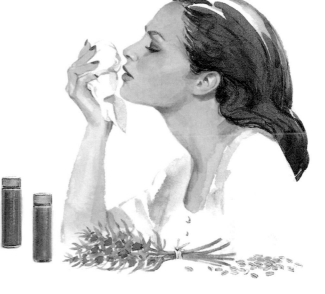

▪ Use airfresheners and ionizers indoors to remove pollen.
▪ Vacuum and dust your home frequently during the pollen season.
▪ Inhale through a handkerchief after impregnating it with a few drops of the essential oils of hyssop or fennel when symptoms are troublesome.
▪ Use small lumps of honeycomb as chewing gum during the hay fever season.
▪ Taking pollen tablets, or grains of Arizona pollen, helps to reduce the likelihood of hay fever, especially if started six to eight weeks before the season begins.

HOMEOPATHY

Homeopathic remedies can be of great help and have been shown to be superior to placebos and antihistamines. *Pulsatilla* or *Phosphorous*, 6x potency, one tablet three times a day, can be tried. *Allium cepa* (the common onion) is the most usual remedy recommended.

CHILDREN: Can take the same dose as adults. Hay fever is unusual in children under three or four years of age, and a proper medical diagnosis should be made if symptoms present themselves.

ACUPUNCTURE

This has also been helpful, not only in the acute phases but as a preventative measure. If it is successful, it will prove to be so within five or six treatments. Chinese medicine classifies hay fever as an invasion of heat and wind, and several points are used to treat this condition. Stress reduction exercises, meditation and hypnotherapy have also all proved successful.

ORTHODOX TREATMENT

Doctors will use a series of different antihistamines. The newer ones on the market are both safe and do not cause drowsiness. The regular use of certain eye drops and nasal inhalers have been tested; they can prevent the symptoms occurring if they are used before the season begins. In severe cases, cortisone eye drops and nasal inhalers can be helpful, but should not be used regularly.

INFLUENZA

Influenza is one of the most common virus infections that can occur as an epidemic each year leading to severe illness and death among vulnerable people (the elderly and people with chronic respiratory disease). It is highly contagious and is transmitted through tiny water droplets caused by coughing or sneezing. Symptoms appear one to four days after contact. They are usually confined to the respiratory system, but can also involve the intestinal system (see below). The infection usually lasts about a week, but can persist much longer if secondary infection or other complications occur. The body's immune system can be depleted by an attack of 'flu and many people suffer with fatigue and tiredness for several weeks.

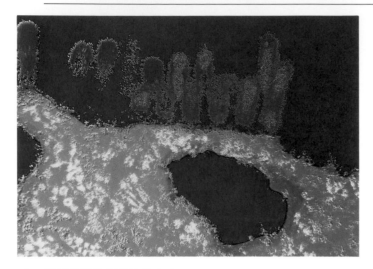

Above: *This is the culprit where influenza is concerned. This virus, magnified x38,000, is releasing more virus particles (shown in red).*

CAUSES

Influenza is caused by a group of viruses. There are many of them, and because they change each year, it is not possible to develop immunity. Classically there are three types of influenza virus: A, B and C. The most common are the Group A viruses (Hong Kong 'flu, Russian 'flu, Bejing 'flu). Viruses invade the body's cells and eventually destroy them, after forcing the cells to produce more virus particles. Because the virus particles live in the cell, the body's natural defence mechanisms – antibodies – are not very effective against them. Antibiotics will not normally be effective either.

SYMPTOMS

▪ The common symptoms of a cold: catarrh, and a cough with sputum.
▪ High temperature and characteristic muscle aches.
▪ Fatigue and a feeling of heaviness in the body.
▪ Sweating and shivering attacks.
▪ Cold, clammy skin with goose pimples.
▪ Dry, sore throat with pain on coughing.
▪ Breathing difficulties and secondary infection of the respiratory system.
▪ Severe headaches and pain behind the eyes.

PREVENTION AND SELF-HELP

▪ General good health measures to boost immunity, i.e. eat a sensible wholefood diet, make sure you exercise adequately, try to avoid getting stressed or run-down.
▪ Take extra Vitamin C and zinc in the form of tablets.
▪ Annual immunization will give 60 to 70 percent protection.
▪ Vitamin B complex will help with convalescence – take one tablet three times a day. One tablet daily for children.
▪ Hot honey and lemon drinks will ease the pain of a sore throat.
▪ Take garlic capsules, one four times a day during an attack. One twice a day for children.
▪ Steam inhalations with a few drops of an essential oil (such as eucalyptus, tea tree, thyme, chamomile, camphor, peppermint, rosemary or lavender) soothe a cough and other troubling symptoms.
▪ Cut out smoking.

HOMEOPATHY

Homeopathic self-help measures include:
Baptisia – for gastric symptoms and severe weakness.
Gelsemium – headaches and painful eyes.
Eupatorium perf. – for "boney" aches and pain.
Arsenicum album – restlessness and irritability.
Bryonia – painful cough and thirst.
All these 6x, take one tablet every two hours for up to six doses. Repeat for three days.

CHILDREN: Children can take a similar dose, but as tincture if under three years of age when tablets are hard to swallow.

HERBAL MEDICINE

Useful herbal remedies include:
▪ Garlic, for the throat symptoms and infections. Take garlic capsules, one four times a day.
▪ Meadowsweet, for muscle aches and pains and headaches. Take as a tea, one cup a day.
▪ Chamomile infusion to bring down temperature. Take as a tea, one cup a day.
▪ Wild cherry bark for the cough and catarrh. Take as a tea, one cup a day.

CHILDREN: Aged between two and 12 years of age should take half the adult dose. Children under two do not get influenza as described.

BIOCHEMIC TISSUE SALTS

Recommended preparations include *Ferr. phos.* and *Kali mur.* Take one tablet every six hours for three days.

NATUROPATHY

Naturopaths recommend fasting for a period of 48 hours, drinking plenty of fluids, rest, and hot baths, hot packs and compresses. Lemon balm tea will help with the process of convalescence – take one cup of this twice a day for up to one week.

CHILDREN: One cup daily for children between two and 12 years; half a cup for children under two.

ORTHODOX TREATMENT

There is no specific cure for the influenza virus, and so doctors will recommend specific symptom treatment (such as a gargle with soluble aspirin), plenty of fluids and rest. Occasionally antibiotics may be prescribed to prevent secondary infection, such as bronchitis or pneumonia, and to protect the elderly and those with chronic respiratory disease.

NOSE BLEEDS

The nose is the first gateway for respiration as well as being the sense organ of smell. It is divided into two parts, one made up of bone and the other of cartilage. The nose is lined by mucous membrane which contains cells that have minute hairy fronds called cilla that act as filters preventing particles of dust and pollutants from entering the lungs. The lining of the nose is very well supplied with blood vessels, especially in the nostril area, and it is bleeding from one of these that produces a nose bleed.

CAUSES

Often there is no specific cause, but a common cold, picking the nose, vigorous blowing or sinusitis may all be a cause. Occasionally these bleeds are associated with high blood pressure or blood disorders. The bleeding usually comes from the superficial blood vessel on the septum separating the two nostrils.

PREVENTION AND SELF-HELP

▪ Do not pick or put foreign objects like cotton buds up your nose.
▪ Regular nasal washes can help keep the nose clean (see pages 66-67).

Below: *Over-vigorous blowing of the nose is one of the commonest causes of troublesome nosebleeds.*

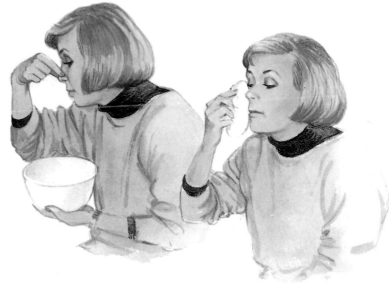

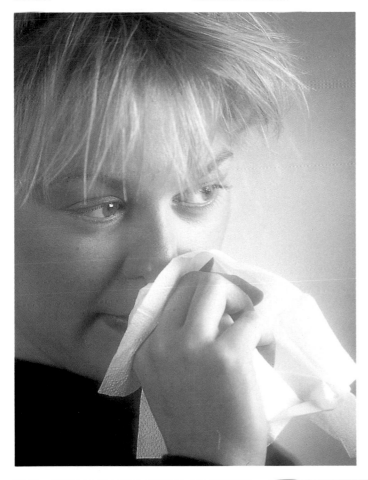

Above: *Pinching the nostrils shut and breathing through the mouth is an effective way of halting a bleed.*

Above: *An ice compress applied to the side of the face or the back of the neck can help staunch the flow.*

▪ Most nose bleeds can be stopped by direct pressure on the side of the nose that is bleeding: sit up straight, lean slightly forward and gently pinch the side of the nostril.
▪ Hold steady for at least fifteen minutes.
▪ Spit out any blood through the mouth.
▪ Breathe slowly through the mouth.
▪ Release pressure and repeat again if bleeding persists.
▪ An ice compress over the side of the face or to the back of the neck can also help.

Right: *The inner lining of the nose is well supplied with blood vessels that warm inhaled air. When one of these vessels ruptures, a nosebleed ensues.*

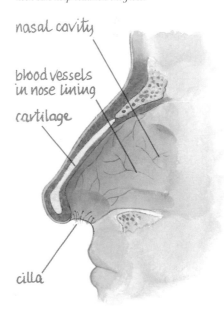

nasal cavity

blood vessels in nose lining

cartilage

cilla

ORTHODOX TREATMENT

If simple measures have not helped, the doctor may anaesthetize the lining of the nose with a simple anaesthetic and then cauterize the bleeding vessel. Alternatively if bleeding is persistent, the nostril may be packed with gauze to staunch the flow. It is important to have a medical check-up if the nose bleed is very severe or if it persists and is recurrent.

POOR SIGHT

The eye is a very complex and sensitive sense-organ. The light from outside passes through the lens and is focused on to the back of the eye (retina). The image formed there is then relayed through the optic nerve to the brain (visual cortex) and is interpreted into an image. Quite rightly any condition affecting its function is viewed with great concern, and should always be treated by an optician.

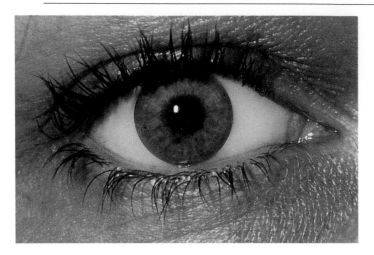

Above: *The eye is our gateway to the world. Conditions affecting sight naturally give cause for concern.*

CAUSES

Although damage to and disorders of the retina and optic nerve occur, the most common causes of poor sight are what are called refractive errors, where, because of some dysfunction, focusing is difficult and blurred vision occurs. The four main types are:
Myopia (short sightedness) Difficulty in seeing distant objects; clear focusing only possible on close-up objects. Possible to read a book but not distinguish writing on a blackboard.
Hypermetropia (long sightedness) Difficulty in focusing on near objects but patient can see objects further away. This problem may become more apparent as the child grows up.
Presbyopia (long sightedness of middle-age) This is the most common problem affecting people of 40-45 years of age and is the result of the lens getting slightly harder, and the focusing power of the eyes thus weakening.

Astigmatism (distortion of vision) This is due to the cornea (the very front part of the eye) not being of the correct diameter so that light waves are "bent" as they pass through the lens.
Other common causes of poor sight include cataracts where the lens contains opacities and loses its translucency. Again this is a development of old age

Right: *Simple massage over the bridge of the nose for a few minutes will often ease painful eyestrain.*

although it can be the result of infection or poor nutrition.

SYMPTOMS

Each of these conditions will have its own pattern of visual disturbance which will be picked up by proper eyesight testing. What most people will notice is *blurring of vision* and *inability to focus*. These may lead to aching eyes or headaches, but it is usually symptomless. Eyestrain, which comes from regular close work, sitting for hours in front of VDU screens, or watching television in poor light, may lead to aching eyes and poor focusing as well.

PREVENTION AND SELF-HELP

■ Ensure your close work is done in good light.
■ If there is a family history of poor sight, have regular eyesight checks.

■ Once you are over 45, if you have any difficulty, get your eyes checked.
■ Never use other people's glasses.
■ Ensure you have a VDU screen anti-glare filter if you carry out a lot of computer work.
■ Regular Bates exercises will both prevent eyestrain and improve eyesight (see pages 60-61).
■ Only wear spectacles if absolutely necessary.
For eyestrain, the following therapies may help:

HOMEOPATHY

Bathe eyes with four drops of Euphrasia mother-tincture in 15cl (¼ pint) pint of lukewarm water.

ACUPRESSURE

Massaging over the face and nose will help relieve pain and aches. Use the thumb and index finger and massage the bridge of the nose up and down for between five and ten minutes.

HERBAL MEDICINE

Cold compresses over your eyes will help. The easiest is a cold slice of cucumber or a cold chamomile tea-bag which is slightly wet – leave the compresses on your eyes for about ten minutes.

CRANIAL OSTEOPATHY

To balance and normalize circulation and drainage around the eyes.

ORTHODOX TREATMENT

Eyestrain will be treated only after proper investigation, but bathing the eyes with any proprietary medication will be advised. Most visual and refractive errors will be referred to an optician for proper testing, and spectacles or contact lenses will be prescribed. Recently, laser treatment has been used to correct deformities in the cornea (astigmatism) which then no longer require spectacles to be worn. Doctors do not believe eye-muscle exercises help, and will not usually recommend them.

RED EYE

The lining of the surface of the eye is known as the conjunctiva and an infection, inflammation, allergy or a foreign body in the eye may cause an irritation that will lead to conjunctivitis (pink eye). More seriously, the coloured part of the eye (iris) may be affected by disease or infection and this can also present as a red eye. Usually vision is not disturbed in conjunctivitis but it can be in iritis. A stye is a "boil" or infected cyst on the edge of the eyelid, and does not affect the eye itself if treated early. Because it can be difficult to be sure what the exact problem is, it is best to consult a doctor early on. Once an accurate diagnosis has been made, it may be possible to use one of the treatments suggested below.

CAUSES

Pink eye is usually the result of a bacterial infection and, in young babies, often a blocked tear duct. The infection is very contagious and a whole school can develop the symptoms if one child has it. Red eye is also a symptom of other infections e.g. measles or viral infections, and will also occur in allergic conditions, especially hay fever. Styes are often the result of rubbing the eyes with dirty hands or towels, or may be a sign of general poor immunity. Occasionally a small piece of dirt, an eye lash or, more seriously, a metal splinter will enter the eye and be the cause of an infection.

Below: *This is what happens when the conjunctiva covering the surface of the eye becomes infected and inflamed.*

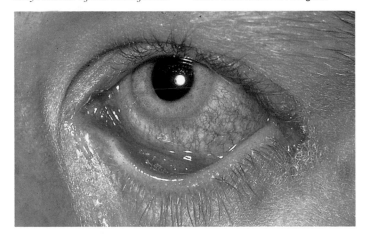

SYMPTOMS

▪ Red eye with swelling and yellow/green pus which often stops the eye opening.
▪ Feeling of grittiness or sand in the eye.
▪ Ache and pain over the eye.
▪ Itchiness and watery running of the eyes.

GENERAL PRECAUTIONS

Do not cover the eye unless told to by a doctor. It can spread infection. Try not to rub your eyes as this will spread the infection also.
It is recommended that no alternative treatment be tried unless an accurate diagnosis by a suitably trained practitioner has been arrived at first. Regular bathing of the eyes before sleeping with a weak salty solution (half a teaspoon of salt in a cup of warm water) can be helpful.

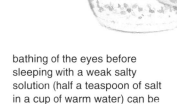

Right: *An eyebath with a weak salty solution is helpful, but do seek qualified advice if you have problems.*

HOMEOPATHY

▪ *Euphrasia* – make a solution of four drops of *Euphrasia* mother tincture in 15cl (¼ pint) of lukewarm water. Bathe the eye in the solution three times a day.
▪ *Ferrum phosphoricum* 6x potency – take five tablets dissolved in warm water four times for three days.
▪ *Aconitum napellus* – red eyes, hot, gritty and swollen.
▪ *Apis mellifica* – stinging, itching eyes.
▪ *Mercurius corrosovis* – lids are painful and stuck together.
For the latter three remedies, take the same dosage as for *Ferrum phosphoricum*.

CHILDREN: Take two tablets of the above remedies a day for three days.

HERBAL MEDICINE

A herbalist may well recommend a compress or poultice to be put over the eye but this should be done only after consultation. Bathing the eye with warm salty water (half a teaspoon of salt in a cup of warm water) may help with an infection, or dislodge a foreign object in the eye. **Do not** try to remove the object unless you have been trained to do so.

ORTHODOX TREATMENT

As with all problems with the eye, most doctors would feel unhappy about the use of alternative treatments unless an accurate diagnosis had been made. Simple conjunctivitis responds well to antibiotic eye drops or eye ointment – a warm poultice soaked in salty water will reduce the swelling of a stye. Foreign bodies will be removed and if there is any doubt about the damage, the eye will be stained with a fluorescent dye to ensure no scarring has occurred. Allergic conjunctivitis, common in the hay fever season, will respond to antihistamines or, if very troublesome, cortisone eye drops. Any more serious eye condition will usually be referred to hospital for proper assessment.

TOOTHACHE AND TEETHING

Careful and appropriate diet together with regular dental care (see page 76) will help prevent most dental problems but toothache which occurs as a result of dental caries (tooth decay) which can go on to develop into a dental abscess, will require the attention of a dentist.

CAUSES

Teething in small children can cause much distress to everyone and can produce a very fretful child who refuses his or her feeds, and may develop a temperature. This condition is often associated with loose motions and foul-smelling diarrhoea.

Teeth-grinding, usually at night and almost always a sign of tension, may produce not only pain and discomfort of the jaw but will go on, if untreated, to develop into further complications: an uneven bite, misaligned jaw, clicking of the temporomandibular joint (jaw joint) and potentially arthritis. Caries (and resulting tooth decay) and abscesses can also cause pain. The consumption of sweets, cakes, sugary drinks etc. should be avoided. Plaque – a mixture of "sugars" and bacteria in the mouth – sticks to teeth causing damage and decay. A proper regime of cleaning teeth is essential to eliminate this.

PREVENTION AND SELF-HELP

■ Poor dental hygiene and poor diet can easily be addressed and will go a long way to preventing and improving the condition of the teeth.

Below: *Teeth only renew themselves once in your life – so make sure children learn dental hygiene early.*

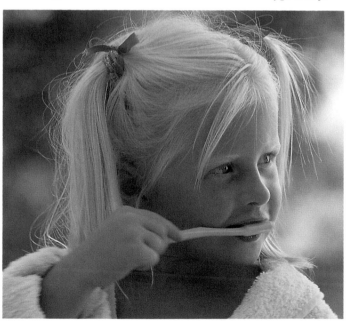

■ If tooth-grinding is a problem, regular relaxation, especially before bed-time, with massage of the face and jaw muscles, will help to reduce the build-up of tension in the jaw muscles.
■ Regular dental check-ups are vital.
■ Avoid all concentrated sweeteners for young babies and infants.

HOMEOPATHY

For toothache in adults:
Aconite 30x – take three hours before extraction and three hours after, repeat up to six times.
Hypericum 30x – If there is any infection.
Dosage: one tablet every three hours.
Hypericum 30x – As a mouthwash (ten drops of mother tincture in a wine glass of warm water). This can also be used for gingivitis.

CHILDREN: For teething in infants and babies:
Chamomilla 6x – One cheek flushed and pale, with diarrhoea.
Aconite 6x – If acute and accompanied by fever.
Belladonna 6x – Flushed cheeks and high temperature.
Calcarea fluor. 6x – Slimy diarrhoea and delay in teething
Dosage: three drops every two hours.

HERBAL MEDICINE

General guidance on good diet and supplementary vitamins would be a mainstay of herbal treatment. A mouthwash of marigold, myrrh and wild indigo will act as a good antiseptic measure. Steep a bunch of each of these herbs in two pints of boiling water. Allow them to infuse for half an hour, strain, and allow the mixture to cool. Then swill the liquid around the mouth liberally and rinse out.

ACUPUNCTURE

Toothgrinding can be helped with acupuncture as can toothache. Dental extraction has been undertaken using acupuncture but it is necessary to identify an expert in the field to undertake this. For the general tension involved in toothgrinding, treatment is given along several meridians.

ACUPRESSURE

Apply pressure two fingers' width in front of the ear in the hollow under the cheekbone, pressing inwards for up to two minutes.

OSTEOPATHY

Realignment of the jaw joint together with checking for vertebral malalignment in the neck and spine have all proved very successful in this particular condition.

FOLK REMEDY

A traditional remedy involves chewing cloves or rubbing oil of cloves on the painful gum to combat toothache and sore gums.

ORTHODOX TREATMENT

Teething is considered a troublesome but not a serious condition and an analgesic (liquid paracetamol) is usually prescribed together with antiseptic and anaesthetic oral jelly that is spread on the gum. All problems with tooth decay and infection will be referred to a dentist, although the doctor may prescribe antibiotics if required. Teeth grinding and temporomandibular dysfunction is commonly treated with pain-killers or anti-inflammatory medication. Occasionally exercises will be prescribed.

DEAFNESS

The complex and sensitive mechanism involved with sound transmission and hearing works almost perfectly almost all of the time for almost all of us. When it does not work well, we can develop symptoms of deafness, vertigo (dizziness) and tinnitus (noises in the ear). Occasionally some children are born deaf, but the two most common modes of deafness are conductive and nerve deafness.

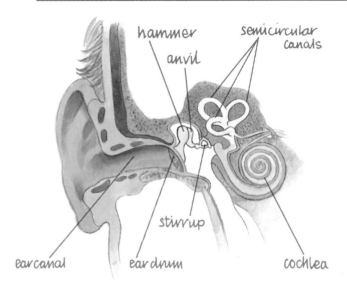

Above: *The ear is a complex organism, responsible for both our sense of hearing and balance.*

CAUSES

Conductive deafness occurs where there is an obstruction (infection, wax, a foreign object) that blocks the sound waves from reaching the middle ear. Damage to the middle ear itself, and otosclerosis (a fusion of the small bones in the middle ear) will also cause conductive deafness. This form of deafness can be cured. **Nerve deafness** occurs as a result of damage to the auditory nerve from virus infections (measles, mumps, German measles), as a result of ageing (deafness of old age), or because of long and constant exposure to loud noise. This form of deafness is usually not curable.

SYMPTOMS

Depending on the type of deafness, certain sounds (high pitch/low pitch) will become inaudible. Listening to the telephone will become difficult, a child will not turn his head when you call him, there may be delayed speech, which can be serious. Other symptoms, including tinnitus and dizziness, should be reported to your doctor as they may be indications of disease of the inner ear (the balancing mechanism).

PREVENTION AND SELF-HELP

▪ Avoid sticking match-sticks or cotton buds in your ear in an attempt to remove foreign objects yourself.
▪ If it is earwax causing obstruction, soften it with oil. You can make a preparation by adding a few drops of olive oil or almond oil to a cup of water and heating it to body heat. Add a few drops of lemon juice and then, using a dropper, apply two or three drops in the affected ear three times a day.
▪ Always wear ear mufflers if using loud machinery or working in a noisy factory.
▪ Do not play your hi-fi very loudly or put your ear close to the loudspeakers. Be careful to regulate the volume of personal stereos carefully.
▪ Ice packs applied over the ear will help with any pain in the ear.

BIOCHEMIC TISSUE SALTS

Deafness caused by persistent catarrh following a cold can be helped with *Kali phos.* and *Kali sulph.* Adults may take four

Below: *Obstinate earwax can be softened by dropping into the ear a preparation made from olive or almond oil, warm water and lemon juice.*

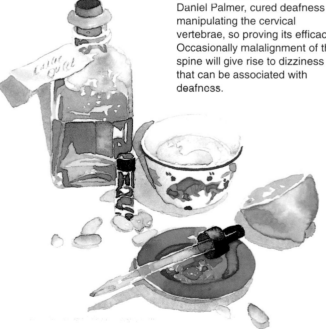

tablets, three times a day for three days.

CHILDREN: Two tablets, three times a day for three days. Babies may have one tablet, three times a day for three days.

ACUPUNCTURE

It has been reported in China that this may help with nerve deafness but no report of this has been confirmed in the West. It can, however, help with symptoms associated with catarrh and tinnitus, which can be very troublesome. Moxibustion (the burning of the herb moxa on the ends of acupuncture needles) is used as well.

CHIROPRACTIC

The founder of this branch of alternative medicine, David Daniel Palmer, cured deafness by manipulating the cervical vertebrae, so proving its efficacy. Occasionally malalignment of the spine will give rise to dizziness that can be associated with deafness.

ORTHODOX TREATMENT

Warm oil is used to soften obstructive earwax and syringing of ears may need to be undertaken to remove all the debris. Deafness is usually treated only after accurate diagnosis, and it may require the wearing of hearing aids. More recently, correction has been possible in some cases following micro-surgery inside the middle ear.

BAD BREATH

DESCRIPTION

The noticeable release of smelly and unpleasant breath which occurs because of poor oral hygiene, poor diet or internal disease.

PREVENTION AND SELF-HELP

- A proper review of diet is called for; avoid onions, garlic and spicy foods.
- Exercise to increase circulation also benefits your respiratory system.
- Fasting for 24 hours and reduction in consumption of coffee/tea and meat helps.
- Proper and regular evacuation of bowels is important.
- Lactobacillus acidophilus will help restore bowel flora (micro-organisms present in the gut).

ALTERNATIVE THERAPIES

Herbal medicine Chewing parsley, drinking infusions of peppermint, and chlorophyll tablets can all help.
Homeopathy *Kali phos.* 6x and *Merc. sol.* 6x – one tablet on waking for up to one week.

CHILDREN: Same dose as for adults.

ORTHODOX TREATMENT

Known as halitosis, this condition is not usually taken particularly seriously and is often referred to a dentist. Mouthwashes or lozenges may be prescribed.

CATARACTS

DESCRIPTION

Cloudy deposits in the lens of the eye leading to misty vision, frequently affecting elderly people. Often both eyes are affected. They can occur as a congenital problem and as a complication of measles in an undernourished child.

PREVENTION AND SELF-HELP

- Avoidance of damage to the eyes from glaring sunlight, and attention to proper visual correction of sight defects is important.
- Bates eye exercises may help to improve eye sight (see page 60).

ALTERNATIVE THERAPIES

Once a cataract has formed, there is no evidence that any form of alternative therapy will help. Occasionally, if associated with poor nutrition, a good diet with supplemental vitamins (B$_2$ and C) will be recommended.

ORTHODOX TREATMENT

Often, if the vision can be corrected, cataracts are left to "mature" before being removed by a simple operation. The lens is replaced or a contact lens implanted instead.

COLD SORE

DESCRIPTION

A small vesicle, spot or blister on the corner of the mouth or lips

Below: *This person has developed a cataract in the right eye as a complication of eczema. It will have to be removed surgically, and replaced by an artificial implant.*

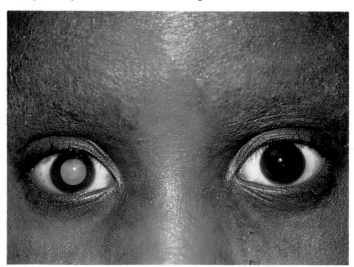

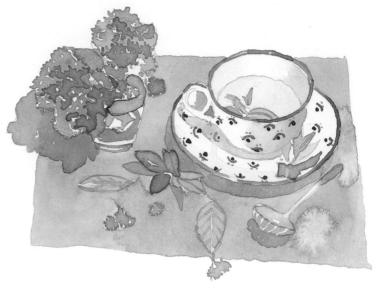

Above: *Chewing parsley is an old folk remedy for bad breath, particularly that caused by eating garlic. Peppermint infusions are also helpful.*

caused by the virus *Herpes simplex.* It can affect other parts of the body, e.g. the genitals. It is often infectious and lies dormant in the skin, becoming obvious at times of stress, periods, colds or other infectious conditions.

PREVENTION AND SELF-HELP

- Avoid kissing someone with a cold sore.
- Use your own towel and face flannel.
- Try not to touch the blisters as they may spread.
- Review your diet, reduce your levels of stress and take some regular exercise.

- Mix equal parts of lemon juice and water, and apply to the cold sore.

ALTERNATIVE THERAPIES

Naturopathy Vitamin supplements (A, B complex and C) will be suggested. A daily dose of zinc and the amino-acid lysine is recommended. Daily garlic capsules are also suggested.
Homeopathy *Rhus tox.* 6x and *Nat. mur.* 6x help. Take one tablet every four hours for two days then twice a day for four days. Calendula cream will soothe and dry out the sore.

CHILDREN: Same dose as for adults.

ORTHODOX TREATMENT

Cold sores are seen as a minor irritant and not often treated unless severe. Vaseline or a soothing cream is suggested. An anti-viral cream is now commercially available.

CRACKED LIPS

DESCRIPTION

Angular cheilitis is the medical name for this condition and it can be a sign of vitamin deficiencies, an over-arching upper jaw, ill-fitting dentures or long-standing illness.

- Check mouth and tooth hygiene.
- Check diet, and seek to remedy any Vitamin B_2 deficiency (B_2 is found in dairy produce and liver).
- Use a mouthwash of ½ part lemon juice to ½ part lukewarm water, and swill around the mouth liberally.
- The biochemical tissue salt *Kali mur.* is useful. Take one tablet twice a day – half this dose for children.
- Eat a liquorice stick twice a day.

Seek medical advice if these measures do not help.

ALTERNATIVE THERAPIES

A thorough exploration of diet and supplements will be undertaken. Vitamin B, Vitamin C, Vitamin A and zinc will be suggested. Iron supplements and dental care will also be recommended. Daily Lactobacillus acidophilus to restore bowel flora is another recommendation.

ORTHODOX TREATMENT

Investigations are usually undertaken to determine the cause and the appropriate treatment. Vitamin or iron supplements are commonly prescribed.

MOUTH ULCERS

DESCRIPTION

These are small ulcerated areas of the mouth and gums with a grey base, which cause pain and soreness. They are associated with viral disease, vitamin deficiency, stress and mechanical problems of dentition.

PREVENTION AND SELF-HELP

Recurrent ulcers are usually a sign of stress and proper measures to promote relaxation are encouraged, such as
- Massage and relaxation exercises.

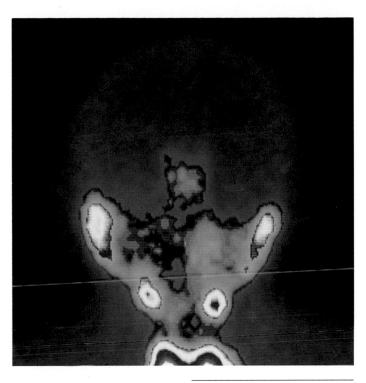

Above: *This gamma scan of a head shows the parotid glands at ear level and the smaller salivary glands under the jaw, which are both affected by mumps.*

- Enjoy a bath with rosemary oil, or take a sauna.
- Check your diet.
- Make sure your toothbrush is not too hard; it may be causing abrasions in your mouth.

ALTERNATIVE THERAPIES

Herbal medicine Chewing liquorice or using a mouthwash made with myrrh is recommended.
Naturopathy A naturopath will check the diet and suggest vitamin supplements (B and C) and zinc. Relaxation and stress relief are also emphasized.
Homeopathy *Merc. sol.* 6x or *Nitric ac.* 6x are the mainstays – one tablet three times a day for one week.

CHILDREN: Same dose as for adults.

ORTHODOX TREATMENT

Because they tend to heal rapidly, normally in three to six days, little is done other than prescribing mouthwashes. Recurrent ulcers will be investigated.

MUMPS

DESCRIPTION

A condition of the salivary (porotid) glands (on the angle of the jaw and under the jaw) caused by a virus which may also affect the testes (causing orchitis) and occasionally meningitis. Usually a mild disease of childhood.

PREVENTION AND SELF-HELP

The only certain way of preventing mumps is through being immunized as a child. The injection carries little, if any, risk.
- Frequent mouthwashes and the biochemic tissue salt, *Kali mur.* one tablet every two hours, will help if you develop mumps.

ALTERNATIVE THERAPIES

Herbal medicine Drink an infusion of yarrow or elderflower every four hours.
Naturopathy A cold compress to reduce the swelling, and garlic perles to prevent further infection are recommended.
Homeopathy *Aconite* 30x will help with pain; *Belladonna* 6x with temperature – take one

tablet four-hourly, adults and children, for as long as there is a fever.

ORTHODOX TREATMENT

No treatment is given other than rest and pain-killers. For complications, steroids may be used. Immunization in childhood is always advised.

SNORING

DESCRIPTION

A troublesome noise during sleep as a result of irregular breathing through the mouth, which has recently been associated with sleep apnoea (cessation of breathing for brief periods) and possible cardiac problems.

PREVENTION AND SELF-HELP

- Yoga is the therapy that helps most, especially if re-breathing exercises are practised before sleeping.
- A hot bath with a few drops of oil of basil will promote peaceful sleep.
- Autogenic exercises may help.
- Sew a small object into the snorer's nightwear, in the small of the back, making it uncomfortable for them to sleep flat on their back.

ALTERNATIVE THERAPIES

Hypnotherapy has been of some help but the underlying breathing pattern needs to be addressed.
Homeopathy Try *Aconite* 30x before sleeping or *Nat. mur.* 30x. Take one tablet before bedtime.
Bach flower remedy The Rescue Remedy may help – take the dose recommended on the bottle.

ORTHODOX TREATMENT

Underlying causes such as obesity and excessive alcohol consumption will be identified. More recently sleep laboratories have explored the use of breathing exercises.

ANAEMIA

Anaemia is the name given to a series of conditions where the amount of haemoglobin (an oxygen-carrying pigment) in the red blood cells is reduced. The haemoglobin combines with the oxygen breathed in through the lungs and acts as a carrier of oxygen to the body tissues – it is the fuel supply needed to maintain all the body's processes. There are several different kinds of anaemia and it is important to have an accurate diagnosis before embarking on treatment. This can usually be done by a series of simple blood tests and, occasionally, through a bone-marrow examination. Some anaemias are hereditary and are due to a malformation of the haemoglobin molecule itself, which restricts its capacity to carry oxygen. Again, this can usually be picked up by a simple blood test, but it may require detailed examination of the haemoglobin molecule.

CAUSES

Iron deficiency This is the most common form of anaemia. Iron is required to carry the oxygen on the haemoglobin and if there is insufficient in the blood, the cells appear pale and "empty". The cause is usually poor nutrition or the body's inability to absorb iron from the intestine because of damage or infection.

Blood loss Commonly through heavy periods, this will deplete the body's store of iron and produce an iron-deficiency anaemia. This also occurs during or after pregnancy when a greater amount of iron is required. Any major loss of blood following an accident or operation will require careful follow-up to ensure there is an adequate supply of iron in the blood stream. Persistent bleeding, such as that associated with haemorrhoids, is another common cause of blood loss requiring extra iron.

Pernicious anaemia This occurs in individuals who do not have an adequate supply of Vitamin B_{12} (strict vegans) or where B_{12} is not absorbed well following gastric surgery or because of a deficiency in the lining of the intestine. This leads to anaemia but can also lead to nervous complications and paralysis.

Megaloblastic anaemia This is the result of poor folic acid (Vitamin B) intake, again either through poor diet or malabsorption because of an intestinal problem.

Sickle cell anaemia Very common among West Indian and Mediterranean communities, this is the main heriditary form of anaemia that occurs because of a malfunctioning gene producing abnormal haemoglobin. Most individuals have partial malformation only (sickle cell trait) and do not suffer at all. Others who have inherited the defective gene from both father and mother have the full blown disease which can be fatal.

Below: *Malformation of the haemoglobin molecule in blood also causes anaemia. These blood cells, magnified x900, are from someone with sickle cell anaemia.*

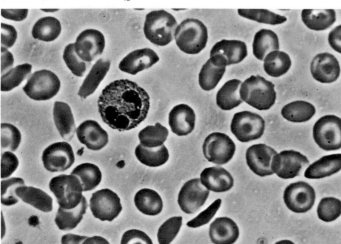

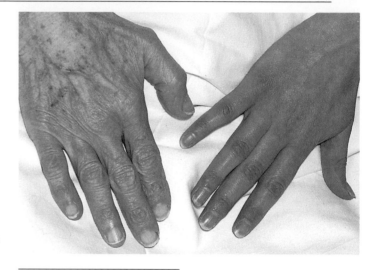

SYMPTOMS

- Dizziness, fainting, tiredness, pale features.
- Sore tongue and cracked lips.
- Shortness of breath, swelling of the ankles, and palpitations.
- Loss of appetite, indigestion.
- Dry, brittle nails (iron deficiency).
- Tingling in fingers and toes, uncontrolled gait (B_{12} deficiency).
- Slight yellow coloration of eyes, jaundice (sickle-cell).
- Pain, temperature and blood clots (sickle-cell).
- Dullness of hair and loss of hair.

PREVENTION AND SELF-HELP

- It is important to consult a doctor for proper investigation and diagnosis.
- A proper wholefood diet will ensure plenty of iron which is to be found in dark green leafy vegetables, walnuts, raisins, wheatgerm, red meat and kidneys.
- B_{12} is found in dairy products

Above: *The pallid hand of a patient suffering from iron-deficiency anaemia (left) is here contrasted with the pink hand of a healthy woman.*

such as eggs, and liver and kidneys.
- All forms of anaemia will be helped by extra Vitamin C, which is found in citrus juices, and Vitamin A, found in carrot juice.
- If you are a vegan and do not take meat or dairy products, supplement your diet with fresh brewer's yeast or wheatgerm.
- Seek help early if your periods become heavier or if you notice you are bleeding from the rectum. Such symptoms require investigation in their own right, but may also lead to anaemia.
- Extra iron tablets are not usually required if you are eating a healthy diet and have no difficulty absorbing iron. In certain circumstances, it is advisable to have extra iron to build up your body stores.
- Tonic wines, which have a high content of iron, are a traditional form of treatment and can be both pleasant to make and take.

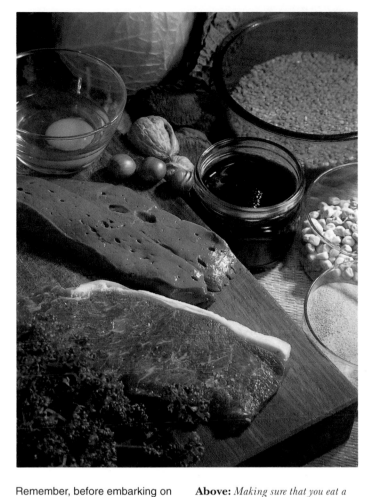

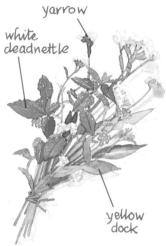

ACUPUNCTURE

Acupuncture will not usually help where there is deficiency but it may aid the process of absorption and will certainly be of value if there is heavy loss of blood

Below: *Herbalists prescribe yellow dock, white deadnettle and yarrow, but only take them under expert guidance.*

yarrow

white deadnettle

yellow dock

Below: *A relaxing body massage with the essential oils of Roman chamomile and lemon is a recommended therapy.*

through menstruation. Additional iron-rich foods including watercress and honey will be prescribed. Moxibustion is said to help "tonify" the circulatory system.

HOMEOPATHY

Homeopathy will not help with the deficiency itself but may aid with some of the troublesome symptoms and may be used in conjuction with replacement therapy.
Arsenicum for pernicious anaemia – 6x, one tablet twice a day for seven days.
Phosphorus for weakness, tiredness, breathlessness – same dosage as above.

AROMATHERAPY

Essential oils of Roman chamomile and lemon may be recommended. They can be taken either as a tea – two drops of lemon and one drop of Roman chamomile in a mug of hot water – or as a lotion – ten drops of each mixed with 60ml (2 fl. oz.) of bland lotion and used to rub over the body.

Remember, before embarking on alternative therapies for anaemia, it is important to have had appropriate investigations and an accurate diagnosis undertaken. It is possible to mask severe disease by partial treatment, and this can lead to long-term problems.

NATUROPATHY

Naturopaths would want to make an accurate diagnosis and would concentrate on your diet, prescribing adequate supplements in the form of extra iron or herbal preparations. Advice on lifestyle including exercise and relaxation would be given if appropriate.

Above: *Making sure that you eat a wholesome diet which includes foods that are rich in iron, such as these, is important in cases of anaemia.*

HERBAL MEDICINE

Again, accurate diagnosis would help determine the appropriate herbal medication and some of these may be prescribed:
Yellow dock: Improves liver function and is rich in iron.
White deadnettle: Will help with heavy periods by reducing congestion.
Yarrow: Repairs damaged blood vessels and improves absorption.
Do not use these preparations unless given specific guidance by an herbal practitioner.

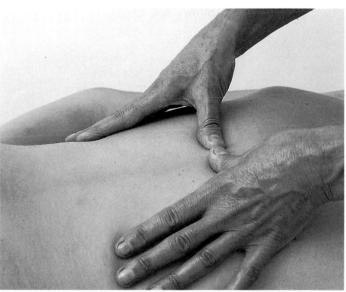

ORTHODOX TREATMENT

No treatment would be suggested before a proper diagnosis has been made. None of the alternative therapies suggested are of themselves harmful, but most doctors would prefer to treat anaemia with iron tablets or folic acid tablets if necessary. B_{12} is usually given in the form of an injection as it is not easy for adequate absorption to take place through the stomach. Careful monitoring would be undertaken to ensure that the haemoglobin is rising satisfactorily. Sickle-cell anaemia cannot be cured and is not usually helped very much by supplemental treatment. Blood transfusions are required to ensure the blood level is maintained sufficiently high.

HYPERTENSION

High blood pressure is one of the commonest problems identified in Western medicine and can be a causative factor in heart attacks, strokes, brain haemorrages and kidney disease. Severe forms of high blood pressure can lead to blindness. The level of your blood pressure determines how hard your heart has to work to pump blood round your body. If it is too high, it will lead to enlargement of the heart and its eventual failure. "Normal" blood pressure varies with age and sex and is usually expressed in two figures – 140/90 or 200/120. (The units of measure are millimetres of mercury or mm Hg.) The first figure is the systolic blood pressure – the peak pressure at the point of the heart beating – and the second figure or diastolic level is the lowest level that occurs between heart beats. The diastolic level is usually considered the more important and a figure of over 105 is considered necessary to treat. Between 90-105 treatment is dependent on age and other factors. The systolic pressure rises with age and most doctors consider a figure of 100+ your age as a "normal" reading, i.e. 170 for a 70-year-old.

CAUSES

In the majority of cases of high blood pressure, it is not possible to identify a specific cause although certain factors are known to be significant. These include being overweight, smoking, lack of exercise, a family history of hypertension, poor diet, stress and tension, high alcohol intake. This form of hypertension is known as essential hypertension and may require medical treatment if the figures are high enough. Some cases of high blood pressure are caused by specific hormonal disturbance. It can be a side-effect of the oral contraceptive pill, and it occurs during pregnancy, and as a result of kidney disorders and rare metabolic defects.

Below: *Fatty foods like this can contribute to the development of high blood pressure or hypertension.*

SYMPTOMS

Contrary to popular opinion, headaches are a very rare symptom of high blood pressure, and by far the most common way that high blood pressure is identified is through a routine medical check, either during ante-natal care, life insurance examination or at your family doctor. Symptoms, when they do occur, are the result of damage to other structures (kidney, heart, eyes, brain) and it suggests the problem has been present for many years, so routine checks are important.

WARNING Alternative therapies have a part to play in the management of high blood pressure because the factors causing the problems may be related to lifestyle. Nevertheless it is important to seek medical advice and ensure that your blood pressure is actually being reduced, because even if you *feel*

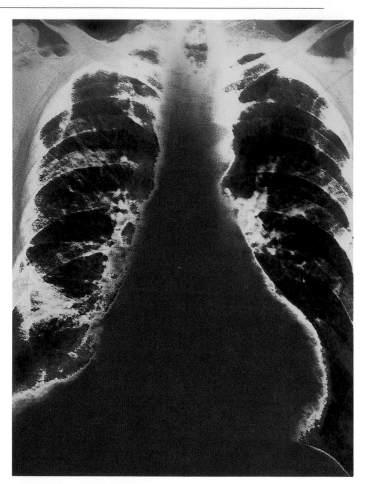

better, it does not mean that your blood pressure has been lowered.

PREVENTION AND SELF-HELP

Essential hypertension is one of those conditions where self-help can be of particular value as so many of the causative factors can be changed.

▪ Establish a wholefood diet, rich in fibre, brown rice and green, leafy vegetables.

Above: *A false-colour chest X-ray of a person suffering from high blood pressure. The heart is enlarged.*

▪ Lose weight by reducing your calorie intake.
▪ Increase your exercise routine gradually.
▪ Practice a regular relaxation and meditation routine. The use of the Yoga "Corpse posture" for ten minutes, twice a day, has been shown to be a very effective way of reducing blood pressure.

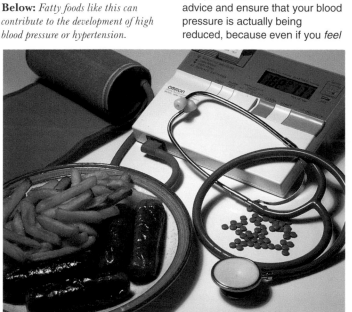

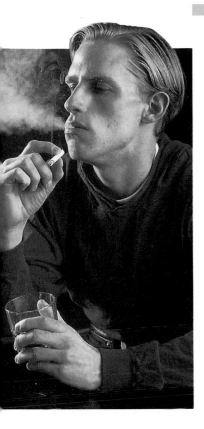

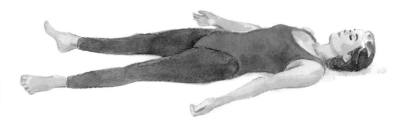

- Stroking, being touched and pursuing an active and guilt-free sex life will help towards a healthy body and mind.
- If you are taking oral contraceptives, make sure you have your blood pressure checked regularly.

NATUROPATHY

Practitioners would advise most of what has been listed in the self-help guide and may add a controlled fast – for 48 hours to begin with, but under guidance this may be extended for longer.

HERBAL MEDICINE

Certain herbal preparations are known to affect blood pressure and restore heart rhythm. They may also be used for improving circulation. They should be taken in the form of teas – one cup a day.
- Lime blossom dilates peripheral vessels and reduces blood pressure.
- Dandelion root acts as a

diuretic reducing fluid in the system and lowering blood pressure.

HOMEOPATHY

The causes leading to high blood pressure will respond to homeopathic treatment, but a whole-person approach needs to be pursued with regular monitoring of blood pressure. *Do not prescribe for yourself* and always see a practitioner.

ACUPUNCTURE

This can have a positive result on blood pressure, probably through its relaxing results, but a full and comprehensive Chinese

Above: *Adopting the Corpse posture for ten minutes twice a day helps to reduce blood pressure. Taking time to ease stress out of the system is an important health measure.*

diagnosis is needed to allow the therapist to determine which points to use. In Chinese terms, high blood pressure occurs when there is an imbalance between the liver and kidney. If the Yang of the liver is excessive, or the Yin of the kidney is too low, corrective measures on each meridian are applied.

BACH REMEDIES

These preparations can be used as a self-help measure, especially for stress and tension but it is important to remember that feeling better is no indication of a change in blood pressure (see Bach remedy chart on page 52 for guidance).

RELAXATION THERAPIES

Hydrotherapy, massage, autogenic training, and reflexology all have a beneficial effect in combating raised blood pressure by reducing levels of anxiety and arousal. For more information about them see the relevant sections in Part Two of this book (pages 36-61).

Above: *Stop smoking and cut down on your alcohol intake. Both habits can lead to hypertension.*

Other relaxation exercises described in the Healthy Living section will also help.
- Reduce your salt intake; avoid adding salt to food.
- Cut down and eventually exclude smoking.
- Stop taking stimulant drinks (coffee – maximum two cups a day).
- Cut down on your sugar intake and cola drinks.
- Eat an onion or a garlic a day. This will not only reduce the blood pressure but reduce your risk of strokes and heart attacks.
- Slow down your pace of life and understand your limitations.
- Cut down on alcohol – a glass of wine a day (one unit of alcohol) is the maximum if you have high blood pressure.

Below: *This high-fibre diet, rich in rice and pulses, green vegetables and fruit, is definitely good for you.*

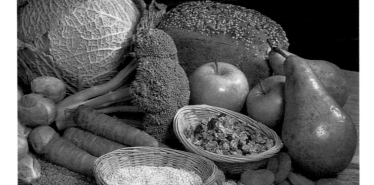

ORTHODOX TREATMENT

Hypertension is a common and occasionally serious condition. It should be taken seriously and treated if necessary. For a young person this may mean many years of medication, and increasingly doctors are looking to alternative therapies to avoid having to prescribe an extended regime of medication which may have short- and long-term side-effects. The first line of orthodox medical treatment involves the diuretic group of drugs which reduce

blood pressure by reducing the fluid status of the body. The second group are the beta-blockers, which reduce the rate of the heart. A third group, the vasodilators, increase the diameter of the blood vessels, thus reducing the blood pressure. All these drugs have minor side-effects; some have serious side effects (such as impotence and tiredness). They all need to be taken regularly and it is important that blood pressure is monitored to ensure the level of therapy is right.

ANGINA

Angina is the name given to the condition resulting from lack of oxygen supply to the heart muscle that causes severe chest pain, usually across the upper part of the body or felt centrally behind the breastbone. The pain comes on suddenly during exercise, very occasionally at rest, and can be viewed as similar to "cramp" in muscles elsewhere. The pain can also be felt in the neck and jaw. It stops once the exercise ceases and rarely lasts for more than a few minutes. Severe angina can be very distressing but is not fatal, and is different from a heart attack when the pain lasts longer, occurs when the patient is at rest and is the result of actual death or infection of muscle tissue. Angina is a symptom of poor circulation to the heart muscle. It must be taken seriously for if untreated it can lead to heart attacks.

CAUSES

Angina occurs either because of blockage to the arteries supplying the heart muscle, the coronary arteria, or because of spasm of these arteries resulting in narrowing of the vessels and thus reduction in blood flow. It can occur as a result of severe anaemia when not enough oxygen is delivered to the heart muscle. It occurs in middle-aged men more than women and is commoner in those who smoke. Blockage of the arteries is the result of "furring up" of the tiny vessels from the deposit of atheroma – a fatty substance related to high cholesterol and other lipid (fatty) substances in the blood. Spasm of the arteries can occur from sudden emotional tension – fear or anger – or as the result of long-term stress, and is thought to be common in those individuals classed as having an "A" type personality. These are competitive, aggressive, ambitious, time-conscious people: "fiery" individuals who very rarely relax and take things easily.

SYMPTOMS

▪ Pain in the chest, jaw, neck and at times radiating down the left arm.
▪ The pain is described as "tight", "heavy", constricting. It is not knife-like or stabbing.

▪ The pain lasts for a few seconds or, at most, five to ten minutes.
▪ Pain occurs during exercise or after a heavy meal and passes with rest.

PREVENTION AND SELF-HELP

It is important that a proper medical examination and diagnosis is made before you embark on a self-help programme, but such a programme can be of great benefit and be complementary to any medical treatment.
▪ If you have an attack, stop all activity and lie down to rest, taking slow, regular, diaphragmatic breaths.
▪ Stop smoking and cut down your alcohol intake.

▪ Reduce weight and go on a wholefood, caffeine-free diet. Avoid heavy meals.
▪ Learn a relaxation exercise and practise it at least once a day.
▪ Avoid anger-inducing situations and try not to lose your temper.
▪ Start a gentle, gradual, regular exercise programme. Avoid sudden intense aerobic exercises (squash, aerobics, competitive sports).
▪ Take up Yoga or T'ai-chi.
▪ Eat an onion or garlic a day to thin the blood of "sticky" platelets.
WARNING Alternative practitioners should not treat angina or other heart problems without the co-operation of a qualified medical practitioner.

Below: *The cause of angina: a blockage in the coronary artery (top right) shows up in this X-ray image.*

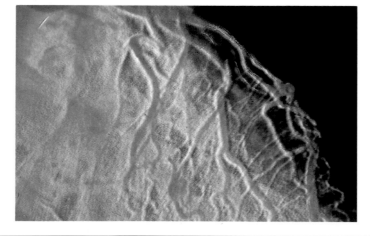

NATUROPATHY

A practitioner will advise a course of weight reduction, diet, exercise and relaxation. Raw juice fasting and hydrotherapy will help generally, but avoid very cold baths or very hot saunas that may put undue stress on the heart.

ACUPUNCTURE

This may help by reducing Yang activity and helping you to achieve relaxation. A course of acupuncture may also help by relieving the pain of an angina attack.

OSTEOPATHY AND CHIROPRACTIC

This may be useful to reduce misalignment of the spine, which is thought will help with blood circulation generally.

HERBAL MEDICINE

A herbalist will aim to help by reducing cholesterol through the use of garlic capsules (one capsule taken twice a day) or an infusion of lime blossom. To make this, add two handfuls of lime blossom to one litre (35 fl. oz.) of hot water and allow it to soak for one hour. Pass the mixture through a sieve and take one cup a day.

ORTHODOX TREATMENT

Proper examination and investigation includes blood tests, X-rays and an electrocardiogram which may be taken throughout the day (24-hour electrocardiogram). Special X-rays of the coronary arteries may be taken to ascertain their state (this is called angiography). Initially you will be given medication to take during an attack and beta-blockers to prevent an attack. If the blockage of the arteries is severe, a balloon catheter may be passed into the coronary arteries and then inflated a few times to clear them. If this is not successful, a coronary artery bypass graft is undertaken and a "new" set of arteries are implanted in the heart muscle – bypassing the blockage. Although this operation may initially be successful, the blockage may recur if the preventative measures outlined above are not undertaken.

ATHEROSCLEROSIS

Arteriosclerosis or hardening of the arteries occurs as part of the natural process of ageing, as the arteries lose their elasticity and become more rigid and "hard". If this is accompanied by the deposit of cholesterol and other fatty substances on the artery walls, it may lead to atherosclerosis which will reduce blood circulation to different parts of the body, leading to angina or strokes. Narrowing of the arteries in the legs leads to cramp on walking or ulcers on the legs and eventually gangrene.

CAUSES

Part of the reason for the development of hardening of the arteries is a "natural" ageing process. Severe atheroma blockage results from abnormal cholesterol and fatty substances being deposited in the blood vessels. This can be an inherited condition but is most commonly caused by a high fatty diet. Both smoking and alcohol consumption increase atheroma

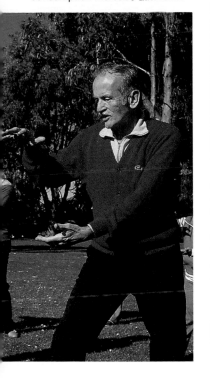

Above: *Learning the slow, rhythmic movements of T'ai-chi is an ideal way to bring relaxation into your life.*

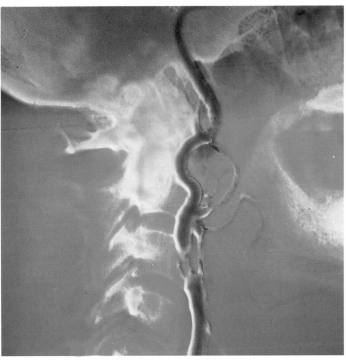

Above: *Potentially fatal, we see here a blockage in the carotid artery caused by the build-up of atheroma.*

development. Cholesterol is a normal and necessary part of the diet essential for the manufacture of hormones and liver salts. Proper medical advice on its reduction must be obtained.

SYMPTOMS

There are usually no symptoms of atherosclerosis per se, except when it impedes circulation and produces the complications described above.

PREVENTION AND SELF-HELP

Much has been described in the section on angina opposite, but it may be important to follow a strict diet to help reduce your cholesterol. You should also take plenty of exercise, cut out smoking, and learn to relax or meditate.

NATUROPATHY

A naturopath would help you find a suitable diet and possibly prescribe some of the herbal remedies known to help with fatty deposits, such as infusions of yarrow and lime flower to improve circulation. It is believed that onions and garlic help to reduce cholesterol levels in the blood, as does a high-fibre diet, so plenty of pulses, beans and bran would be recommended.

Foods to avoid	Healthy option
Butter, animal fats	Vegetable oils
Lard	Margarine
Milk, cream	Semi-skimmed milk, yoghurt (live), soya milk
Meat (especially red)	Fish, pulses, chicken, tofu/soya
High fat cheese	Cottage cheese, curd cheese
Fried food	Grilled and boiled food
White bread, cakes and biscuits	Wholemeal bread, oats
White sugar	Honey or molasses
Salt	Low sodium salt
Too much alcohol	Only one or two glasses a day.
	Add onion and garlic to your diet

ORTHODOX TREATMENT

Doctors would follow the same approach as outlined for angina, but further detailed testing of your lipid profile would indicate whether medication to reduce cholesterol was necessary. If the individual is suffering from intermittent claudication (cramps in the calves after walking or exercise), then X-rays of the blood vessels in the legs would help determine whether surgery is required to replace blocked sections. More recently the daily dosage of half an aspirin tablet a day has been found to cut down the risk of further strokes or heart attacks that may occur as a result of the atherosclerosis blockage to the blood supply to the heart and brain.

HEART FAILURE

This is a serious but treatable consequence of a number of different complaints, some the direct result of heart disease, others as a consequence of disease elsewhere in the body. When the heart "fails", its pumping mechanism is disrupted and two major consequences are the reduction in blood flow through the body and the collection of fluid behind the pump (heart), because the pumping mechanism is deficient. Heart failure will not only affect the body generally, but may have serious consequences because it can affect other organs of the body, such as the kidney, brain, lungs and liver.

CAUSES

There are numerous causes but the main ones include
Hypertension High blood pressure – the heart has to pump harder and eventually fails.
Heart valve disease Narrowing or faulty valve mechanisms will interfere with blood flow.
Anaemia The blood will not produce enough oxygen to the heart muscle for it to work efficiently.
Heart attacks Will destroy muscle tissue.
Atheromatous coronary arteries Will obstruct blood flow to the heart muscle.
Severe lung disease (bronchitis/emphysema) Will eventually reduce blood flow to the heart.
Carditis or cardiomyopathy Diseases of the heart muscles.
Congenital heart disease Usually because of malformation of heart valves or the heart, such as "hole-in-the-heart".

Below: *A hole-in-the-heart is revealed here. The catheter used to produce the image is seen passing through a hole between the two heart ventricles.*

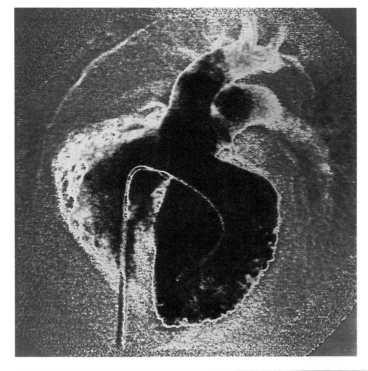

SYMPTOMS

▪ General symptoms of fatigue, breathlessness, especially on exertion.
▪ Rapid palpitations are because the heart beats faster in an attempt to compensate.
▪ Fluid accumulation in the ankles or liver.
▪ Fluid accumulation in the lungs which will produce a cough and lots of phlegm.
▪ Needing to sleep upright to reduce fluid pressure on the lungs.

PREVENTION AND SELF-HELP

It is unwise to proceed without proper medical attention and diagnosis but many of the preventative measures described in the angina and hypertension sections will be of value, especially the following:
▪ Reduce weight – less amount of blood is then required to circulate.
▪ Cut out smoking.
▪ Avoid excessive or unnecessary physical activity.
▪ Sleep in a raised position propped up with pillows.
▪ Keep your feet raised to help with circulation and reduce swelling at the ankles.
▪ Reduce your salt intake and avoid excessive fluid intake.
▪ Avoid experiencing extremes of temperature.
▪ Follow medical advice, including medication, carefully.

Above: *Digitalis drugs are used to treat heart conditions; they are derived from the foxglove plant.*

Additional preparations that are natural diuretics that help eliminate excessive fluid include infusions of yarrow root or chamomile tea. Coffee and tea are also diuretics and will help with eliminating fluid, but they can have a deleterious effect on blood pressure and heart rate and so should be avoided.

NATUROPATHY

Naturopathic treatment of heart failure will limit itself to general lifestyle advice. Most responsible alternative practitioners would not embark on treating heart failure without the co-operation of a trained doctor.

ORTHODOX TREATMENT

An orthodox doctor would undertake a series of investigations to ascertain the right diagnosis. Diuretics would be prescribed to increase the fluid output together with digoxin (a remedy derived from the foxglove plant). Abnormality of the valves may require heart surgery. High blood pressure will be treated with medication and any anaemia corrected. In severe cases, oxygen will be given to improve the quantity of oxygen being delivered to the heart. Carditis and cardiomyopathy are difficult to treat, and in very severe cases a heart transplant operation may be recommended. In all cases of heart failure, once the problem has been corrected or controlled, it is important during convalescence to address lifestyle issues that may prevent further damage to and deterioration of the heart.

VARICOSE VEINS

These are deformities or varicosities of the veins of the lower limbs resulting in distended and tortuous enlargements of the veins under the surface of the skin. They can occur on one leg only, but usually affect both. They are more common in women, especially over the age of fifty. Similar varicosities occur on other parts of the body (i.e. the anus, where they are called haemorrhoids.)

CAUSES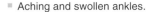

This is usually due to a chronic obstruction of venous blood flow as a result of pressure, which can be caused by pregnancy or chronic constipation. It is thought that chronic straining on defecation raises the pressure in the abdomen and restricts the flow of blood, especially in people who are obese or who take insufficient exercise. A low-fibre diet will reduce the bulk in the faeces and this may lead to constipation. The increased pressure eventually deforms or ruptures small valves in the veins that are present to prevent pooling of blood in the legs because of the pull of gravity during the course of it being pumped back to the heart. If blood does pool in the veins of the legs, varicosities appear.

SYMPTOMS

■ Unsightly swellings along the course of the veins together with discoloration.

■ Aching and swollen ankles.
■ Fatigue when walking.
■ Ulcers may appear around the ankles if the skin becomes very thin or injured.

PREVENTION AND SELF-HELP

■ Avoid constipation and eat a high fibre diet.
■ Avoid standing still for long periods of time.
■ If your job entails standing, keep compressing your calf muscles (i.e. by moving your feet up and down for five minutes every hour).
■ Lie down with your ankles raised above chest level for at least half-an-hour to aid circulation.
■ Take plenty of exercise and avoid being overweight.
■ Avoid tight undergarments or garters.

Below: *Constipation and straining to defecate are bad for the blood flow in your legs. Switch to a high-fibre diet and try to avoid being overweight.*

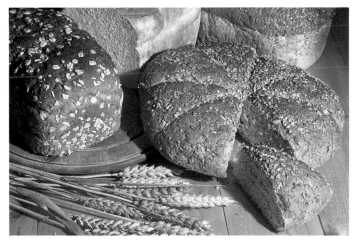

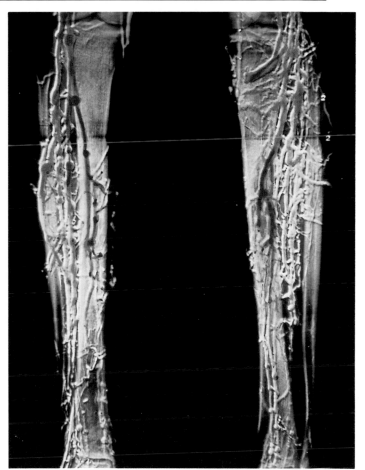

Above: *This is a venogram – an X-ray image that reveals the condition of the body's veins. This patient suffers from varicose veins, which show up as knots of colour in the legs.*

NATUROPATHY

A good wholefood diet, plenty of exercise and hot and cold baths to aid blood circulation will be suggested. Some extra Vitamin E and Vitamin C may be recommended.

HOMEOPATHY

Homeopathic remedies are aimed at improving circulation. Once the veins are distended it is unlikely that any medicines can help.
Pulsatilla: If veins appear during pregnancy. Take one tablet, 6x, three times a day.
Carbo vegetabilis: For general improvement of circulation. Take one tablet, 6x, twice a day for three days; repeat for three months.

ORTHODOX TREATMENT

The most helpful advice will be the provision of support stockings which help prevent the veins from distending and blood from pooling. Small varicosities can be injected and destroyed. Most moderate cases of varicose veins will be treated with a "stripping" operation which surgically removes the whole vein. Blood then circulates in other veins, which, however, unfortunately may then become distended themselves in years to come.

BRUISING

DESCRIPTION

This occurs when a blood vessel ruptures either because of an injury or blow. Spontaneous bruising is due to a fragile blood vessel, as in the elderly, or because of a blood-clotting abnormality, such as haemophilia.

PREVENTION AND SELF-HELP

- Follow the orthodox advice given below (RICE).
- If bruising is extensive, seek medical help.
- Avoid "raw steak" treatment; it is not beneficial.
- Take painkillers if necessary.
- Make sure your diet is adequate – especially green vegetables. They contain substances that promote blood clotting.

ALTERNATIVE THERAPIES

Homeopathy *Arnica* ointment or oil rubbed on the area is recommended. *Arnica* 6x will help with pain and swelling – take one tablet every two hours; same dose for children.
Herbal medicine Apply a cold compress with a few drops of comfrey oil added or soaked in an infusion. Lavender or comfrey ointment will also help.

Naturopathy will recommend cold water treatment and if the bruising is spontaneous will suggest added Vitamin K obtained by eating live yoghurt and green vegetables daily.

ORTHODOX TREATMENT

Bruising following an injury or blow may need to be examined to exclude underlying ligament or bone fracture. The first aid treatment centres on RICE: Rest, Ice, Compression, Elevation (see entry on Joint Strains in Complementary First Aid section, page 210).

CHAPPING

DESCRIPTION

Flaking of skin around the face, hands and ears due to cold weather, or frequent washing and a consequent reaction to soap and water.

PREVENTION AND SELF-HELP

- Many preparations, such as lotions and salves, are available from chemists.
- Pay attention to your diet and take regular exercise.

Below: *Green vegetables contain substances that promote blood clotting. If you bruise easily, make sure that you eat plenty of them.*

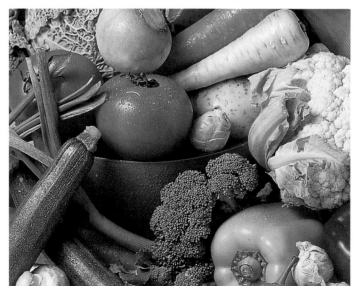

- Regular skin care of areas exposed to wind and cold is sensible.
- Avoid nicotine and caffeine.

ALTERNATIVE THERAPIES

Aromatherapy Add benzoin or patchouli oil to some carrier oil (20 drops to 100ml, 3½ fl. oz.) and apply to the skin.
Hydrotherapy Toughening the skin with alternate hot and cold showers, saunas and mud-packs is recommended.

ORTHODOX TREATMENT

Covering exposed skin with cream or ointments (such as vaseline), lanolin or lip salve – all obtainable from chemists – is the normal recommendation.

CHILBLAINS

DESCRIPTION

Discoloration of the the skin (reddish-blue) or areas of skin (toes, feet, hands, ears, shins) which cause pain, itchiness, swelling and can sometimes become inflamed. Caused by cold weather and poor circulation.

PREVENTION AND SELF-HELP

- Precautions should be taken against the cold by wearing warm clothing.
- Regular exercise improves circulation.

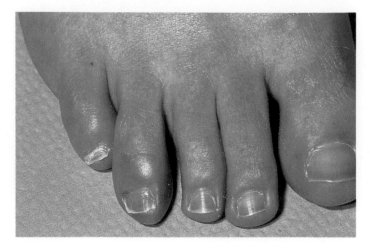

Above: *Chilblains such as this usually occur in cold weather, and often afflict people with poor circulation who suffer from cold hands and feet.*

- Warm your bedroom and use hot water bottles to warm the bed.
- Make sure you enjoy a good diet.
- Deep breathing exercise routines practised daily help to warm the body's extremities.
- Folklore suggests a paste made with equal quantities of glycerine, flour, and honey mixed with the white of an egg, placed on the chilblain and covered up with a bandage for 24 hours will alleviate the pain.

ALTERNATIVE THERAPIES

Naturopathy Recommendations include bathing extremities in warm water, then cold water alternately (three minutes in warm and one minute in cold repeated five times), adding some gentle massage with lavender oil.
Homeopathy *Tamus* ointment rubbed in gently can help.
Rhus tox. 6x – one tablet four times a day for a week.

CHILDREN: One tablet twice a day for a week.

Carbo veg. ointment or tablets 6x – three times a day.
Aromatherapy Massage with lavender or lemon oil can relieve the pain of chilblains.

ORTHODOX TREATMENT

A commonsense approach to cold weather (warm underwear,

socks, gloves to be worn at night if necessary) is encouraged. Pain-killing drugs and occasionally medication to improve circulation may be prescribed.

HYPOTENSION

DESCRIPTION

This is the medical term for low blood pressure. It is not recognized as an entity by many Western doctors other than in acute situations, e.g. shock. However, some physicians see it as a problem as much as hypertension or raised blood pressure.

PREVENTION AND SELF-HELP

This is a common diagnosis for the causation of fainting, dizziness and fatigue because blood flow to the head is reduced.
- General measures include regular exercise, breathing and relaxation routines including autogenic training.

ALTERNATIVE THERAPIES

This is not an uncommon diagnosis in some alternative therapies.
Acupuncture An acupuncturist will see this as the result of

Below: Herbalists tackle hypotension by recommending that you take regular infusions of broom and rosemary.

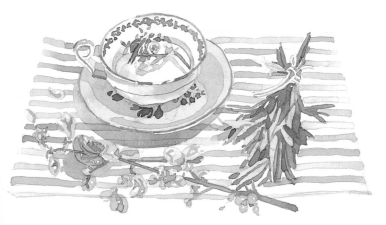

having low Chi and treat accordingly.
Naturopathy Naturopaths normally prescribe exercise and cold water treatment, and suggest excluding stimulants like tea, coffee and alcohol from the diet.
Herbal medicine Infusions of broom and rosemary are recommended by herbalists to regulate the heart and raise low blood pressure.

ORTHODOX TREATMENT

Where this is recognized as a genuine medical condition, tablets are given to raise the blood pressure, or if caused by the over-treatment of hypertension, the level of drugs is correspondingly reduced.

PHLEBITIS

DESCRIPTION

Superficial inflammation of or clotting (thrombophlebitis) in a vein in the legs, usually associated with varicose veins or after pregnancy. Sometimes caused by the pill or immobility following an operation. It gives rise to pain, swelling, tenderness, sometimes change in colour – "white leg".

PREVENTION AND SELF-HELP

- Avoid tight bandages, stockings and underwear.

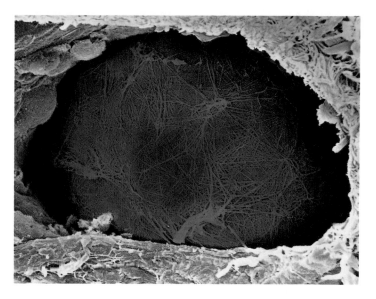

- Avoid chronic constipation. Straining to defecate puts pressure on the veins in the legs.
- If you have developed phlebitis, take the weight off your legs, elevate them, and avoid any direct pressure on the vein until you seek medical advice.

ALTERNATIVE THERAPIES

Medical attention should be sought initially to ensure a potentially serious condition is excluded. Local treatment is best left to the guidance of a qualified nurse or doctor but a hydrotherapy approach may be suggested if there is no breakage of skin.

ORTHODOX TREATMENT

If the phlebitis is superficial, local treatment with dressings, pain relief, and antibiotics will be prescribed, usually in association with rest and elevation of the limb. If the phlebitis is associated with a clot (thrombosis) then drugs to thin the blood (anti-coagulants) will be prescribed.

THROMBOSIS

DESCRIPTION

This is a term used to denote the formation of a clot in the vascular system. Venous thrombosis is the most common (see above). Arterial thrombosis is much more

Above: *This remarkable image shows a thrombus, or clot, blocking one of the small blood vessels in the lung. It is here magnified 1,750 times.*

serious and can lead to heart attack (coronary thrombosis), or strokes, or gangrene if it affects the blood supply to the limbs.

PREVENTION AND SELF-HELP

- Acute thrombosis is a medical emergency.
- Call for an ambulance or your own doctor.
- Make the patient comfortable and warm.
- Avoid giving the patient any drinks or food.
- Do not move unless you have expert help.

ALTERNATIVE THERAPIES

No alternative therapy should be tried until orthodox medical opinion is sought. Long-term help and prevention of further thrombosis will be helped by advice on a good diet, exercise and reduction in tobacco and caffeine consumption. Obesity will be clearly discouraged.

ORTHODOX TREATMENT

A thrombosis will require immediate treatment with anti-coagulants prescribed to thin the blood, and occasionally surgery will be undertaken to by-pass the blockage.

ALLERGIES

A number of ailments including hay fever, eczema, asthma, migraine, skin rashes and chronic catarrh can be caused by an allergic reaction of the body. This reaction can be due to something you eat, such as a chemical additive to the food, or a reaction to the environment e.g. pollen or air pollution. The terms allergy, intolerance and sensitivity are often used as if they mean the same thing, but allergy entails a specific reaction of the immune system when the substance causing the allergy – known as an allergen – stimulates the body to produce an abnormal response – the allergic response which results in the release not only of antibodies known as IgE, but also histamine and other chemical substances which cause the reactions commonly observed. Sensitivity and intolerance do not involve an allergic reaction and may be related to the quality of the food itself, i.e. you cannot take spicy curries or you have a psychological inability to eat snails. There is no doubt that allergic diseases are becoming more widespread and some alternative practitioners believe that this is the result of the practice of mass immunization in childhood, the use of antibiotics, the presence of chemical additives in food, together with an increase in air pollution. Although usually minor in their effects, severe allergic reactions can cause both long-term illness and death. So large is the increase in allergic disease that a new branch of specialist expertise has developed within the ranks of alternative practitioners – clinical ecology.

CAUSES

Almost any substance can trigger off an allergic reaction, but the cause is usually a small protein or vegetable complex. Chemical additives may be actually toxic rather than stimulating an allergic reaction, i.e. smoking is harmful to the body but does not cause allergies. Common allergenic substances include milk protein and other dairy products, eggs, wheat (gluten), nuts, fish (especially shell fish), chocolate, red wine. Additives such as tartrazine and benzoate (found in sweet colourings and cake preservatives) may lead to problems in small children. Environmental allergens include the pollen of grass, flowers and trees, house dust, animal fur, feathers etc.

SYMPTOMS

- Red wheals and itchy rash – a condition known as urticaria, or nettle rash.
- Red running eyes, itchy nose and mouth.
- Swelling of the lips, eyes or other parts of the body.
- Cough, dry with wheezy chest breathing, asthma.
- Diarrhoea, swelling of stomach, occasional constipation.
- Eczema – weeping, raw rash on hands and legs.
- Headaches, migraine.
- Feeling tired and depression (not always caused by allergies).
- Hyperactivity and insomnia especially in children.

Below: *Oil seed rape is an attractive and useful crop, but the plant's pollen is a major cause of hay fever.*

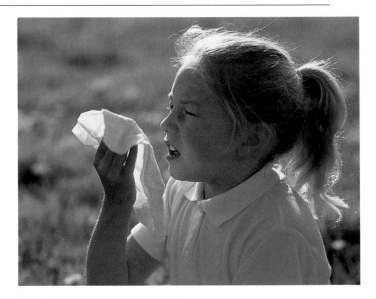

Above: *Sneezing is one of the typical allergic responses to the presence of allergens (such as pollen and dust) floating about in the air.*

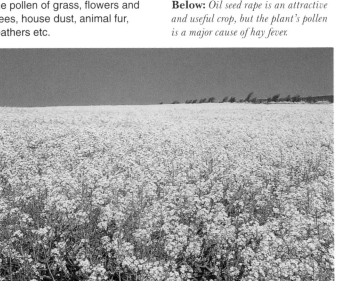

PREVENTION AND SELF-HELP

Keep a diary. The most effective way of identifying the substance to which you are allergic is by checking when you get the symptoms and trying to identify what brings them on, e.g. a headache after wine, wheezing when doing housework, diarrhoea after a particular food.
- Avoid some of the commonly known allergens as a first step. Omit all dairy products, or eggs, or wheat-based products. These are probably the commonest cause of allergies and it is well worth checking if one of these is the cause, especially in the case of young children.
- Avoid the allergen once identified. Check food labels carefully and choose household goods with care, especially soap powders and detergents (biological detergents are well known to produce allergic skin reactions). Vacuum frequently to remove all dusty pockets, especially in the bedroom and the bed itself (you can get special mattresses and pillow covers that may help here). If you suffer from hay fever or plant allergies, you may need to check your garden.
- Breast feeding babies in the first six months of their lives will help protect them from cow-milk protein allergies and will strengthen their immune systems.

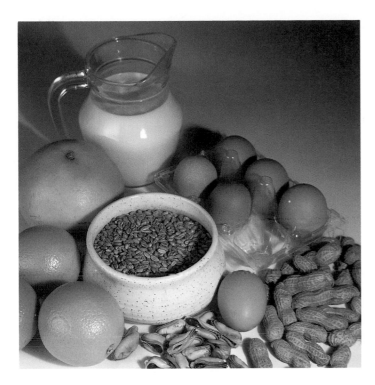

■ General measures to improve the way you deal with stress, anxiety and tension are particularly important if you have long term allergic problems.
■ Be wary of expensive "alternative allergy clinics" as they are not always reliable, and the treatment can be expensive and not helpful. Check with a medical practitioner who is sympathetic to alternative medicine generally.

ALTERNATIVE METHODS FOR IDENTIFYING ALLERGIES

Recently medical doctors interested in alternative medicine have developed new techniques for identifying specific allergies. These include blood tests, electrical testing of certain

Above: *Some common allergenic foods are shown here. Approach them with caution if you are a sufferer.*

responses to the allergies, and kinesiology (muscle testing with a series of potential allergens, see page 48). Practitioners claim to be able to identify much more accurately the course of the allergic symptoms, but these tests are thought to be unreliable by orthodox doctors.

HOMEOPATHY

A homeopath will take an extensive history and be particularly interested in your immunization record and dietary history. A number of specific remedies will be prescribed depending on your symptom picture. First aid homeopathic

remedies for allergic symptoms include:
Apis mel. 6x, one tablet every two hours for three days.
Sulphuricum 6x, one tablet every two hours for three days.

CHILDREN: The same dose can be used for children over two years of age.

NATUROPATHY

Naturopaths would supervise, with great care, your diet and nutrition history and may start with a controlled fast, introducing specific foods one by one. They may add specific mineral and vitamin supplements, especially B complex, to correct any imbalances and strengthen the immune system. Pollen tablets (one daily) for several months before the hay fever season can be helpful.

ACUPUNCTURE

The use of Chinese herbs together with needling has proved very effective in a number of allergic states (e.g. eczema,

asthma). The practitioner would measure through pulses and tongue diagnosis your normal level of Chi (energy) and identify ways of strengthening this, usually with needles placed along the lung meridian.

HERBAL MEDICINE

Practitioners would primarily concentrate on identifying and eliminating the allergen, but would also look towards specific herbal preparations to counteract the symptoms.

OTHER THERAPIES

Other helpful alternative approaches would be those aimed at strengthening general resistance and decreasing stress (relaxation, meditation and hypnotherapy may be of particular use here). Bach remedies, particularly clematis, mimulus and impatiens are all useful to try to control symptoms.

Below: *Hypnotherapy remains a rather controversial therapy, but it may help in certain circumstances.*

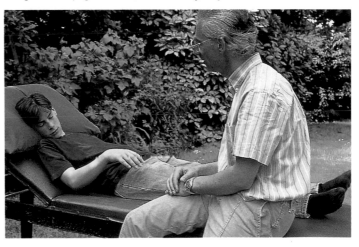

ORTHODOX TREATMENT

Elimination diets and allergy testing form part of the medical approach, but most doctors will rely on medication to suppress and control symptoms, such as anti-histamines, cortisone cream and sprays. Desensitizing injections to the allergen are rarely undertaken now, although at one time it was very popular. A new drug (sodium cromoglycate) has been used to prevent the development of allergic reaction and can be of some use in the treatment of hay fever and asthma.

WARNING

It has become very popular to attribute many mental and nervous conditions to allergies, a diagnosis which has become known as "total allergy syndrome". This condition is not recognized by orthodox medicine. It is important not to ignore psychological issues that may be relevant to your life, and instead blame all the negative experiences and distress on "allergies".

CANDIDA

Candida is a yeast infection which occurs naturally in the human body and generally causes no problems. In certain circumstances the infection can spread throughout the body and produce a number of non-specific and troublesome problems. Although orthodox medicine recognizes candida as a cause of infection (thrush in the vagina, and oral thrush in the mouth), it has not accepted the view that generalized candida, as described by alternative practitioners, actually exists, so that controversy surrounds what treatment is appropriate for this condition.

CAUSES

Vaginal thrush Candida is normally found in the vagina and rarely gives rise to problems. Women taking oral contraceptives, or antibiotics, pregnant women and those with diabetes are more prone to developing widespread infection.
Oral thrush Oral thrush is often transmitted to an infant by the mother transferring the infection onto the bottle or directly by touch. This condition is rarely seen in adults.
Generalized candida Will certainly occur when people have low immunity, e.g. as a result of AIDS or long-term cortisone treatment. Long-term use of antibiotics will allow the fungus to grow in the alimentary tract, as antibiotics kill the bacteria in the body that naturally keep candida under control.
Skin thrush This will occur in moist folds (under the breast, between the buttocks and in the groin). Candida likes to grow in warm moist areas of the body, and can be transmitted by

Below: *The rash on this child's buttocks is caused by candida, which favours moist areas of the body.*

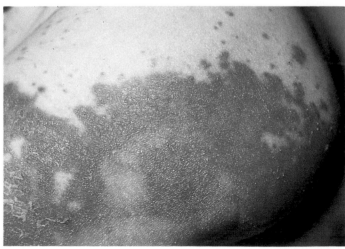

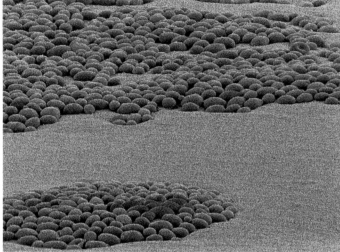

physical contact. Sexual intercourse is a common way in which thrush is transmitted.

SYMPTOMS

These will depend on the site of infection but it will usually produce red inflamed areas with a white cheesy discharge or nappy rash. The skin becomes inflamed and itchy. Those people who frequently have their hands in water may develop chronic thrush of the nail beds. Severe infection in immune-deficient people may

Above: *Not a modern sculpture, but colonies of the* Candida albicans *fungus magnified 1,650 times.*

result in serious chest infections, e.g. pneumonia and occasional severe diarrhoea. Candida as understood by alternative practitioners has a number of symptoms which include:
▪ Tiredness, fatigue, mood swings, depression, loss of control.
▪ Diarrhoea and constipation, feelings of bloatedness.
▪ Bulky stools which fail to flush down the toilet.
▪ Irregular and heavy periods. These symptoms may be accompanied by the local symptoms described above.

PREVENTION AND SELF-HELP

There are a number of precautions that women can take to avoid the onset of vaginal thrush:
▪ Avoid wearing tights, nylon pants or tight trousers.
▪ Use sanitary pads not tampons.
▪ Avoid perfumed soaps and deodorants.
▪ Avoid disinfectants in the bath.

▪ Avoid strong detergents, particularly biological ones.
▪ Avoid using soap on the vulva if there is irritation.
▪ Avoid antibiotic use, if possible.
▪ Avoid bad toilet habits and wash your hands after use.
▪ Pay attention to your diet.
▪ Reduce your intake of sugar and starchy foods.
▪ Eating live yoghurt will help restore intestinal flora.
▪ Apply live yoghurt on a pad to the vagina.
▪ Avoid intercourse when you have infection.
▪ Reduce stress levels and develop a relaxation programme.
▪ If you have to take antibiotics, make sure you take acidophilus capsules at the same time.

NATUROPATHY

This is probably one of the commonest diagnoses made by naturopaths and they have a systematic and clear approach to its treatment. It will involve:
Dietary changes
▪ Cut out sugar and starchy products.

Below: *Naturopaths will suggest that you cut out mould-containing foods, such as mushrooms, to combat candida.*

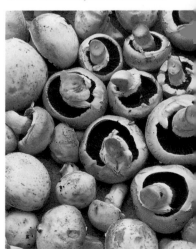

- Stop all alcohol.
- Avoid mould-containing foods (cheese, mushrooms).
- Eat no fruits for the first two weeks.
- Introduce lactobacillus acidophilus and bifidobacillus (one tablet twice a day). These are the useful bacteria killed off by antibiotics which control the spread of candida.
- Vitamin B tablets (Biotin) will also help to control candida.

Killing the yeast
Some practitioners will prescribe natural anti-fungoides e.g. tea-tree oil, garlic, chlorophyll (aloe-vera juice).

Detoxify the body
You may be advised to undertake colonic lavage (irrigation, enema), but this should be done only after advice and in the knowledge that most doctors consider it to be useless. Other ways of cleansing the body may be by the ingestion of vegetable juices (celery, water-cress, cucumber).

Rebuilding the immune system
Useful mineral supplements include zinc, selenium, manganese, Vitamin B complex (pantothenic acid, pyridoxine, nicotinic acid). Amino acids: cysteine, tyrosine, glutamine. Herbs: echinacea, red clover, yellow dock. It is possible to obtain a multi-vitamin/mineral complex tablet that contains all these ingredients. Take one a day.

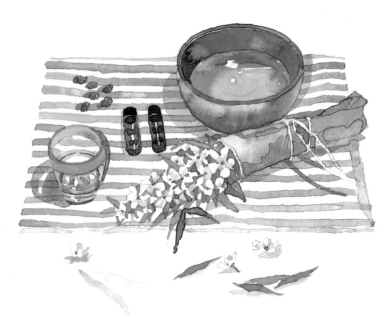

Below: *These foods are rich in Vitamin B (the jar contains molasses). By eating them you increase your chances of controlling troublesome candida infections.*

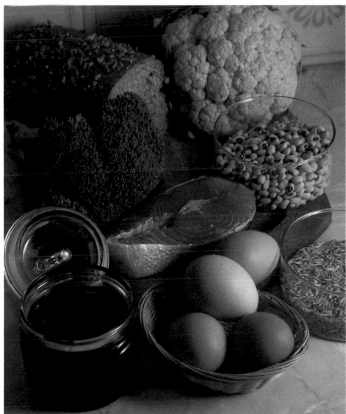

Stress reduction exercise
Relaxation, meditation and breathing exercises are all considered valuable.

HERBAL MEDICINE

Tinctures of myrth or marigold can be used as a mouthwash. A vaginal wash can be made by dissolving one tablespoon of salt in 600ml (one pint) of water.

AROMATHERAPY

There are various ways in which essential oils may be useful. For instance, put three drops of tea tree oil and one drop of myrrh in a glass of water and use it as mouthwash. (Not appropriate for children).

Dampen the end of a tampon, add three drops of tea tree oil to it and insert in the vagina for up to two hours.

Regular sitz baths (three to four drops) or conventional baths (six to eight drops) with the above oils can relieve the symptoms of vaginal thrush.

Above: *A mouthwash made from three drops of tea tree essential oil and one drop of myrrh in a glass of water can help deal with oral thrush.*

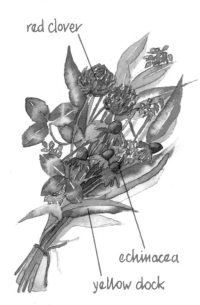

red clover

echinacea

yellow dock

Above: *Echinacea, red clover and yellow dock are all herbs that help rebuild the immune system.*

ORTHODOX TREATMENT
General hygiene measures will be advised, but the mainstay of treatment will be anti-fungal treatments. Swabs will be taken to identify the fungus and treatments may involve pessaries, creams and tablets. The infection can also cause inflammation of the skin, so some of the creams may contain a cortisone to help reduce the itchiness. Treatment may need to be taken for at least two weeks, but more recent medication can be effective in three days and some single dose medications are also available. Recurrent vaginal infection is common if a sexual partner has the infection, and both people may need to be treated.

M.E.
(MYALGIC ENCEPHALOMYELITIS)

Although not a new disease, this condition has become much more common in the last ten years, and it is estimated that more than 500,000 people suffer with it in America and Western Europe alone. It is now more accurately known as post-viral fatigue syndrome, but was known as the Royal Free disease in the 1960s, and has also been called Iceland disease, and epidemic neuromyasthenia. Because many of the symptoms are non-specific, such as tiredness, depression, and aches and pains, it has often been labelled as "hysteria" or "all in the mind", and many sufferers have had great difficulty in getting acceptance that they are actually ill. They have often received hostility and unsympathetic treatment from their doctors. Like all new diagnoses, it is certainly true that not all who suffer from tiredness have M.E. Nevertheless, it is now increasingly accepted that this condition does exist and does have a physical basis as part of its cause, which is usually a viral illness of some sort. Typically, the condition will start within a few days or weeks of a "flu-like" illness, possibly glandular fever, followed by weeks, months and sometimes years of debilitating fatigue where patients are unable to undertake everyday activities without experiencing a recurrence of their symptoms. It can affect old and young alike but typically is a condition of young adults. It has been diagnosed in people as young as ten years old, however. Laboratory tests have, as yet, not proved reliable enough to make an accurate diagnosis possible but testing of the immune system can be helpful in indicating problems. Recently, brain scans of the hypothalamus (the relay station in the brain) have suggested there is a malfunction due to diminished blood circulation.

CAUSES

Many viruses have been . identified that trigger off the problem, including Epstein-Barr (glandular fever), the Cocksackie viruses (attacking muscles) and entero-viruses (which live in the gut).
▪ People who get M.E. do have a pattern of stressful job or personal relationships – they can be over-ambitious and suffering from emotional or psychological stress. This factor resulted in the condition being nicknamed "yuppie-flu".
▪ Disturbance of the immune system and poor nutrition have also been thought to predispose to its development.

SYMPTOMS

They can be wide-ranging but tend to have a typical pattern:
▪ Fatigue, extreme tiredness, depression, poor concentration, loss of memory, disturbed sleep pattern including hypersomnia (sleeping too much).
▪ Aches, pains and tenderness of muscles including those in the arms, legs and shoulders. These can be made worse by the slightest exertion.
▪ Itchy, prickly skin with rashes.
▪ Swollen tender glands, sore throat and headaches.
▪ Sickness, dizziness, abdominal discomfort, loss of appetite, diarrhoea and constipation.
▪ Fever and shivery fits.
▪ Difficulty passing urine, strong smelling urine.
▪ Aversion from certain foods.
▪ Ringing in the ears and visual disturbances.

Below: *Extreme tiredness and depression are characteristic symptoms of M.E. It often strikes young adult "over-achievers".*

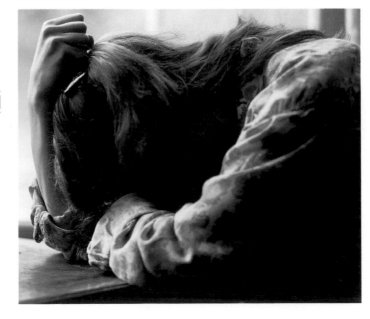

▪ Bloating and bowel disturbance.

PREVENTION AND SELF-HELP

▪ If you do catch a 'flu-like illness, ensure you take plenty of rest and do not return to work before you are fully fit.
▪ Review your lifestyle. Are you in the "characteristic band" of M.E. sufferers: over-ambitious, not taking enough relaxation, keeping late nights? If so, take adequate steps to improve your stress management routine.
▪ Try to seek the advice of a sympathetic doctor and obtain an accurate diagnosis. Remember, not all tiredness and depression is M.E.
▪ Seek the help of an alternative practitioner, if you fail to get medical support.
▪ Join your national M.E. society which produces pamphlets, newsletters and maintains support groups.
▪ If you have been diagnosed as having M.E., rest is very important; do not push yourself.
▪ Avoid undue stresses, both personal and dietary.
▪ Cut down on alcohol and stop smoking.
▪ Keep a diary of your symptoms with a numerical grade against each one ranging from 0 to 10 (0 = no symptoms, 10 = very bad). This will allow you to chart the course of your condition.
▪ Learn about a healthy lifestyle and the diet you need to take. Professional advice may be needed but wholefood and fresh juices are important for everyone.
▪ Many supplements are suggested by alternative practitioners to boost the immune system. Avoid taking them unless you are monitoring your symptoms or are under supervision.

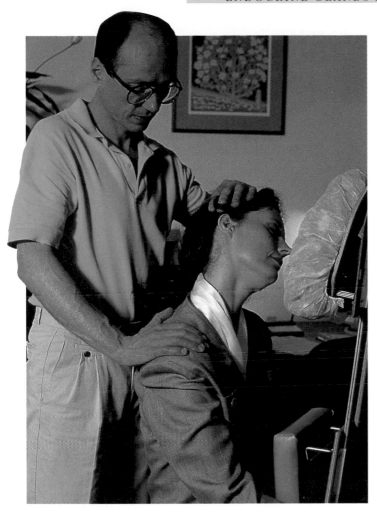

traditional Chinese approach, which focuses on "balancing energies" in the body can be of particular help. Treatment may be required weekly and can last up to six months. However, good results are obtained in a proportion of cases.

HOMEOPATHY

Homeopathic remedies do not usually help if taken in a self-help symptomatic way. An experienced homeopath may, however, be able to pin-point a specific symptom pattern and prescribe remedies specific to you. This can have excellent results.

HERBAL MEDICINE

A herbalist will aim to relieve some of the symptoms by aiding a calmer sleep, helping to relax the body and addressing any nutritional imbalances. *Ginkgo biloba* (the maidenhair tree) helps the blood circulation to the brain.

Below: *Hydrotherapy does have something to offer M.E. sufferers. This woman is finding deep and restorative relaxation in a pool.*

HYDROTHERAPY

Other alternative therapies that can help include hydrotherapy, especially the taking of a cold bath every day. Recent reports have shown how this simple and easy routine can help to boost the immune system and assist the individual recover his or her ability to overcome the low-level viral infection. Hot baths and saunas can also be tried as a soothing and relaxing way of reducing muscle pains.

Below: *M.E. may be related to the blood supply to the brain; the herb ginkgo is thought to improve this.*

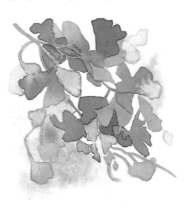

■ Take up meditation to allow you to get through your most difficult times.
■ Consider counselling if you feel your lifestyle may have precipitated this attack. M.E. can be a time when you reassess your career and personal goals, and learn more about your strengths and limitations.
■ Almost everyone recovers from M.E., even if it takes a year or two.

NATUROPATHY

All the above self-help measures will be emphasized together with a more detailed analysis of your diet. If candida is suspected, which can often develop in

Above: *A busy office worker receives an on-site massage. Simple routines like this can improve your lifestyle and reduce stress levels.*

someone with M.E., treatment will be offered specifically for this problem. Vitamin, mineral and enzyme supplements will be suggested. The most common are Vitamin B complex, zinc and magnesium, one tablet daily of each. Breathing retraining plus bodywork to normalize tense muscles which will "burn" energy uselessly are also recommended.

ACUPUNCTURE

Because M.E. affects energy levels so dramatically, the

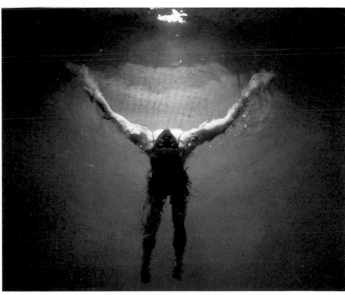

ORTHODOX TREATMENT

Initially hostile, certainly sceptical, the medical profession has slowly come round to recognize this condition as a distinct clinical entity. Much research is being undertaken, but as yet few positive results have occurred. Treatment is usually symptomatic: rest, vitamins, counselling and, more recently, a small dose of anti-depressant at night has been found to help greatly, partly because of its anti-depressant effect but also because it aids the chemical transmission in brain cells which seem to cause many of the mental symptoms associated with M.E.

STRESS DISORDERS

In the section on stress and lifestyle (pages 14-17) we looked at the causes of stress and the symptoms and signs that are the early warning signals of stress. Such early warning signals, if not properly attended to, will turn into stress disorders or diseases in their own right. Many of these disorders and diseases are dealt with separately in other sections of the book. The following table is a guide to how unrelieved stress can affect the muscles and organs of your body in a variety of unwelcome ways.

Muscle groups affected	Symptoms produced by tension
Voluntary muscles	
Eye	Eye strain
Back of neck	Tension headache
Back	Back pain
Involuntary muscles	
Around arteries	High blood pressure
Around bowel	Irritable bowel syndrome (constipation/diarrhoea)
Around stomach	Passing wind

TYPES OF DISORDER

In the early work on psychosomatic disease, various commonly occurring conditions were grouped together and described as the classic seven. These were *migraine, high blood pressure, irritable bowel syndrome, peptic ulcer* (gastric and duodenal), *asthma, rheumatoid arthritis* and *ulcerative colitis*. It is now accepted that although stress may play a part in the causation of these conditions, other factors, including pollution, allergies, diet and hereditary factors all have a causative role.

Recently a bacteria (heliobatier) has been identified as a major factor in the causation of duodenal ulcers.
As well as the classic seven, stress will undoubtedly make many chronic conditions not normally associated with stress worse. People who suffer with *arthritis* or *diabetes* or even *epilepsy* will often comment that their condition is a lot worse when they are under stress. More recently the connection between

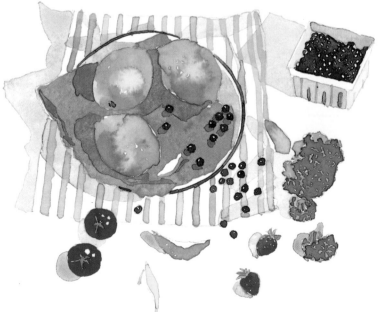

Below: *These fruits and vegetables are rich sources of Vitamin C, which may help boost the body's immune system.*

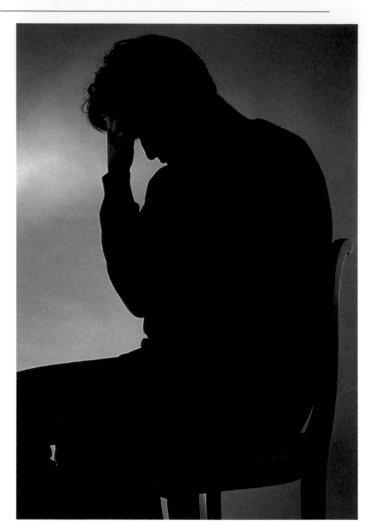

Above: *"Stressed out." One of the most common symptoms associated with stress is listlessness and lack of energy.*

stress and *cancer* has been extensively investigated. Although it is as yet not proven that stress itself will cause cancer, many women with breast cancer who have been successfully treated with surgery and radiotherapy, often associate the recurrence of their cancer with a stressful period of their life (husband dying, family turmoil, or financial hardship).
At the other end of seriousness, many of the *minor recurrent infections* to which we are prone (sore throat, coughs and colds) have been shown to occur more frequently when we are under

stress, and *allergic conditions* (hay fever, skin rashes, diarrhoea) are also more prone to deteriorate when the general level of well-being is reduced. More recently, the condition known as M.E., or chronic fatigue syndrome, has been linked to a preceding period of chronic stress, followed by a viral infection which stays in the body and produces the post-viral myalgia (muscle pain) so commonly found in this condition.

CAUSES

It is now generally accepted that one way that stress results in increased infection or disease is through the immune system, which is that part of our bodily processes that protects us against attack from outside forces. The immune system consists of several specialized cells – the lymphocytes and their products, antibodies. Lymphocytes are of two basic types: "B" cells which are connected with bone-marrow and will attack invading bacteria, and "T" cells which are linked with the thymus gland in the chest and are responsible for dealing with parasites, viruses and fungi, as well as cancer cells. Another important cell of the immune system are the macrophage or scavenger cells which circulate in the blood acting as policemen against invading bacteria.

In addition to these cells, the lymph glands, liver and other specialized areas of the body will produce special proteins called immunoproteins or antibodies. There are five types of antibodies, IgG, IgA, IgE etc., all with special functions, e.g. IgA is found in the secretions of the nose and throat and is there to protect us from invading viruses and bacteria. IgA is our first line of defence.

STRESS AND THE IMMUNE SYSTEM

In recent years exciting discoveries have been made as to how the brain and mental functioning can affect the immune system. Messages from the brain to the immune system are carried not by the nervous system but by chemical messengers. This new science has developed its own name, psycho-neuro-immunology. Thus science has been able to identify how unhappiness, or stress of some kind, can "get into the cell" and affect its capacity to deal with infection. Even more exciting discoveries are being made that suggest that we are able to improve our immune system through a series of physical, mental and visualization exercises. In addition, dietary factors such as Vitamin A, zinc and Vitamin C appear to be important in ensuring that our immune system is operating effectively. Regular exercise is known to improve the "T" cells count, as is meditation.

AN ALTERNATIVE VIEW OF STRESS

An alternative view of stress and one shared by many complementary therapies is that of impairment of "energy" or the vital force. This often links in well with the most common complaint of people suffering from stress, that of having no energy. Energy is the central concept in traditional Chinese medicine, homeopathy, spiritual healing, and cranial osteopathy. These therapies aim to improve energy flow and through a combination of diet, exercise, meditation and breathing exercises endeavour to

Below: *Regular exercise improves the body's "T" cell count, which is vital for combating infections.*

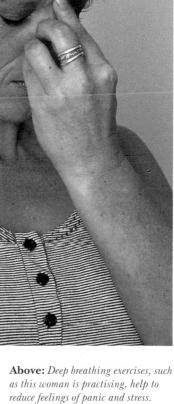

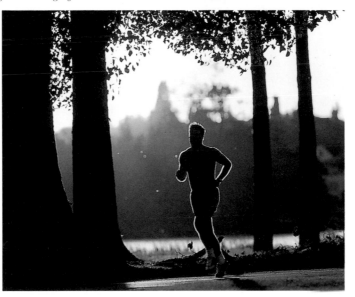

Above: *Deep breathing exercises, such as this woman is practising, help to reduce feelings of panic and stress.*

restore a natural balance. This "Eastern" view of stress is finally booming more acceptable among Western scientists.

PREVENTION AND SELF-HELP

Self-help measures to prevent stress and to boost energy levels are described in the section on healthy lifestyle (pages 14-31). Successful management of stress is one of the most positive contributions that you can make towards achieving a healthier lifestyle.

ORTHODOX TREATMENT

Orthodox medicine has mostly relied on the prescribing of tranquillizers, anti-depressants and sleeping tablets, together with counselling. There has, however, been an increasing reluctance to use these drugs recently, due to the possibility of damaging side effects and the danger of possible addiction if they are taken for a prolonged period.

DIABETES

Diabetes is a condition whereby the body is unable properly to process the metabolism of sugar. This results in an increased sugar level in the body which produces many of the symptoms described. The condition also affects the micro-circulation of the blood in the small blood vessels giving rise to complications affecting other organ systems, including the kidneys, eyes, nervous system, the heart and the brain. Sugar is metabolized by the hormone insulin which is produced by the pancreas, a small glandular tissue behind the stomach. Two forms of diabetes occur: that affecting young people which is due to pancreas malfunction and very little production of insulin, and adult-onset diabetes which is often associated with poor diet and obesity. This latter is the result of over-use of the pancreas which produces insufficient insulin to process the excess carbohydrate intake. Diabetes is a life-long condition and as yet no cure has been found, although the symptoms can be controlled by diet and medication.

CAUSES

Both forms of diabetes have a hereditary tendency. If both parents have diabetes, the risk of a child developing it is greatly increased. Late-onset diabetes is definitely brought about by a high sugar/starch diet, but this is not the case in the early onset type where sufferers are usually thin. Certain drugs can precipitate diabetes – steroids and some of the oral contraceptives are examples of these.

SYMPTOMS

▪ Thirst and the passing of copious dilute urine is the most common early sign due to the high level of sugar in the blood.
▪ Loss of weight in early onset type is common together with tiredness.
▪ Skin infections (thrush) and itchiness of penis and vagina are common.
▪ Disturbance in menstruation is common.
▪ Pins and needles in advanced cases, together with leg ulcers.
▪ Difficulty with focusing and disturbance of vision.
Complications of long-term diabetes include more serious problems including blindness, loss of mobility, failed circulation and gangrene, thickening of the arteries and an increased risk of heart-attacks, kidney infections and eventually kidney failure.

PREVENTION AND SELF-HELP

▪ A wholefood diet incorporating *complex* carbohydrates (oats, wholewheat) and the avoidance of all refined sugar products not only prevents but helps to eradicate late-onset diabetes.
▪ Keep to the recommended bodyweight for your height and age.

Below: *A young diabetic girl is taught how to give herself insulin injections to maintain her blood sugar balance.*

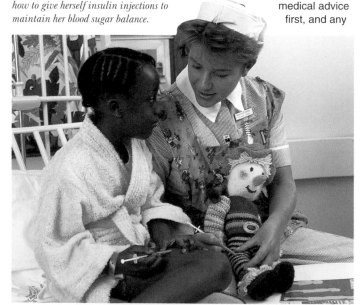

▪ If you have diabetes, keep it under good control and have regular check-ups.
▪ Hypoglycaemia attacks (when the sugar level in the blood is too low because of over-treatment) can be controlled by proper monitoring and having barley sugar sweets available to eat when the warning signs of an attack appear.
▪ Regular exercise will help as well as special Yoga breathing exercises.
WARNING All responsible alternative practitioners will suggest you obtain medical advice first, and any therapies they suggest are complementary to adequate medical treatment. No alternative therapy can cure diabetes, although control can be improved and medication reduced if you follow good naturopathic advice regarding diet. Herbal medicines are sometimes given to improve the working of the pancreas. Goats rue and gentian are thought to stimulate insulin. Garlic taken raw or in the form of garlic capsules, will reduce the effects of fatty imbalance and protect the heart. Daily porridge (oats) will help stabilize sugar levels and a high-fibre diet may reduce the need for medication. All are worth trying under medical supervision.

ACUPUNCTURE

Needling will form a small part of traditional Chinese treatment where the emphasis will be on diet and herbs. In general, a wholefood diet with plenty of fresh fruit and green vegetables is recommended.

HOMEOPATHY

This has little to offer the management of diabetes but may help with individual or constitutional symptoms *Phosphorus* is often prescribed to reduce symptoms. Take one tablet 6x, twice a day.

ORTHODOX TREATMENT

Orthodox doctors will undertake a series of base line tests, then prescribe a specific diet (both early and late-onset diabetes respond well). You may be asked to see a dietician and be given a list of foods to avoid and those to eat. Joining your national diabetic association will allow you access to many useful guide books. If you need insulin injections, you will be taught how to administer these yourself and how regularly to test your blood and urine to help you monitor your own blood sugar levels. Regular checks are important to pick up early complications. Oral medication (tablets) will be prescribed for most cases of adult-onset diabetes and these are perfectly safe to take regularly.

GLANDULAR FEVER

Glandular fever (or infectious mononucleosis) is a common condition among the young. It is often caught through kissing or mouth to mouth contact. Usually there is an incubation period of up to seven weeks before the symptoms develop. It is not a serious condition but it can take a long time to recover from, and is one of the predisposing viral infections that can cause M.E. or post-viral fatigue syndrome.

CAUSES

A small virus particle called Epstein-Barr Virus (EBV) is the culprit, although other viruses have been identified. Viruses are very small particles that live inside cells and chiefly infect the white cells of the body. Thus glandular fever can occur when there is low immunity following a stressful period, for instance, pre- or post-exams. The virus is transmitted through saliva and is not particularly infectious, so that isolation of the patient is not necessary.

SYMPTOMS

▪ Sore throat, difficulty in swallowing, and bad breath.
▪ Swollen lymph glands in the neck and also in the armpits and groin.
▪ Fever and a rash (faint pink that may resemble German measles).

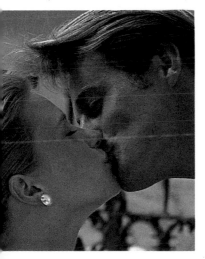

Above: *Glandular fever or "the kissing disease" can be contracted through mouth-to-mouth contact.*

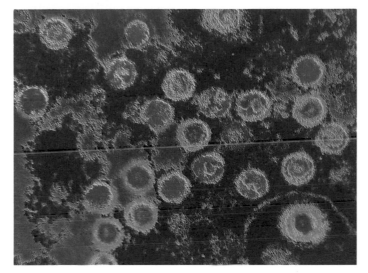

Above: *The tiny cause of glandular fever: the Epstein-Barr virus is here seen magnified 47,000 times.*

▪ Headache which can be severe.
▪ Jaundice, abdominal upsets and pain (swollen spleen or glands).
▪ Occasional damage to nerves.
▪ Tiredness, fatigue and depression.

PREVENTION AND SELF-HELP

▪ No vaccine exists and other than avoiding close physical contact with a patient, it is difficult to prevent yourself catching glandular fever. Attention to your stress levels and avoiding getting run-down will ensure your immunity is sufficiently high.
▪ Once you have been diagnosed as having the illness, take plenty of rest, especially in the dark.
▪ Fluids may be difficult to swallow but you can try using a wide-bore straw.

NATUROPATHY

Infusions of yarrow and elderflower will reduce sweating and temperature. Other recommendations are:
▪ A light but nourishing diet (such as soup) together with plentiful fruit juices.
▪ A 36-hour water-only fast.
▪ Extra vitamins B and C may help to boost your defences; take one tablet twice a day. (For children take half the adult dose).
▪ Gargling with honey and lemon will ease the discomfort in the throat.
▪ Rosemary tea will be refreshing.
▪ Natural antibiotics such as garlic may be tried.
▪ Echinacea – take one tablet twice a day.

HOMEOPATHY

Remedies to help with the symptoms include:
Belladonna, 6x – one tablet every three hours for six doses if the symptoms include a temperature, sweating and swollen glands. *Baryta carbonica* is good if you have red inflamed tonsils. (Dosage as above).
A homeopathic remedy derived from infected tissue (Glandular Fever Nosode) is available and it is claimed to protect other members of the family.

BIOCHEMIC TISSUE SALTS

Ferr. phos. – one tablet taken hourly for two days may reduce the severity of the attack as does *Kali mur.*
It is important to take great care during the convalescence period, especially if the liver has been involved, and a good rule of thumb is to double the days of infection before you return to full-time work, and to avoid alcohol for six months after infection.

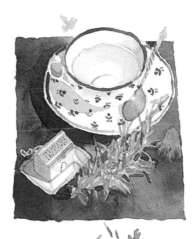

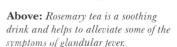

Above: *Rosemary tea is a soothing drink and helps to alleviate some of the symptoms of glandular fever.*

ORTHODOX TREATMENT

At times difficult to differentiate from an ordinary sore throat, the diagnosis of glandular fever is easily made by a simple blood test. Treatment is usually symptomatic – antibiotics do not help and indeed may make the condition worse. Very occasionally in severe cases cortisone has to be used to reduce the severe swelling of the tonsils that can otherwise cause obstruction to breathing. If the liver is involved, then a close follow-up is maintained to ensure recovery is complete.

CIRRHOSIS

DESCRIPTION

A condition of the liver almost always caused by excessive and prolonged alcohol intake which leads to liver failure, jaundice and metabolic disturbances (oedema, tremors, skin changes, infertility). It is characterized by damage to the liver cells and the accumulation of scar tissue in the liver itself.

PREVENTION AND SELF-HELP

Stop consuming
- Alcohol.
- Red meat.
- Fatty foods.
- Coffee.

Do
- Drink plenty of liquids.
- Increase Vitamin B supplements.
- Reduce weight.
- Reduce your intake of salt-containing foods.

ALTERNATIVE THERAPIES

A strict dietary routine is suggested with a large supplementation of vitamins and minerals.
Acupuncture can help with overcoming addiction, as well as restoring liver function.
Homeopathy will help with symptoms (nausea, pain) and may restore metabolic function. Specific recommendations include *Nux vomica* 6x – one tablet twice a week for one month.

ORTHODOX TREATMENT

Strict cessation of alcohol is essential to stop the progress of disease. Vitamin supplementation and treatment of complications will help symptoms. Occasionally a liver transplant is required.

Below: *In the case of alcohol, the road of excess can lead to cirrhosis. Alternative therapies need to address the mental problems of addiction.*

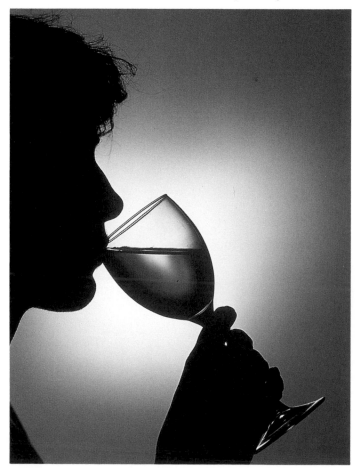

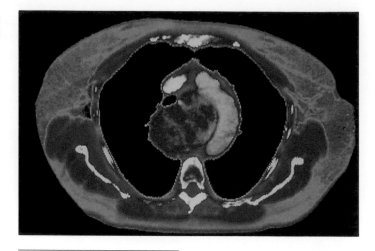

Above: *CT scanning enables doctors to see transverse "slices" through a body. The red circle in the middle is a goitre affecting the thyroid gland.*

GOITRE

DESCRIPTION

A swelling of the thyroid gland, sometimes hereditary, sometimes due to diet (insufficient iodine), and sometimes associated with endocrine disturbance and malignant growths.

PREVENTION AND SELF-HELP

- An adequate diet is important, but it is unusual with iodized salt so commonly available for this now to be a problem caused by dietary deficiency.
- Seek medical help.
- Reduce stress.
- Practise relaxation and meditation.

ALTERNATIVE THERAPIES

Herbal medicine If due to lack of iodine, seaweed such as bladderwrack will be prescribed.
Homeopathy Precise medical diagnosis is important but some homeopaths may use *Fucus vesiculosis* or *Iodium* 30.
Acupuncture can help to restore the thyroid to normal functioning.

ORTHODOX TREATMENT

Treatment will depend on diagnosis following thyroid scans. Usually goitres are treated with thyroid supplements. Sometimes they occur at times of stress or physiological demand. Sometimes surgery is required.

GOUT

DESCRIPTION

A condition affecting the joints which is caused by a high level of uric acid in the blood depositing crystals in the lining of the joints, especially those of the big toe, foot, ankle, knee and hand. Crystals can also be deposited in the kidneys which leads to kidney stones.

PREVENTION AND SELF-HELP

- Cold green clay poultices (mix with water and apply as paste on the affected joint for the acute phase) help relieve pain.
- Rest and elevation of legs will help.
- Painkillers obviously help with the pain.
- Follow a prescribed diet regime.
- Try this infusion: put four slices of lemon and a pinch of lavender in a glass of warm water. Allow to infuse and take four times a day.
- Seek medical advice.

ALTERNATIVE THERAPIES

Although commonly thought to be related to a rich diet (alcohol, sweetmeats, meat and oysters), it is unusual for this to be the case.
Naturopaths would recommend fasting (48-hour fluid only) with a

vegetarian diet and reduction in sugar, coffee and alcohol. Cold compresses are used to reduce pain.

Homeopathy *Arnica, Colchicum* and *Belladonna* 6x are all used, one tablet two hourly for 12 doses.

Acupuncture will help reduce pain and inflammation and also improve kidney function.

ORTHODOX TREATMENT

Gout is a well-recognized form of arthritis, sometimes caused by diuretics or accompanying blood disorders, but mostly as a result of an enzyme deficiency. The acute phase is treated with painkillers and anti-inflammatory drugs. Then a drug to reduce the uric acid level of the blood is prescribed.

JAUNDICE

DESCRIPTION

A condition where excess production of bile or a blockage of the bile duct causes yellowing of the eyes, skin and nails because of an accumulation of a pigment in the blood. It is associated with liver disorders (hepatitis), gall stones, and blood disorders. It can be a side effect of drugs.

PREVENTION AND SELF-HELP

See Hepatitis (pages 122-123).
▪ Generally a healthy, vegetarian diet with minimal fat, meat,

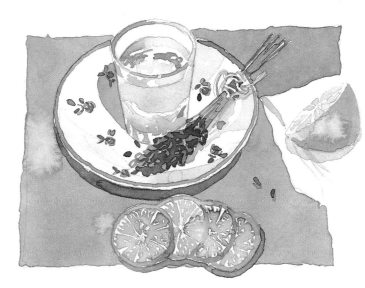

Above: *One way to ward off painful attacks of gout is regularly to take infusions of lavender and slices of lemon in a glass of warm water.*

alcohol and sugar will reduce the risk of gall stones.
▪ Jaundice should be immediately reported to a medical practitioner so that appropriate diagnosis is made.

ALTERNATIVE THERAPIES

Unless a definitive diagnosis of hepatitis is made, most alternative practitioners will suggest medical treatment. Diet therapy is of great help and recommendations may include fasting, juice-only diets and vitamin supplements.
Herbal treatments to boost liver function include balmony, dandelion and golden seal. They should be taken under expert guidance.

Below: *If you suffer from gout, this is what is causing the pain: crystals of uric acid that collect in joints.*

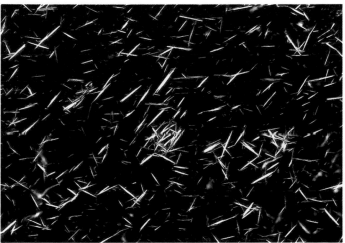

ORTHODOX TREATMENT

Diagnosis will be arrived at through examination and blood tests, a liver scan and occasionally liver biopsy. Treatment will depend on the cause. It may require hospitalization and special medication.

OVERACTIVE AND UNDERACTIVE THYROID

DESCRIPTION

Both these conditions may be accompanied by a goitre, but need not necessarily be so. Symptoms may include:
▪ Overactive: loss of weight, bulging eyes, anxiety, diarrhoea, fast heart beat.
▪ Underactive: weight gain, fatigue, depression, constipation, change in facial features.

PREVENTION AND SELF-HELP

▪ Check family history – there is an hereditary link.
▪ Keep a record of symptoms.
▪ Ask for regular blood tests to check thyroid levels.
▪ Keep on medication if prescribed.

▪ Tackle excess stress in your life – try to relax and take more exercise.

ALTERNATIVE THERAPIES

As for Goitre, but most alternative practitioners will refer to an orthodox medical doctor.

ORTHODOX TREATMENT

This condition is much more common in women than men and can be linked to menstrual irregularity. Diagnosis is undertaken with blood tests and treatment includes thyroid tablets if underactive, or radio iodine to damp the thyroid down if overactive.

PANCREATITIS

DESCRIPTION

A severe condition of the pancreas (the gland behind the stomach that secretes digestive enzymes and hormones) that causes acute pain, peritonitis and pancreatic failure leading to digestive disturbance and diabetes.

PREVENTION AND SELF-HELP

Prevention is the golden rule in this condition.
▪ Avoid excess dietary intake of alcohol, caffeine and red meat.

ALTERNATIVE THERAPIES

Acupuncture may help with pain and digestive disturbance.
Naturopaths would prescribe a strict diet regime including periods of fasting, and enzyme, vitamin and mineral supplements.

ORTHODOX TREATMENT

Normally treated with bed-rest and fluids. The condition is usually associated with high alcohol intake, which is forbidden. Pancreatic enzymes and insulin may be required to treat the chronic state.

CONSTIPATION

Constipation is one of the commonest complaints encountered in Western cultures. It can usually be easily corrected through dietary means and is more often than not caused by poor diet. Bowel movements vary in frequency and number between individuals, so it is important to clarify that constipation exists in the first place. Some people have a motion once every three days, others three times a day. More important than the frequency is the consistency of the faeces which, if they are hard and difficult to evacuate, can cause painful anal problems including haemorrhoids. Chronic constipation has been identified as one of the factors causing several common Western diseases including appendicitis, hiatus hernia, varicose veins, haemorrhoids and gall-bladder disease.

CAUSES

Most commonly it is due to low fibre content in the diet, which reduces the bulk of the motion so making it more difficult to evacuate. Fibre is made up of a number of different constituents in the diet which are not absorbed by the processes of digestion. Vegetables, fruits and wholewheat bread are good natural sources of fibre. If the diet is low in fibre, food takes longer to pass through the intestines and can release harmful toxins in the

Below: Putting a new slant on the term "regular" exercise, it is clear that a regime of fitness and exercise also helps maintain daily bowel mobility.

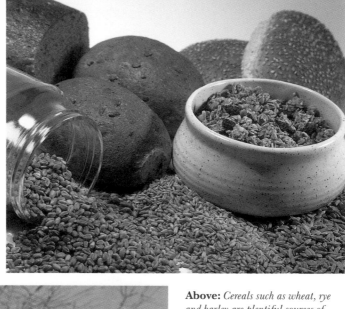

Above: Cereals such as wheat, rye and barley are plentiful sources of carbohydrates and dietary fibre. Fibre is essential to a healthy bowel.

colon which are thought to predispose to cancer of the bowel. Other possible causes of constipation are:

▪ Long illnesses associated with fever producing dehydration can cause constipation, because of the dehydration which affects the consistency of the faeces.

▪ Bowel condition can be a factor; commonly irritable bowel syndrome, where the movement and muscular contractions of the bowel are disturbed, is to blame.

▪ Elderly people can lose mobility of the bowels.

▪ Lack of exercise is another cause.

▪ Anatomical obstruction from defective bowel formation in children and cancer in adults.

▪ Certain thyroid disorders.

▪ Pregnancy, due to the changing levels of hormones and their effect on bowel mobility.

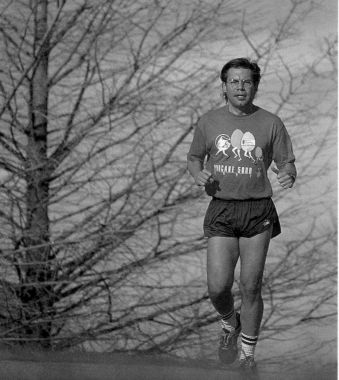

SYMPTOMS

▪ Difficult or infrequent motions.
▪ Hard pellet-like motions.
▪ Occasionally diarrhoea may signal long-standing constipation, especially in the elderly.
▪ Painful cracked fissures around the anus.
▪ Bleeding from the anus, which must be investigated medically.
▪ Stress, anxiety and tension.

PREVENTION AND SELF-HELP

▪ Take extra fluids and eat plenty of vegetables and stewed fruits.
▪ Change to wholemeal bread and try a tablespoon of bran sprinkled over your cereal.
▪ If your baby is constipated, increase the sugar content of each feed – one teaspoon (5ml) will help to loosen the motions.
▪ Hot baths will relax muscles and aid defecation.
▪ Use one of the natural laxatives (see recommendations below).
▪ Increase your daily exercise.
▪ Visit your doctor if none of these measures helps, if you have lost weight, if there is blood in the motion, if you experience abdominal pain or have a discharge from the anus.
▪ Occasionally a glycerine suppository will help both adults and babies to pass extremely hard faeces.
▪ Do not rely on laxatives long term as they may mask underlying problems and make the bowel lazy.
▪ Ensure your diet has a high fibre content which is acceptable to you.

NATUROPATHY

Naturopaths will focus on the diet and recommend a natural laxative

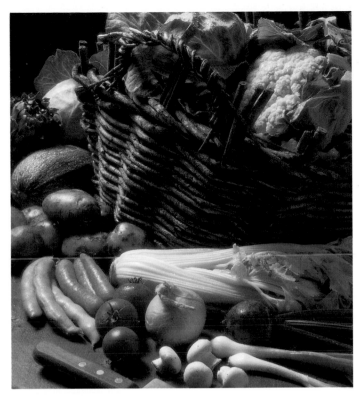

Above: *Vegetables are another valuable source of dietary fibre. They are particularly beneficial if eaten raw.*

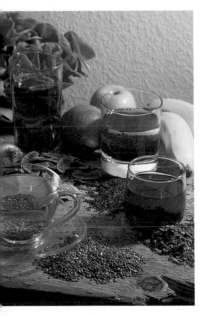

Above: *Remedies from nature's medicine chest: senna, linseed and psyllium are effective laxatives.*

regularly. To make a laxative drink, soak a half to one teaspoon of cascara bark in a cup of hot water for 60 minutes. Strain and drink the liquid at night.

With all these natural products you may experience wind and griping abdominal pain. It is important not to proceed with the remedy if this happens, and to rely instead on the bulk laxatives that do not stimulate bowel activity but help to increase the amount of motion, and act as "softage" rather than roughage.

HERBAL MEDICINE

Herbal mixtures that help bowel mobility include chamomile, fennel and hops. All may be taken as teas or infusions.

HOMEOPATHY

Homeopaths would want to take a detailed medical history and prescribe according to the

Below: *Gentle massage of the large intestine point on the sole of the foot can ease constipation.*

such as linseed. Some will suggest a colonic lavage in severe cases, but it is unwise to rely on this as a regular method of dealing with constipation. Naturopaths may recommend a raw food diet for a few days and if you find this difficult to digest you may ask to rely on stewed fruit/prunes, apples. Other sources of fibre include peas, beans, dried fruits, brown rice, jacket potatoes.

Natural laxatives (not to be used for children)

Crush up to six senna pods in a cup of boiling water and add a small piece of liquorice root. Allow the mixture to stand and cool for ten minutes. Strain and drink at night. This may take up to six or eight hours to work.

■ Linseed is a gentler laxative providing bulk in the gut. Soak a tablespoon of seeds in 150ml (¼ pint) of cold water overnight and add them to your breakfast cereal.

■ Cascara is a strong bowel laxative and should not be taken

symptom picture. Remedies often used include *Bryonia, Lycopodium, Alumina* and *Plumbum metallicum.*

MASSAGE AND REFLEXOLOGY

Both can be of great help in reducing tension and pain in the lower bowel, thus aiding bowel movements. Pressing on the large intestine point on the sole of the foot and gently massaging that area for ten minutes is a self-help measure that often is effective.

ACUPUNCTURE

Constipation is classified as the result of too much dryness or heat in the system or because of weakness of Chi, especially Yang. Attention would be paid to diet but needling along the large intestine meridian may help the large intestine regain its function.

ORTHODOX TREATMENT

For simple constipation general dietary advice and mild laxatives would be suggested. However, all chronic problems would be examined rectally and if necessary with a flexible tube viewing instrument to exclude serious problems. An X-ray of the bowel (barium enema) might be undertaken to check there is no underlying blockage further up the bowel.

DIARRHOEA

Diarrhoea is an extremely common symptom involving the passage of frequent runny and watery stools. It can be acute, lasting three to seven days, or part of a long-standing problem usually related to digestive and intestinal problems. Its seriousness as a symptom is minor if it is of short duration, but because of the very heavy loss of fluids and body salts associated with it, it can lead to dehydration and weakness fairly quickly. It is of particular importance in young babies, who cannot afford to lose too much fluid and can get dehydrated very quickly, especially if they are not taking fluids or are vomiting what they have been given. In acute cases, one can afford to take a symptomatic approach initially, but diarrhoea lasting more than three days should be investigated and treated by a medical practitioner, although many naturopaths are also able to manage the problem.

CAUSES

These can be many and various:
Acute diarrhoea is usually the result of an intolerance to certain foods or an infection, ranging from mild non-specific viral conditions (gippy tummy) to dysentery, typhoid and amoebic dysentery. Young babies are very prone to infective diarrhoea and epidemics can spread very rapidly through nurseries or hospitals. Cholera is still the most serious cause of diarrhoea, but is not found in the Western world. However, careful attention should be paid if diarrhoea occurs after visits to foreign countries. Acute diarrhoea can also be the presentation of allergic response to food, especially shellfish.
Chronic diarrhoea Again, this may be caused by dietary problems, the most common being irritable bowel syndrome (see pages 112-113) which is often associated with bouts of constipation. Cystic fibrosis is a condition where lack of appropriate enzymes produces fatty unformed stools, and there is a noticeable lack of growth in children. Gluten sensitivity or coeliac disease, when the lining of the small intestine is damaged by the protein gluten, is another common cause of intermittent diarrhoea. Inflammation of the lower bowel (colitis and diverticulitis), common in the elderly, will produce diarrhoea, as does the malabsorption syndrome (bulky, foul-smelling stools which fail to flush). Lastly, more serious causes include polyps in the bowel, and cancer.

SYMPTOMS

- Loose, frequent, at times "explosive" bowel motions.
- Abdominal pain which can be intermittent (gripes).
- Vomiting and nausea.

Below: *This is a* Salmonella *bacterium, the cause of food poisoning. Infection of the gastro-intestinal tract leads to severe diarrhoea and nausea.*

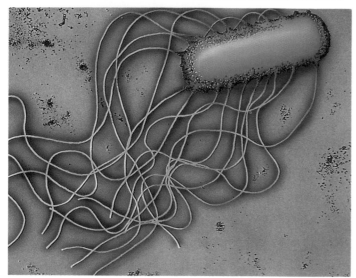

- Slimy mucus or blood in the motions (report to your doctor).
- Dehydration – dry tongue, sunken eyes, loss of elasticity of skin.
- Tiredness and fatigue from lack of minerals.

PREVENTION AND SELF-HELP

- Cleanliness in the kitchen, especially in making sure babies' feeding bottles are properly sterilized, is very important.
- If you are visiting a very hot climate, you may wish to drink only bottled water.
- Avoid shellfish if at all possible.
- Make sure you drink lots of fluid to replace fluid loss. Initially this can be only water, but if diarrhoea persists you may have to replace the lost "salts". To one part of water add one tablespoon of sugar and one teaspoon of salt, and drink the mixture. Another very helpful drink is rice water. Boil some rice but use double the quantity of water that you normally would. Once the rice has boiled, strain off the water, let it

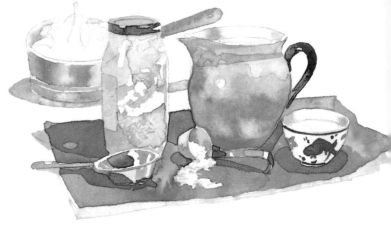

Above: *Rice water is not the world's tastiest drink, but it can alleviate the symptoms of diarrhoea.*

cool and drink one cup every hour, or more if the diarrhoea is very runny.
- Bed-rest will help, and certainly avoid eating any solid food.
- A hot water bottle will help ease a gripey abdominal pain.
- Peppermint tea will also ease the abdominal discomfort.
- Avoid "stopping mixtures" like kaolin as they will only prevent the infective material from being passed and so allow it to be absorbed in the body.
- Avoid self-medication with sulphonamides or other antibiotics, unless you are unable to seek medical advice.
- Chronic diarrhoea will require precise diagnosis so as to give specific treatment. You will need to seek medical advice, but if the problem is an allergy or irritable bowel syndrome, keeping a diary and increasing the fibre content of your diet may be very helpful.
- Do not eat solid food during an attack; stick to liquids.

NATUROPATHY

Treatment will allow the diarrhoea to be eliminated (the body getting rid of toxins) and not prescribe suppressants. Boiled rice, live yoghurt, acidophilus capsules and bifidobacteria powders may be prescribed. In chronic diarrhoea a detailed history will reveal any allergies and candida may be found to be the cause (see pages 98-99). Once the diarrhoea attack is over, a gradual return to solid foods will be advised. Raw foods should be avoided but eating boiled carrots and bananas will be recommended.

CHILDREN: A bout of diarrhoea may make babies and children sensitive to the milk protein for a few weeks afterwards, and it is best to feed them soya milk for a while.

HOMEOPATHY

For acute infectious diarrhoea, *Arsenicum album* or *Carbo veg.* can be taken, 6x potency, one tablet ever half hour for six hours. If associated with temperature

Below: *Aromatherapists recommend a "tea" made of peppermint, cypress and sandalwood oils in warm water.*

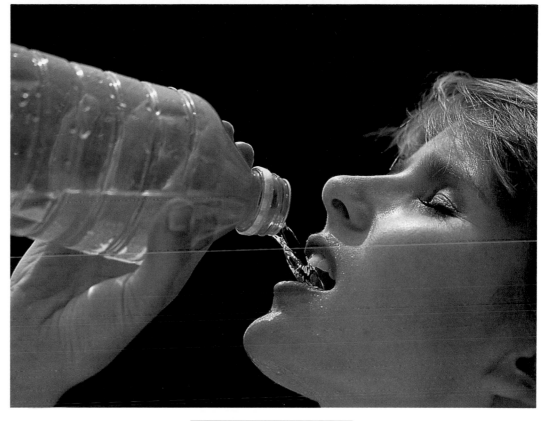

and cold sweats, *Veratrum album* is recommended (dosage as above).

CHILDREN: Children and babies can take the same dosage, but as a tincture rather than as tablets.

HERBAL MEDICINE

Herbalists advise taking a garlic oil capsule three times a day. An infusion of agrimony, plantain or geranium will also help to reduce the diarrhoea.

CHILDREN: Should take half the adult dose prescribed above.

AROMATHERAPY

One drop of peppermint oil on a sugar lump every two hours will help in young children. Alternatively, make a tea mixture (one drop of peppermint, cypress and sandalwood oils in a cup of warm water). Chamomile tea can also help in this condition. If the diarrhoea is very severe, many practitioners will suggest hot baths with three drops of rosemary or lemonbalm oils to soothe both the pain and the soreness around the anus.

Above: *A bout of diarrhoea is very dehydrating – make sure you drink lots of water to make up fluid loss.*

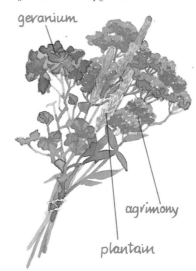

geranium

agrimony

plantain

Above: *An herbal remedy suggests an infusion of agrimony, plantain or rosemary to soothe the aching gut*

ORTHODOX TREATMENT

General advice for acute diarrhoea includes avoiding all solid foods and remaining on clear fluids. Packets of "replacement salts" are now available that can be diluted and given to children to counteract the loss of these important minerals. It is no longer usual to prescribe

antibiotics, as they rarely are effective. Nevertheless, in severe cases, they may be necessary, as may an intravenous fluid replacement if the individual is very dehydrated or has severe vomiting. Chronic diarrhoea will be investigated and the treatment will depend on the cause.

IRRITABLE BOWEL SYNDROME

This is one of the most common causes of gastro-intestinal disorders. It is said to be the cause of over 50 percent of abdominal symptoms and is one of the most frequent referrals to hospital from general practice doctors. It produces recurrent pain, abdominal swelling, diarrhoea and constipation. IBS is one of the classic psychosomatic diseases (disorders caused by psychological factors) and has attracted much attention from complementary therapists. It has also been labelled mucous colitis, spastic colon, functional bowel disorder, nervous diarrhoea, chronic catarrhal colitis, vegetative neurosis.

CAUSES

The different names given to this syndrome suggest that the causes are not specifically known. The colon is the name given to the large bowel in which the end products of digestion are deposited. The colon, like other parts of the bowel, is encircled by a thin ring of muscles that contract and relax – a motion called peristalsis. This movement is normally regular and causes a wave of contractions to pass down the bowel, thus pushing the faeces towards the rectum and anus. The condition is caused by the irregular and defective muscle contraction of the large bowel. The muscles of the bowel are supplied by a parasympathetic nerve supply (i.e. one controlling the involuntary activities of the body's organs), and it is thought that emotional tension and anxiety leads to inappropriate and ineffective muscle contractions.

Other causes are thought to be dietary factors which cause defective contraction from the inside of the bowel. By passing catheters and balloons into the colon, it has been possible to measure these jerky and rapid contractions. IBS is common in young people: it is commonly found between the ages of 20-45. It is always important to exclude other causes such as lactose intolerance or cancer of the bowel when diagnosing this condition.

SYMPTOMS

Spasmodic pain, distension and swelling of the abdomen, excessive passing of wind (eructations and flatus), together with bouts of diarrhoea and constipation. Blood is not a symptom of IBS and usually indicates more serious conditions. IBS is not a disorder of the elderly and it is important to exclude

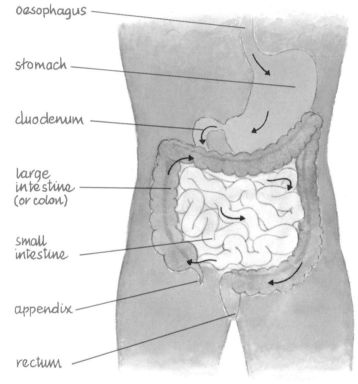

oesophagus

stomach

duodenum

large intestine (or colon)

small intestine

appendix

rectum

Above: *IBS interferes with the muscle contractions that cause waste matter to move through the large intestine.*

other conditions if such symptoms occur in elderly people.

PREVENTION AND SELF-HELP

It is important to ensure that an appropriate medical examination is undertaken before following the measures described below.
Dietary habits It is important to establish if there is any link between what you eat and other symptoms. Keep a diary of all your food and drink and list all your symptoms for at least one week, noting every bowel movement and the consistency of

stool as well as the amount of pain you experience. It is also important to take note of your mood and whether your bowel movements are in any way linked to your mental state. Diet is important in managing IBS and the following foods should be avoided:
- Dairy products, wheat and gluten-based products (biscuits, cakes), sugar, coffee, alcohol, fried foods and red meat.
- Tomatoes and seed-containing foods should also be avoided.
- You may also need to avoid pulses and beans, but it is important to try these first to see if you are intolerant of them.
Certain foods are helpful:
- Gluten-free whole grain (rice, millet, buckwheat), live yoghurt, green vegetables, fish, chicken. It is not only the types of food you eat, but how you eat that is important. Eating quickly, and failing to chew your food properly will make it more likely that the

Below: *They look tempting, but tomatoes and seed-containing foods should be avoided if you have IBS.*

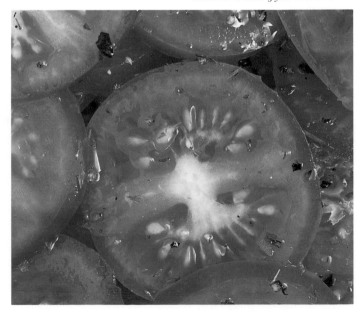

bowel will react to the undigested products. Dietary supplements, including Vitamin B_1 (thiamine), Vitamin B_6 (pyridoxine) and Vitamin C (ascorbic acid) may be helpful. These can be taken as separate tablets (one twice a day) or as a multivitamin (same dose). **Massage and relaxation** will reduce the level of stress and tension, and learning to breathe with your diaphragm will help to reduce the abnormal parasympathetic activity causing irregular bowel contractions.

HERBAL MEDICINE

Herbal treatments that have been most successful include peppermint oil (either taken as peppermint tea or peppermint oil capsules, three to six capsules daily). For constipation, prune or fig juice in warm water will help, while diarrhoea responds well to

Below: *Massaging the abdomen with essence of sassafras mixed with alcohol is a pleasurable remedy.*

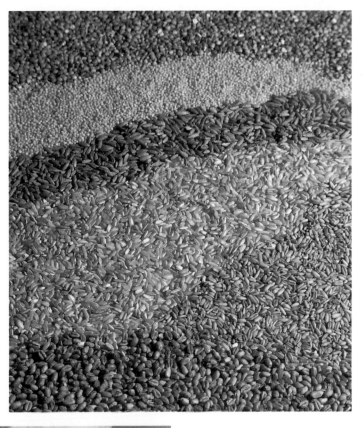

Above: *Gluten-free whole grains are sensible dietary choices for sufferers of irritable bowel syndrome.*

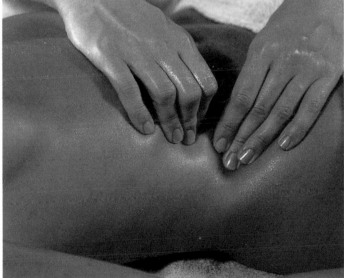

foot and hand baths in the following concoction: two litres (three and a half pints) of warm water in which a small cup of the following herbs are infused – mallow flowers, nettle leaves and meadowsweet flowers. Soak the feet or hands in the bath for up to 15 minutes.

AROMATHERAPY

A few drops of valerian essence taken on brown sugar will reduce tension and anxiety. Intestinal spasm can be treated with essence of savory (three drops

on a teaspoon of sugar) between meals. Rubbing the abdomen with essence of sassafras in pure alcohol (two teaspoons in 100ml/3 fl.oz.) can also help.

HOMEOPATHY

Homeopaths will suggest *Nux vomica* 30x (one tablet three times a day for three days) for flatulence and colic. If you note much trouble with tension, *Aconite* 6x (one tablet twice a day for one week) is suggested. *Argentum nit.* 6x (one tablet twice a day) will help reduce the mucous diarrhoea.

OTHER THERAPIES

Counselling and psychotherapy and, at times, hypnotherapy all help to reduce the stress associated with this condition. Acupuncture will also help to restore balance in the autonomic nervous system which appears to be the cause of the abnormal muscle contraction.

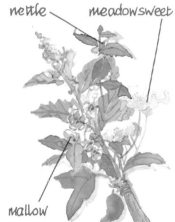

nettle   meadowsweet

mallow

Above: *These herbs infused in warm water make a foot and hand bath that helps with symptoms like diarrhoea.*

ORTHODOX TREATMENT

A full history of the symptom is taken and physical examination will exclude other causes. It may be necessary to examine the inside of the large bowel using a special viewing instrument called a sigmoidoscope. A barium enema is a form of X-ray that shows the large bowel and allows the doctor to exclude serious disorders (cancer and polyps). Motility studies which measure the level of contractions of the bowel are undertaken in special circumstances, and examination of the stools will exclude infections or allergic conditions (gluten sensitivity). Treatments with dietary

interventions and the prescribing of bulk agents that ensure there is a formed stool (lactulose, fybogel) may be recommended. Medication to control the motility of the bowel (anti-spasmodics) will decrease the spasm and reduce the pain. Side effects of these drugs include a dry mouth, flushing and occasional difficulty with passing urine. IBS usually ceases during middle age and most people need to be reassured that it is a benign condition and does not lead to serious bowel disease. The key to managing this condition is reduction of stress and improving your diet.

EATING DISORDERS

These consist of a range of problems related to food, body-shape, self-image and dieting. They primarily affect young women who, consciously or unconsciously, develop an obsession about "how they look" and usually embark on a relentless pursuit of thinness. Even in the most extreme cases of anorexia, where the individual may weigh less than five stone (32kg), she may still consider herself to be overweight and refuse food. The prevalence of this condition has increased substantially over the last decade and it is thought by many feminists to be a result of the social and cultural pressure on women to be thin and beautiful. The three major problems are compulsive eating, anorexia nervosa and bulimia, although the commonest form of eating disorder is, paradoxically, compulsive dieting because of perceived obesity.

TYPES OF EATING DISORDER

Compulsive eaters These people binge and grow fat. They eat more than they want or need. Then they feel guilty and go on a rigid diet, which is subsequently broken by another compulsive binge. Fat people may actually enjoy their food and the problem here is their greed. In compulsive eating, however, the problem is fear and anxiety, and the eater rarely enjoys the binges. Some of them involve cravings for certain foods. These are often sugar-containing snacks or chocolate (the chocaholic).

Anorexia nervosa This is a much more serious and, at times, fatal disease where there is persistent refusal to eat. It mostly affects adolescent girls. Also known as slimmers' disease, it may begin in the early teens and can soon develop into an obsession with food and dieting. Other common features include loss of weight, the cessation of menstrual periods, loss of interest in sex, severe constipation, depression and anxiety. If the

Below: *The Western preoccupation with dieting and the body beautiful is not a particularly healthy obsession. It can result in women becoming uneasy about their self-image which can lead on to eating disorders.*

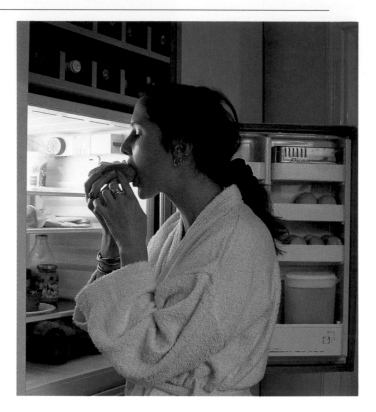

food refusal becomes severe, then metabolic changes and malnutrition can lead to emaciation and eventual death. Anorexics feel under a pressure to succeed, have problems with control and power, and can use food refusal as a way to manage their parents.

Bulimia nervosa A condition (often a well kept secret) whereby after uncontrollable bouts of over-eating, the sufferer attempts forcibly to vomit up the food and takes an excessive amount of laxative to ensure no food is left in the body. Many people with anorexia will go on to develop bulimia, and both conditions can be present at the same time. It is a common symptom in young girls, but the full blown picture is probably present in one or two

Above: *Eating disorders such as bulimia are characterized by bouts of secretive binge eating followed by self-induced vomiting and purgation.*

percent of women. In addition to taking laxatives, other medication, appetite suppressants, amphetamines, and diuretics may be consumed that could lead to excess loss of water and fluctuating bouts of diarrhoea and constipation. Bulimia is characterized by deceit and secretive behaviour, such as going to the lavatory to force vomit while in the middle of a dinner party. A variant of such eating disorders is compulsive exercise (particularly jogging and aerobics), more common in men who have a fixation about "keeping fit".

CAUSES

Much research has been undertaken, both at an individual as well as family level. Hormone tests suggest there may be an abnormality of the body's control mechanisms, but this may be an after-effect rather than a cause of the problem. Psychological explanations suggest disturbed family relationships, where parents are over-controlling and intolerant of the growing adolescent. The child is believed to use food as a way of defying her parents. Food carries several symbolic meanings, which may indicate love and affection, and some therapists believe that food may become a substitute for love where family relationships have been strained or broken. More recently feminists have agreed that the role-models for women portrayed on the T.V. (such as beautiful announcers) or cinema screen (starlets) and in the fashion magazines (models) are all "beautiful" and "thin". Developing adolescents may feel pressure to conform to these models. Together with an obsession with thinness goes an obsession with beauty, which is seen in the billion pound beauty industry which involves make-up, plastic surgery, cosmetic improvement of the body form, beauty clubs, exercise machines etc.

PREVENTION AND SELF-HELP

▪ If you suffer or think you suffer from any of these disorders, it is important to seek help and possibly to join a group where you can share your experiences with other men or women.
▪ If you are obsessed with your body and diet, read some of the feminist literature available and try and put your problem into perspective.
▪ Check your nutritional state. In view of your condition it may need balancing with extra vitamins and minerals.

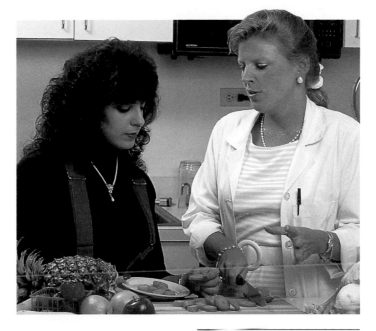

Above: *Eating disorders often go hand in hand with dietary deficiencies. It is important in severe cases to get advice on preparing a balanced diet.*

▪ Build up your confidence and self-esteem; join an assertiveness training group.
▪ Keep a diary of your emotional mood swings and thought patterns relating to yourself and others.
▪ Develop new eating habits and establish new patterns of shopping and cooking.
▪ Exercise less if you are fanatic, and exercise more if you do little or none. Choose an exercise routine which is not focusing on beauty or achieving perfection.

COUNSELLING, PSYCHOTHERAPY AND GROUP THERAPY

These are the commonest forms of intervention that will help with eating disorders. The more contact you have with others who have the same difficulty, the more you may learn about yourself. Many of the other alternative therapies will help and give support, but it is important to establish a "talking therapy" to enable you to understand and overcome the difficulties.

ACUPUNCTURE

A course of acupuncture can help restore proper energetic balance and can lead to increased self-confidence.

Below: *A course of acupuncture has proved beneficial in some cases. Any therapy that increases the patient's self-esteem is worthwhile.*

NATUROPATHY

Focusing soley on dietary changes will not necessarily help, as the problem is psychological. However, obtaining the right advice regarding a balanced diet will be important in the severe cases.

DANCE AND ART THERAPY

These disciplines can be particularly helpful for those who are shy and unable to express themselves. It is possible to explore your emotional difficulties and express some of the guilt and anger that may be present through dance and by painting and drawing.

BACH REMEDIES

Bach remedies may be helpful as first aid. Try the Rescue Remedy: four drops in a cup of water sipped frequently through the day. However, the problems are often so deep-seated that it is important to try to remedy this complaint with a multi-therapy approach.

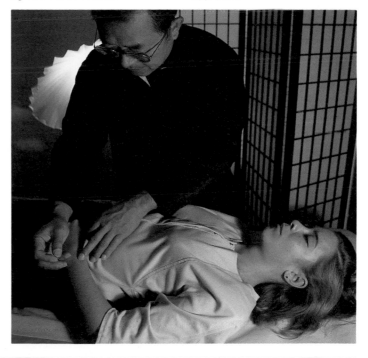

ORTHODOX TREATMENT

Psychiatric help is often sought and there are now several specialized eating-disorder clinics to choose from. Occasionally severe anorexics will have to be admitted to hospital and intravenous therapy or forced feeding can be tried. Anti-depressants and tranquillizers may be prescribed.

STOMACH ULCERS

Peptic ulcers are one of the conditions in a spectrum of problems affecting the lining of the stomach. The term peptic comes from the name of the cells lining the stomach which secrete the enzyme pepsin. Associated problems include gastric irritation (from aspirin), gastritis (indigestion) and duodenal ulcers. All involve an ulceration of the lining of the first part of the digestive tract. The lining, or mucosal layer, contains cells that secrete both hydrochloric acid and enzymes that digest the food. Normally a protective mucus prevents the acid and pepsin eating away at the stomach wall, but if the mucous lining is inadequate, an ulcer may develop. It was a rare condition before the 1900s, but is now becoming more frequent, and women, who hitherto rarely developed ulcers, are now more prone to them. They do occur in children but are rare in the elderly. Symptoms that develop after the age of 50 or 60 should be properly investigated to exclude stomach cancer. There is an element of genetic predisposition, and people with the blood group D seem to be more liable to ulcers. Although it is commonly believed that diet plays a large part in the causation, and acute ulcers do occur after eating hot spicy foods, the significance of diet is still not altogether certain. Many minor ulcers may occur without causing any symptoms: it is the persistence of symptoms that suggest the presence of a deep ulcer that will not heal.

TYPES

Gastritis is a mild everyday variety of "indigestion" that can occur partly as a result of over-eating or eating foods that harm the lining of the stomach. It can also affect the lower part of the oesophagus (gullet) and give rise to irritation and inflammation (heartburn). This is often associated with a weakness of the muscle between the oesophagus and the stomach – a hiatus hernia.

Below: An "ulcer personality" has been described by psychiatrists: typically a youngish male executive striving for success at work.

Gastric ulcers occur more commonly in men in the middle-age range and are signalled by acute pain in the upper part of the abdomen relatively soon (0-30 minutes) after eating a meal. The pain can be associated with vomiting and nausea and more seriously will cause some bleeding, which will either be vomited or passed in the faeces which will appear black and tarry. Acute ulcers can occur from severe alcohol intoxication or the use of certain drugs (aspirin, anti-inflammatory drugs and steroids).

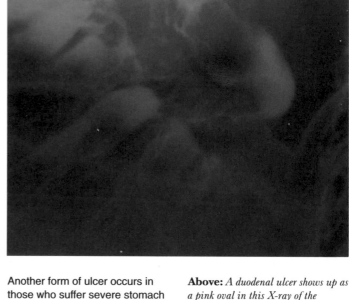

Another form of ulcer occurs in those who suffer severe stomach burns.
Duodenal ulcers are most common in young adults in the 20-40 age group, and affect both men and women. It is estimated that up to 10 percent of the male population in Western countries will suffer from minor duodenal ulcer symptoms at some time in their lives. The pain is felt a little while after eating a meal (30 minutes to two hours) and is usually lower down the abdomen on the left side. It is less acute than gastric ulcer pain but like the latter, if severe, will bleed and cause complications described above. A further serious complication is when the ulcer perforates, leaks digestive juices and bacteria from the digestive tract into the abdomen and

Above: A duodenal ulcer shows up as a pink oval in this X-ray of the intestinal tract. Ulcers are craters in the lining of the stomach or gut.

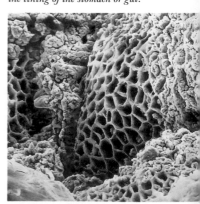

Above: This magnified (x220) view of the lining of the stomach shows a gastric ulcer in pink, while the normal membrane appears green.

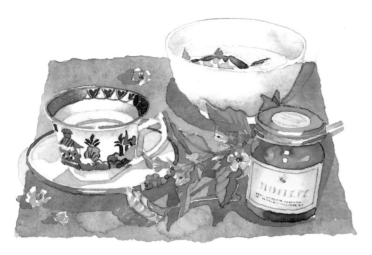

causes peritonitis. In such a case, the patient needs immediate surgical attention.

CAUSES

- Certain foods are known to cause ulcers, including coffee, tea and other gastric irritants such as alcohol.
- Smoking increases your chance of developing an ulcer.
- Overwork, anxiety, stress and tension of any kind will increase the excretion of stomach acid and predispose to ulcers.
- Psychiatrists have described an "ulcer personality" – a young middle-class male executive striving for success with a need to be loved and supported.
- More recently, a bacterium has been isolated that grows in the ulcer crater and prevents the healing process. This also ensures recurrence of the ulcer unless it is eradicated.

PREVENTION AND SELF-HELP

- Keep a careful diary noting symptoms against diet content.
- Cut out alcohol, tobacco, coffee

Above: *A traditional herbal remedy for soothing the stomach is an infusion of marshmallow leaves in water.*

and reduce tea to two cups a day.
- Review your lifestyle regarding tension, stress and anxiety levels.
- If you are a "worrier", learn some relaxation exercises.
- Take up Yoga or meditation.
- Eat regularly and *slowly* – avoid hurried snacks.
- Avoid hot spicy foods and those to which you are allergic.
- Do not leave your stomach empty for long hours and if you have to drink alcohol, make sure it is not on an empty stomach.
- Avoid aspirin and aspirin-containing analgesics.
- Your diet should include plenty of fruit juices and raw vegetables.
- See your doctor if there is any sign of bleeding or if pain persists.

NATUROPATHY

The advice will be to eat a wholefood diet, to eat little and often, and to take the steps outlined above. Grains (oats), pulses and green vegetables are particularly helpful. Liquorice will

help to heal the ulcer – chew up to three liquorice sticks a day.

HERBAL MEDICINE

Coriander, either drunk as a tea or eaten raw, reduces heartburn. Chamomile and lemon balm teas will help with relaxation, and celery sticks or celery juice will aid digestion. A marshmallow infusion is a traditional remedy for soothing the lining of the stomach. Take 30g (1oz.) of dried marshmallow leaves. Allow them to soak in 60cl (one pint) of boiling water, strain, allow to cool, and flavour with honey. Sip from a cup every five minutes or so. Another herb that can help as above is meadowsweet.

ACUPUNCTURE

This can be particularly helpful in chronic duodenal ulcers and will help to reduce acid secretion and increase relaxation. However, any treatment must be accompanied by attention to lifestyle and change of diet.

HOMEOPATHY

Homeopathy will be helpful with symptoms but an accurate constitutional diagnosis needs to be made if the ulcer is to heal properly. Significant relief can be obtained from:
Argentum nit. – flatulence and pain.
Arsenicum album – anxiety and persistent pain.
Nux vomica – for nausea and pain, especially in the early morning.
All the above, take one tablet twice a day for three days, 6x potency.

OTHER THERAPIES

Autogenic training, relaxation, meditation and hypnotherapy will all help in bringing about a state of relaxation, thus reducing acid secretion in the stomach.

Below: *A colourful array of pulses, the edible seeds of plants such as peas, beans and lentils. They are an important part of a wholefood diet.*

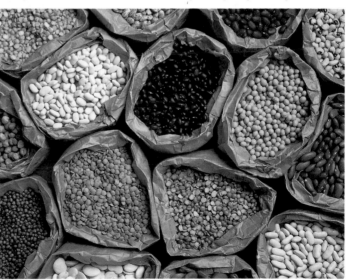

ORTHODOX TREATMENT

The management of peptic ulceration has changed dramatically in the last ten years, both because of better medical technology and the availability of more advanced drugs. Although not everyone with indigestion needs to be investigated, it is now common to pass a flexible endoscope down the gullet to see if an ulcer exists. Other methods include the barium meal when a patient swallows a barium sulphate mixture that shows up in X-rays of the digestive tract. A specific diet is not so frequently prescribed, nor are the alkali mixtures (antacids) that can be bought over the

counter. Most doctors now rely on a new class of drugs called H_2 antagonists that reduce the secretion of acid in the stomach and allow the ulcer to heal. These may need to be taken for a long time and ulcers may recur if the causative factors are not dealt with. More commonly, the addition of antibiotics with H_2 antagonists will eliminate the bacteria that are thought both to predispose and to cause recurrence of the ulcer. Surgery is now rarely performed unless it is needed because of an emergency (blood loss or perforation), or because of severe repeated attacks.

HAEMORRHOIDS

Over 50 percent of adults will develop these small varicose swellings in and around the anus. They feel like lumps which will bleed or itch. There is no connection between varicose veins and haemorrhoids or piles, although both appear to be common in humans (who walk on two legs) as opposed to animals (four legs). There are three degrees of piles.

First degree piles bleed but do not prolapse, or come down outside the anus. Second degree piles prolapse on defecation but can return inside the anus. Third degree piles remain external to the anus. One other form of piles which can be extremely painful is an external pile, which develops rapidly after straining and is felt like a painful lump – a small blood clot.

CAUSES

The most likely explanation for haemorrhoids is the low-fibre diet all too common in Western cultures and the subsequent constipation that ensues. The increased straining required to defecate is felt to increase pressure on the veins in the anal canal, which can destroy their valves. Pregnancy is another common cause partly because of the increased pressure and straining during labour, but also because pregnancy hormones allow the walls of the anal veins to relax.

SYMPTOMS

- Bleeding, usually at the beginning or end of defecation.
- Itchy anus with discharge.
- A little blood on toilet paper.

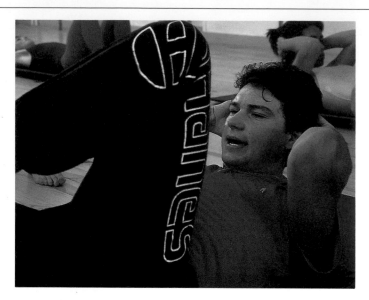

Above: Regular exercise helps prevent constipation, which in turn prevents the formation of haemorrhoids. A healthy lifestyle pays dividends!

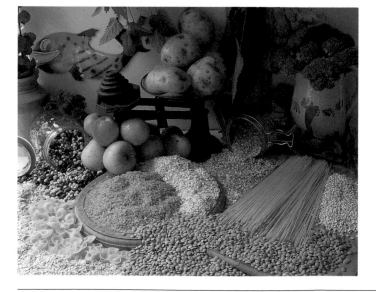

Below: *This food looks great, and it will do you good. The large amount of fibre these items contain will encourage easy bowel motions.*

- Lump around the anus, with or without pain.
- Feeling of fullness and something come down from the anus.
- Grape-like swelling through the anus.

PREVENTION AND SELF-HELP

It is important to have a proper medical diagnosis before embarking on your own treatment. A doctor will perform a rectal examination, as well as examine the inner lining of the anus. Once other conditions have been excluded, then it will be useful to pursue the following measures.

- If in great pain, hot baths and hot compresses pressed on the anus will provide relief.
- Avoid constipation and develop a wholefood diet and regular toilet habits.
- Rutin is an additive felt to be helpful with strengthening the capillaries. (Rutin is found in buckwheat, rose-hips, cherries, blackberries and citrus fruits.)
- Regular exercise will help to prevent constipation.
- Local anaesthetic creams and suppositories are available from chemists.
- Take care with your personal hygiene. Make sure you keep the anal area clean by washing with warm water after defecation.

NATUROPATHY

Increased fibre and linseed oil in the diet will soften the consistency of bowel motions. Try taking a large spoonful of linseed seeds washed down with water at the same time each day, away from mealtimes. Hot baths and a massage gently down the left side of the abdomen will aid defecation.

AROMATHERAPY

Add two drops of an essential oil such as cypress, chamomile, juniper or peppermint to a cup of warm water, and dab this mixture on the piles. It will help to ease discomfort. Alternatively, take a sitz bath by adding four drops of two of the above oils to a washing bowl of warm water and sit in it for five or ten minutes.

ORTHODOX TREATMENT

After appropriate examination, local treatment will include ointment, suppositories or foam which will both ease pain and reduce inflammation. If this does not help, surgical intervention – either by injection, surgical removal or freezing – may be necessary. Dietary advice will be given to avoid constipation.

GALLSTONES

The gall bladder is a pear-shaped organ that lies behind the liver just below the right ribs. Bile produced by the liver is stored in the gall bladder and it is there that gallstones develop. These are solid masses like pebbles. Ten percent are made of cholesterol, ten percent of bile pigments and eighty percent of a mixture that also contains calcium. Gallstones *per se* do not cause any particular problem but if they block the flow of bile they will cause either pain or infection (cholecystitis). Sometimes the blockage will lead to jaundice and serious infection of the liver.

CAUSES

Gallstones occur in between five and ten percent of the population of Western countries and are more common in certain families. They are more frequent in people with diabetes, the obese, and pregnant women. The most common factor in producing gallstones is a high-fat and low-fibre diet.

SYMPTOMS

- Severe intermittent colicky pain, sometimes felt at the hip or the right shoulder.
- Mild upper abdominal discomfort following a meal.
- Bloated feeling in the abdomen with wind.
- Jaundice, temperature and severe illness.
- Paradoxically, often there are no noticeable symptoms.

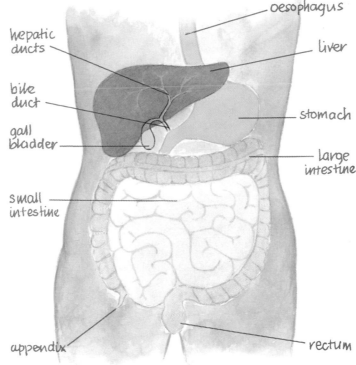

Above: *The gall bladder is a small organ that lies under the liver. It stores bile produced by the liver.*

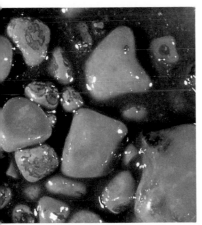

Above: *These are gallstones, hard masses that are made up of calcium salts, cholesterol and bile pigments,*

PREVENTION AND SELF-HELP

Gallstones are primarily a Western affliction, and are often related to an unhealthy diet. If there is a family history of gallstones, do begin to reduce weight if you are obese, move to a wholefood, high-fibre diet and avoid fried foods, red meat, eggs and cheese.

NATUROPATHY

Fasting, a low-fat diet with no dairy products and no animal fats, together with plenty of vegetables

are the main recommendations. Vitamin C as a supplement – two tablets a day – and fresh lemon juice are useful. Garlic and bitter salads, such as chicory, endive and globe artichokes, are also thought to be valuable components of a healthy diet.

HERBAL MEDICINE

A cup of centaury tea a day may help, but the mainstay of herbal medicines are cholagogues,

natural substances that help dissolve bile stones. These include artichoke, rosemary, sage, boldo, dandelion, and golden seal. Take as teas, two cups daily.
WARNING Pregnant women should seek medical advice before taking any herbal prescription.

AROMATHERAPY

To alleviate the pain of gallstones, essence of Scots pine (three drops) is helpful in the bath and, added to a carrier oil, can be used for body massage.

ACUPUNCTURE

This has had some successes in helping dissolve gallstones but should not be relied on if surgery has been recommended.

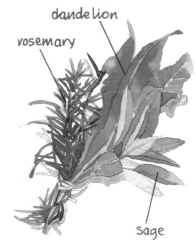

Above: *Cholagogues are substances that dissolve bile stones; they include the herbs shown in this posy.*

ORTHODOX TREATMENT

Gallstones that give rise to no symptoms need no treatment. Most treatment will include antibiotics and surgery. Drugs used to dissolve gallstones have not proved very effective, but more recently ultrasound machines have been used in order to break up the stones into small fragments that are then passed through the gall duct, and so out of the body.

NAUSEA/VOMITING

This is a very common symptom which almost everyone will have experienced from time to time. It is not in itself serious, unless it persists and leads to repeated vomiting when medical attention is required. It may occur as a direct result of a digestive disturbance or a disorder of the balancing mechanism of the ear, such as motion sickness. It can also be a response to a disturbing condition when actual vomiting occurs. It may be important to exclude allergic problems if no immediate cause is found. Vomiting in infants can be more serious if persistent, because of the loss of fluids and potential dehydration.

CAUSES

Digestive problems These can be caused by acute toxic ingestion of food substances, such as shellfish or mouldy meat, resulting in bacterial infections, such as gastro-enteritis or typhoid. Allergic responses to strawberries or dairy products can all produce the symptoms.
Pregnancy Early morning vomiting in the first twelve weeks is fairly common and may be associated with food intolerance or cravings. The problem almost always stops in the second trimester of pregnancy and is associated with changes in hormone level as well as stress.
Ear disorders The inner ear controls the balancing mechanism of the body and can be disturbed by motion sickness, or alcohol intoxication (when

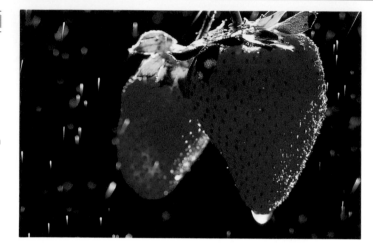

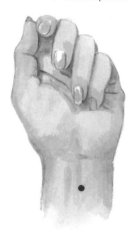

Above: *Firm pressure on the Heart Governor 6 acupoint is a useful self-help measure to deal with nausea.*

there is usually a gastric element involved as well). Positional vertigo, labyrinthitis and Ménière's disease are all disturbances of the inner ear that lead to nausea and vomiting.
Migraine This is often associated with nausea and vomiting, as are head injuries and, more seriously but very rarely, increased pressure on the brain caused by meningitis or a brain tumour. Only recurrent symptoms need to be investigated by a doctor and you should be able to treat yourself if you have only a mild attack. Be sure to seek medical advice if the symptoms persist.

PREVENTION AND SELF-HELP

▪ Avoid all foods that are "old" or doubtful in quality. Do not use foods past their recommended "Sell by …" date.
▪ Rely on fresh vegetables and fruit and make sure that they are washed thoroughly.

Above: *If you are unlucky, you may be allergic to foods such as these delicious-looking strawberries.*

▪ If abroad, drink bottled water if you are uncertain of the purity of the source of tapwater.
▪ If you suffer from migraine, avoid hunger – take a snack or a biscuit before getting up. Peppermint tea will help. Avoid rich fatty foods including chocolate.

HOMEOPATHY

Try *Ipecac.* 6x, *Pulsatilla* 6x, *Arsenicum alb.* 6x. Dosage: in each case one tablet every half-hour until improvement is felt. Homeopathic remedies will not harm the baby if pregnant.

CHILDREN: The adult dose can be given to children between two and 12 years of age. For children under two, use a tincture and administer two drops every half-hour.

ACUPRESSURE

Motion sickness nausea, as well as morning sickness and post-anaesthetic nausea, can be helped by acupressure on the Heart Governor 6 acupoint. This is found on the inner arm three fingers' above the wrist-crease, in line with the middle finger. Apply pressure with a finger tip for two minutes. Special bands can be bought to apply when travelling by sea, etc.

HERBAL MEDICINE

An infusion of ginger, Roman chamomile or black horehound will be helpful. **Do not take** if you are pregnant.

Below: *Sipping a cup of peppermint tea is pleasurable way of countering the acute symptoms of nausea.*

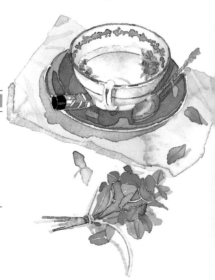

ORTHODOX TREATMENT

Advice to refrain from heavy eating will be given in single cases, but more complex problems will be investigated before any treatment is undertaken. Motion sickness tablets are available and stronger medication is given when the cause arises from problems in the inner ear. It is not wise to take medication in the first three months of pregnancy.

COLIC

Most commonly, this is a symptom of young babies with feeding problems. Although not serious, it may cause great distress to both baby and parents. In adults, it is usually a symptom of intestinal infection or irritability. In both cases, it is associated with gripey, acute abdominal pain – the baby may raise its legs and scream while adults may double up in pain. It usually lasts only a few seconds, rarely longer, and may be associated with nausea, vomiting, diarrhoea, and the sufferer may break out in sweat and feel cold and shiverish at the same time. The abdomen can become very distended, and in both cases there may be the passage of wind which brings instant relief.

CAUSES

Colic in babies This is common in the first six months, worst during the evening (six o'clock colic) or may wake the baby up at night. It is more common in bottle-fed babies but may also occur in the breast-fed. A simple cause may be the swallowing of air while the baby is feeding because either the teat on the bottle is too wide or the baby is so hungry that he or she rapidly sucks in air as well as milk. How the baby is held while feeding is also important. It is customary and enjoyable to help the baby bring up the wind (and occasionally a little milk) by keeping him or her upright after a meal and tapping or rubbing gently on his or her back. Colic in babies occurs partly because the gut has not established its own rhythm, and it should not be seen as a sign of poor mothering. If the child is breast-fed and the mother eats onions, garlic or pulses, this may pass through the breast milk and give rise to colic, so dietary care on the part of the mother is important.

Colic in adults This may simply be the result of over-eating or of eating too many pulses or raw food: some adults cannot digest these. Acute infection and toxic food poisoning account for the majority of cases, but you may also suffer from irritable bowel syndrome (see pages 112-113) where the bowel does not contract properly and produces distension and flatulence. Acute colic occurs in more severe intestinal conditions including appendicitis, obstruction and twisted bowel. In severe cases, a doctor needs to be called immediately.

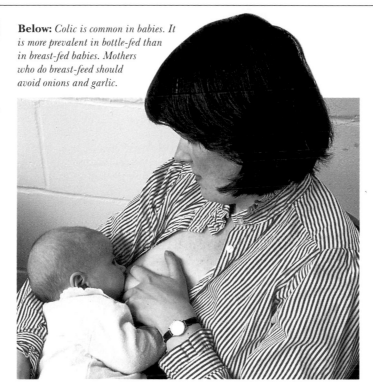

Below: *Colic is common in babies. It is more prevalent in bottle-fed than in breast-fed babies. Mothers who do breast-feed should avoid onions and garlic.*

PREVENTION AND SELF-HELP

In other than the most serious conditions, it is appropriate for self-help to be tried. For babies the following herbal teas are helpful: peppermint, cat-mint, fennel. Give them half a teaspoon every half-hour. In adults a cup of herbal tea or an infusion will help. It is worth trying seed tea: put a teaspoon each of caraway, fennel and aniseed in a cup and cover with hot water. Allow the mixture to infuse for five to ten minutes, strain and drink.

Aromatherapists recommend gripe water (diluted fennel essential oil) and you can make your own by adding one drop of oil to some warm water and taking it with half-a-teaspoon of honey. Fennel essential oil (two drops in half-a-teaspoon of carrier oil) can be tried as a massage gently applied over the abdomen. Adults can be helped with other essential oils to help digestion, notably lavender, camphor, juniper and patchouli. It can be helpful to give babies twice daily half-a-teaspoon of Bifidobacteria infantis (obtainable from healthfood shops) dissolved in a little water to restore the bowel bacterial flora especially in non-breast-fed infants or those who have had antibiotics, which may have killed off the bacteria naturally present in the gut.

HOMEOPATHY

Homeopathic remedies for colic (all 6x potency) include *Colocynth, Dioscorea* and *Magnesia phos.* Adults can take one tablet every two hours for six doses.

CHILDREN: Administer three drops every two hours for up to six doses.

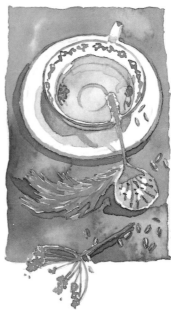

Above: *A cup of seed tea containing fennel, caraway and aniseed will relieve colic in adults.*

ORTHODOX TREATMENT

In simple cases general dietary advice will be given after an examination to exclude any physical abnormalities. Pain-killing drugs may be prescribed, and an antispasmodic which calms the gut is given to adults and occasionally to babies.

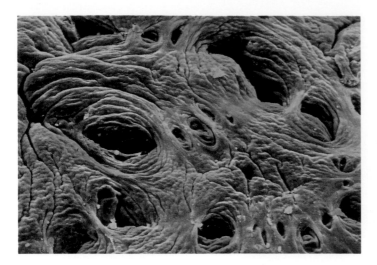

COELIAC DISEASE

DESCRIPTION

A condition where the bowel wall becomes allergic to gluten (the protein in wheat, rye and other cereals) leading to diarrhoea, failure to thrive in children and other nutritional abnormalities. It is often hereditary, but can develop after a bout of gastroenteritis.

PREVENTION AND SELF-HELP

▪ Breast-feed babies if at all possible – there may be a connection between this disease and bottle-feeding.
▪ Restrict cow's milk, especially after a bout of diarrhoea.
▪ Avoid bread, biscuits, cakes and gravy which is thickened with flour. Also avoid processed foods which often contain flour.
▪ Eat lots of fresh vegetables, fruits, fish and nuts.
▪ Join your national Coeliac Society for further advice.

ALTERNATIVE THERAPIES

Naturopathy will adopt the same approach as orthodox medicine and ban wheat-containing foods, but also suggest avoiding milk protein as well. Some naturopaths believe that too much cow's milk protein in early infancy can bring on this condition.
Herbal medicine In addition to the above, herbalists will

Above: This magnified view of the wall of the small intestine shows how coeliac disease has rendered it flat and devoid of the normal hair-like villi.

prescribe marshmallow or slippery elm. Diarrhoea may be helped by chamomile.

ORTHODOX TREATMENT

At one time the cause of this distressing condition was not known, but biopsy of the lining of the wall of the small intestine can help to make a definitive diagnosis. A stool examination is also useful. Treatment is by avoiding all gluten-containing food and by taking vitamin supplements.

COLITIS

DESCRIPTION

Inflammation or infection of the large bowel (colon) which can become longstanding ulcerative colitis and be a precursor for cancer of the bowel. Symptoms are bloody diarrhoea, pain, fever, loss of weight and occasional arthritis.

PREVENTION AND SELF-HELP

Stress is considered to be one of the factors which, if it does not actually cause colitis, certainly exacerbates it, and you will need to learn some relaxation exercises, such as
▪ Yoga.

▪ Autogenic training.
▪ Meditation.
▪ The occasional fast.
▪ Plenty of exercise.
Follow a prescribed diet carefully and treat the mild bouts of diarrhoea with:
Acupressure Press on the point just below the knee on the outside of the leg, pointing downwards, for three minutes. Repeat every two hours, as necessary.

ALTERNATIVE THERAPIES

Naturopathy Naturopaths will suggest an exclusive diet: no milk, wheat, or meat, no seed-containing fruit or vegetables (tomatoes etc.). Cooked vegetables, mashed fruit (bananas) and vitamins and mineral supplements are recommended.
Herbal medicine will treat with slippery elm drinks.
Acupuncture will help direct Chi away from the colon by placing needles in the Gall Bladder meridian.

ORTHODOX TREATMENT

Investigation will include sigmoidoscopy (a tube is passed into the colon via the rectum) with a biopsy. A barium enema (X-ray of the large bowel) will help determine the extent of the condition. Treatment involves diet, local suppositories and enemas (steroids) to reduce inflammation, together with sulphur drugs. Surgery is occasionally necessary to remove portions of diseased bowel.

DIVERTICULITIS

DESCRIPTION

Little "sacs" or diverticulae appear in the lower part of the large bowel (the descending colon) which can retain faecal material, become infected and cause abdominal cramping, diarrhoea and temperature.

Right: *The wavy pattern in this person's colon (left), revealed by a barium X-ray, is evidence of colitis.*

PREVENTION AND SELF-HELP

This is an almost entirely preventable disease as it is rarely found in cultures that habitually eat a high roughage diet.
▪ Drink plenty of fluids to avoid dehydration.
▪ Avoid alcohol, coffee.
▪ Take plenty of exercise and ensure regular bowel movement without straining.
▪ Ensure that your diet contains plenty of fibre.

ALTERNATIVE THERAPIES

Naturopathy This is a disease of dietary imbalance and after an initial fast, a diet will be prescribed to increase roughage (stewed fruit, porridge and mineral supplements). Some will recommend enemas but this should be proceeded with caution.
Acupuncture can help with constipation as can **reflexology** and **herbal medicine**.

ORTHODOX TREATMENT

This is commonly a condition of the elderly, and is felt to be caused by a low roughage diet and constipation. Commonly these diverticulae cause no symptoms at all. Examination with

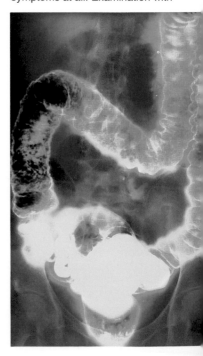

sigmoidoscopy and a barium enema confirms the diagnosis and treatment is initially with antibiotics and a prescribed diet.

FLATULENCE

DESCRIPTION

An excessive build-up of gas in the upper or lower bowel leading to feelings of bloatedness and fullness, and embarrassing release of gas. Not necessarily a symptom of serious disease.

PREVENTION AND SELF-HELP

This is a perfectly preventable condition once its cause is identified. If you swallow air because of irregular breathing, practise:
- Diaphragmatic, regular breathing.
- Chew your food slowly.
- Talk slowly.
- Avoid holding your breath.
- Sit upright when eating.
- Avoid gas-containing foods (beans, pulses etc.) and fizzy drinks.
- Do not drink with meals but *between* meals sip a cup of peppermint or chamomile tea.

ALTERNATIVE THERAPIES

Naturopathy A 24-hour fast will often relieve all symptoms. Garlic perles twice a day and a thorough review of diet are also recommended.
Herbal medicine Cook with thyme, marjoram and sage. Chew caraway seeds or cloves.
Reflexology Pressing on the appropriate point on the foot relating to the large colon will relieve gas.

ORTHODOX TREATMENT

This is not viewed as a serious condition even though it causes much distress. Most commonly caused by air-swallowing associated with tension and anxiety. Often caused by gas-releasing foods – beans, vegetables, fizzy drinks. Generally dietary advice is given.

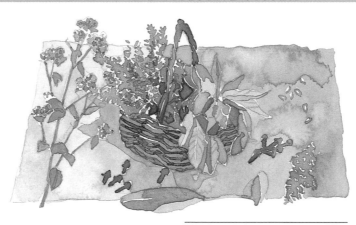

Above: *Carminative herbs dispel wind; they include thyme, majoram, sage, cloves and caraway seeds.*

HEPATITIS

DESCRIPTION

An infectious condition of the liver caused by viruses. The most common, Hep.A is food-borne; Hep.B is blood-borne and caused by anything from a mild viral condition to severe jaundice and liver failure.

PREVENTION AND SELF-HELP

Hepatitis is often caught while travelling abroad. A vaccine is now available and should be considered if you are visiting a high-risk area. When away,
- Boil water or drink mineral water.
- Avoid shellfish.
- Wash your hands carefully before and after eating.
- Do not eat food off someone else's plate.
If you contract hepatitis,
- Consult a doctor and follow dietary advice.
- Avoid all alcohol for at least six months.

ALTERNATIVE THERAPIES

Ensure medical diagnosis is made before embarking on alternative therapy.
Naturopathy Recommendations are fresh vegetable juice, plenty of fluids, avoid fatty foods, red meat and alcohol. Take mineral supplements, zinc and Vitamin B, garlic capsules – one twice a day.
Herbal medicine See Jaundice on pages 106-107.

ORTHODOX TREATMENT

Blood tests will reveal the diagnosis and occasionally a liver biopsy is taken to exclude other possibilities. Rest, plenty of fluids, diet restriction (no fats or meat or alcohol) is often all that is necessary. No specific treatment is given but care is taken not to spread infection.

ITCHING ANUS

DESCRIPTION

A troublesome and common condition often caused by worms (see below) but which can be caused by haemorrhoids, skin conditions, tight-fitting underwear and bowel disease.

PREVENTION AND SELF-HELP

Check you do not have worms or haemorroids.
- Avoid obesity.
- Go on a fluid fast for 24 hours.
- Use sitz baths – one full of warm water and one of cold water: put your bottom in warm, feet in cold for three minutes, then vice versa for a minute.

ALTERNATIVE THERAPIES

Herbal medicine Dry skin can be helped with applications of almond oil; chickweed paste is often prescribed.
Homeopathy *Urtica* 6x, one twice a day, or *Apis mel.* 6x, same dose.

CHILDREN: Same dose as for adults.

Naturopathy Regular bowel motions, colonic lavage and cold water baths are recommended.

ORTHODOX TREATMENT

Examination may reveal the cause of the condition, e.g. worms or haemorrhoids, but often no cause can be found and occasionally this is a stress-related condition. Suppositories, injections and steroid ointments are sometimes prescribed.

WORMS

DESCRIPTION

Worms can quite commonly infest the gut (threadworms, pinworms), especially in children. More serious, tapeworms and hookworms are associated with travel abroad and poor diet.

PREVENTION AND SELF-HELP

- Keep finger nails short to avoid the accidental ingestion of eggs which can be trapped under the nails if hygiene is poor.
- Cook all food thoroughly.
- Treat the whole family if an infestation is diagnosed.
- Avoid raw or undercooked meat.
- Keep separate towels.
- Wash hands before and after eating.

ALTERNATIVE THERAPIES

Naturopathy Various combination of foods are said to get rid of worms (for example, garlic and raw carrots).
Herbal medicine Wormwood and male fern are used, but are potentially dangerous so need to be taken under guidance.

ORTHODOX TREATMENT

Diagnosis is usually easy with the inspection of eggs or the worms themselves. Whole families have to be treated as they can be very infectious. Treatment depends on type of worm involved – a variety of drugs are available.

ARTHRITIS

Arthritis is the most common disorder affecting the joints of the body. There are many different kinds, but the three main varieties are rheumatoid, osteo- and gouty arthritis. The first two are by far the most common. Even now, after many years of research, the actual causes of arthritis are not fully understood and cures are no more likely now than they were 50 years ago. Each joint in the body is lined with synovial membrane which produces a lubricating fluid which allows the joints to function properly with little or no pain. Arthritis of all kinds destroys this process and damages the joint space, leading to bone rubbing against bone, which produces the pain, swelling and discomfort characteristic of the condition. Whereas osteoarthritis is usually considered a function of "wear and tear" and occurs as a result of increasing use and old age, rheumatoid arthritis is a disease of the whole body and can affect other organs as well as the joints. Arthritis can occur in other conditions including Reiter's syndrome, a sexually transmitted disease, ankylosing spondylitis and ulcerative colitis.

CAUSES

Osteoarthritis This is a degenerative condition of the joints resulting from destruction of cartilege and synovial fluid leading to loss of space between the bones. It is a condition of old age, although it can be brought about by previous injury or polio, so that the young can also suffer. It generally involves the large weight-bearing joints – the hips and knees primarily – although any joint in the body can be affected. In the spine it is the major cause of low back pain and neck ache as a result of the loss of vertebral discs that act as shock absorbers in the spinal column. It can affect the hands, particularly the joints of the thumbs. It tends not to spread from one joint to another and is more common in women than men. It is more prevalent in the obese (because weight increases

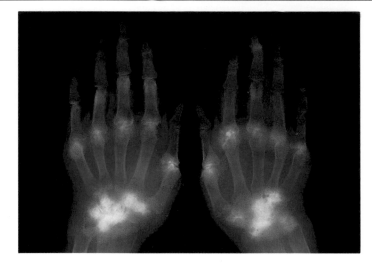

Above: *A false-colour X-ray of a pair of arthritic hands showing typical deformation of the finger joints.*

pressure on the joints) and is also common in athletes who exercise very regularly. Joggers are more prone to arthritis of the feet. No other organs of the body are affected, although the muscles around the joints may become wasted and weak.
Rheumatoid arthritis This is a generalized inflammatory condition affecting young adults and the middle-aged. It occurs commonly in Europe and North America and in temperate climates. A special variety (Still's disease) occurs in young children. It is generally progressive and affects other parts of the body including the muscles, skin, eyes, heart and sometimes lungs. It is associated with low-grade anaemia and is characterized by acute episodes when the joints are swollen, hot and painful. There is also a temperature. Twenty percent of sufferers only experience one episode, but the majority will have relapses and remissions. The most common joints affected are

those of the hands and wrists but, like osteoarthritis, any joint can be involved. The actual cause is unknown but certain factors are thought to play a part, including post-viral infection and stress. An "arthritis personality" has been identified: this is someone who has not expressed grief in the loss of husband/wife/child, or who is bottling up anger. Dietary factors are also felt to be important, and many alternative practitioners will pay great attention to diet (see below). Allergies are also common.
Gouty arthritis This form of arthritis occurs when excess uric acid is circulating in the blood which then crystallizes out into the joints, producing acutely painful and swollen hot joints, typically in the big toe, but also knees and hands. It is generally treatable and does not spread like other forms.

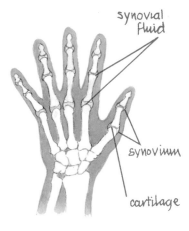

Above: *The body's joints are encased in capsules lined with a membrane that produces a lubricating fluid.*

synovial fluid

synovium

cartilage

SYMPTOMS

▪ Pain, stiffness and redness especially early in the morning.
▪ Weakness and wasting of muscles.
▪ Tiredness and fever.
▪ Coldness of hands and feet.
▪ Trapped nerves in osteo-arthritis can lead to tingling in hands, and the condition called carpal-tunnel syndrome, which causes numbness and pain in the thumb, index and middle fingers.

PREVENTION AND SELF-HELP

Diagnosis is very important to help guide you in your own programme, so a visit to your doctor is essential. Alternative therapies have a large part to play and can help reduce the acute disease as well as prevent recurrences.
▪ Lose weight.
▪ Begin a relaxation and stress reduction programme.
▪ Yoga and gentle exercise, including swimming, will help.
▪ If having difficulty with emotional responses to major life events (death/divorce etc.) consider seeking a counsellor.
▪ Diet can be of vital help.
Anti-arthritis diet
▪ Reduce dairy products.
▪ Cut out red meat and all meat if possible.
▪ Avoid very hot and very cold foods.
▪ Cut out coffee and tea.
▪ Take up herbal teas.
▪ Reduce white flour products.
▪ Fluid fast for one day a week: avoid all solid food and drink clear liquids, such as herbal tea, water, apple juice.

■ Get advice on minerals and vitamin supplements.
■ Avoid acid fruits, including citrus fruits and tomatoes.
■ Take lots of vegetable juice – celery, carrot or beetroot.
■ Experiment with excluding wheat products from your diet.

NATUROPATHY

A naturopathic therapist would explore your lifestyle and prescribe the diet routine outlined above. A controlled fast can be of great help, both in the acute phase and to prevent recurrence, as can a long-term balanced vegan diet. Hydrotherapy has been the mainstay of this approach to arthritis and many sufferers will visit spas to "take the waters". Saunas, steam baths, Epsom Salts baths, mud-packs will all help but care should be taken in the acute phase of the disease. Additional supplements include sulphur-rich foods, Vitamins A, B and C, evening primrose oil, kelp or seaweed and mussel extract which can help in the short term.

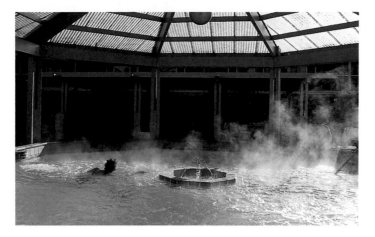

You will be advised to take up gentle stretching exercises, and if your practitioner is trained in cranial osteopathy, this may well be effective.

HOMEOPATHY

Rhus tox. and *Ruta* are two general remedies you may try as a self-help measure, but a proper homeopathic diagnosis will help to suggest more specific remedies. Constitutional remedies would be identified to

Above: *Taking the waters in a health spa is a mainstay of the naturopathic treatment of arthritis.*

help address the underlying problem and *Sepia* and *Pulsatilla* could be tried: take one tablet, 6x, twice a day for four days.

ACUPUNCTURE

A course of acupuncture with moxibustion can help both in the acute phase to reduce inflammation, and also in the chronic phase to reduce pain and stiffness. The Chinese believe arthritis is caused by a blockage in Chi caused by one or other factors (cold, damp, heat or wind) and they will determine treatment depending on which factor is predominant. Attention to diet and the prescribing of herbs (root ginger) will form part of the comprehensive management of the illness.

HERBAL MEDICINE

Devil's claw is the traditional remedy and drug companies have now isolated the chemical believed to be the effective ingredient. Infusions of alfalfa and ginger are prescribed as an addition to the diet, and teas of parsley, willow, primula are all commonly used. Lignum vitae and wild yams are used in acute attacks of rheumatoid arthritis.

ACUPRESSURE

Acupressure to release pain as a first-aid measure should also be tried regularly.

OSTEOPATHY AND CHIROPRACTIC

Manipulative therapies may be useful to relieve stiffness and help mobility, but should not be applied in the acute stages. The practitioner needs careful expertise to avoid causing further damage. Much more helpful is gentle massage and reflexology.

OTHER THERAPIES

All forms of stress reduction (autogenic training, meditation, relaxation, bio-feedback) can be used to reduce pain and alleviate distress. Aromatherapy oils, e.g. chamomile rubbed into the joint, are helpful, and the following can be added to a hot bath – pine, lavender, juniper. Traditional folk medicine is very common in dealing with this complaint. Traditional remedies range from the copper bracelet through to cider-vinegar drinks, honey, pollen and, most importantly, royal jelly.

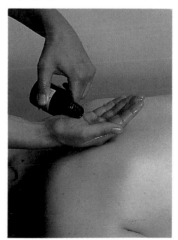

Above: *A massage with aromatherapy oils is a pleasant way to ease the stress and discomfort of arthritis.*

Site of pain	Acupressure point	How to find it
Pain in upper back	Gall Bladder 21	Midway between the shoulder and the spine. Apply pressure angled downwards.
Pain in lower back	Urinary Bladder 23	Two fingers' width from the centre of the spine at the level of the waist. Apply gentle pressure with thumbs.
Pain in hands	Large Intestine 4	Spread out the thumb and forefinger. The point is at the centre of the triangle created by the fold of skin. Apply pressure with the thumb directing it towards the wrist.
Pain in hips	Gall Bladder 30	In the "hollow" on the side of the buttock underneath the thigh bone. Press firmly into the hollow and maintain pressure for two minutes.
Pain in knees	Knee acupoints	There are two depressions on either side of the ligament below the knee cap. These should be pressed firmly with finger and thumb, the pressure being angled towards the knee cap.

ORTHODOX TREATMENT

Rest and analgesics are the mainstay of treatment initially. Physiotherapy, ultrasound treatment and hydrotherapy are then introduced. As far as drug medication is concerned, anti-inflammatories are regularly prescribed, as are steroid tablets, usually in short courses only. Gold injections in very severe cases may also be prescribed. Surgery in osteoarthritis is now common and replacement hip and knee joints can give people a new lease of life.

BACK PAIN

A problem that will affect 80 out of 100 people in any one year, back pain costs 33 million working days annually in the UK alone. The lost working time amounts to billions of dollars in the USA, and the economic effects of this malady are more important to Western economies than all the strikes, go-slows and recession periods of growth put together. It probably accounts also for the rapid growth of alternative therapies in the UK, USA and Europe as it is cited as the most common reason for people turning to complementary therapies by seeking treatment from osteopaths and chiropractors.

CAUSES

There are very many causes of back pain, some having little to do with the spine, so it is important to seek proper diagnosis, especially if the problem is recurrent and causes you to stay off work. The spine can be thought of as the "central pole" holding up the tent of the body, so that if it is stiff or twisted, it can affect all the other organs as well. It is made up of 33 bones in total: 24 small bones called vertebrae (seven in the neck, cervical, 12 in the chest, thoracic, five in the lower back, lumbar). Below these are the sacral bones which consist of five fused bones, and the last one or tail bone is made of four fused vertebrae and is called the coccyx. Each vertebra is made up

of a body, spine and facet joints. The spinal cord runs through the middle and the nerves supplying muscles and skin come out of each side of an opening formed by two vertebrae. Between each vertebra is the "disc" or spongy cushion which acts as a "spring" keeping the spine flexible and absorbing many of the shocks and pressure when we exercise or move. The facetal joints are surrounded by ligaments to which are attached the muscles. Back pain can arise from any of these areas (bone, disc, joint nerves, ligaments, muscles) and an

Below: *The spine consists of a column of 33 vertebrae. Discs made of cartilage are found between vertebrae; they act as shock absorbers.*

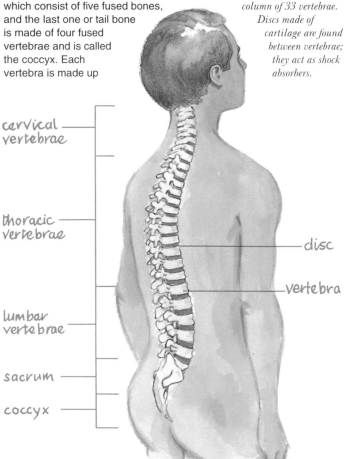

cervical vertebrae

thoracic vertebrae

disc

vertebra

lumbar vertebrae

sacrum

coccyx

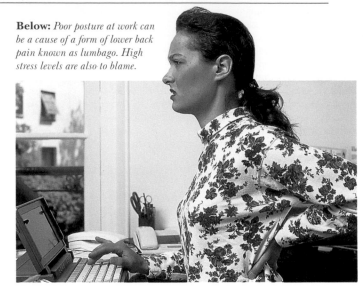

Below: *Poor posture at work can be a cause of a form of lower back pain known as lumbago. High stress levels are also to blame.*

accurate diagnosis will help treatment and recovery. Although everyone is subject to back pain, certain occupations and age groups are more likely to suffer attacks. These include manual workers, clerical workers, sportsmen and women who injure their backs especially in contact sports, people who are obese, because of the pressure on their spines. Arthritis may develop as a consequence. Elderly and extremely tall people are also prone to suffer. Other causes of back pain include referred pain from gynaecological causes, especially in late pregnancy.

The pain may be acute and searing and be referred down the leg as far as the ankle (sciatica), or it can be dull, aching, and made worse by movement or coughing. It can occur when lifting heavy objects, or playing sport, or bending over rapidly to pick something up – even tying your shoe lace. It is often the result of poor posture or an unsupported car seat, office chair or soft mattress. It often arises at times of stress and can be a sign of unresolved mental conflict. Chronic back pain often has a psychological component to it which will need exploring.

Causes of specific back pain		
Lower back	**Upper back**	**Neck**
Fibrositis	Fibrositis	Cervical spondylosis
Kidney trouble	Sprain/strain	Muscle tension
Osteoarthritis	Osteochondritis	Torticollis (wry neck)
Slipped disc	(degeneration of	
Sciatica	growing point in	
Osteoporosis	spine)	
(soft bones)	Pleurisy	
Cancer	Scoliosis (curved	
Ankylosing	spine)	
spondylitis	Shingles	
(brittle spine)	Infections of the spine	

PREVENTION AND SELF-HELP

- Check all your furniture and ensure that your back is supported well.
- Follow a regular exercise routine – try Yoga, T'ai-chi, or the Alexander Technique.
- Take care over everyday activities, like lifting, or bending.
- Treat the acute symptom with rest, heat, hydrotherapy, pain-killers.
- Seek help from an osteopath or chiropractor.
- Approach your doctor for an X-ray if the pain persists, or if there is doubt about the diagnosis.
- Take *Rhus tox.* 6x or *Arnica* 6x, one tablet every two hours in the acute stages (**not appropriate for children**).

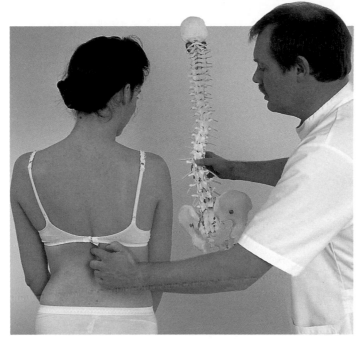

Above: *An osteopath explaining the cause of scoliosis to a patient. Back pain is the commonest reason why people visit osteopaths.*

- Have regular massage and aromatherapy treatment to relax your muscles.
- Seek the help of a counsellor if the problem is recurrent and you have identified a high level of stress or conflict.

OSTEOPATHY AND CHIROPRACTIC

These are the most effective therapies to pursue initially and it is best to seek the help of someone known to you, your friends or your doctor. He/she will examine you, possibly take X-rays and proceed after proper diagnosis to manipulate your spine. Up to six or ten treatments may be necessary and a regular annual check may be advisable. The therapist will suggest a course of exercises or may ask you to attend Alexander classes or take up Yoga.

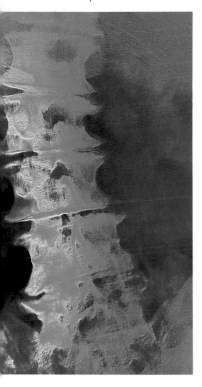

Above: *An X-ray of a patient with scoliosis, curvature of the spine, caused here by osteoarthritis.*

ACUPUNCTURE

This can be equally effective in both acute and chronic cases and can shorten the period of pain and stiffness dramatically. Moxibustion may be used. Treatment will be focused on improving the circulation of Chi and the precise points treated will depend on the type and locality of the pain: again, exercises would be suggested including Yoga.

HERBAL MEDICINE

Herbal prescriptions are unlikely to help greatly other than by relieving the acute symptoms of pain and stiffness, and improving relaxation and circulation.

HOMEOPATHY

Homeopathy would only be used as a first aid measure and continued until an accurate constitutional remedy is identified. It is better to seek the help of an osteopath or chiropractor or Chinese practitioner.

MASSAGE AND AROMATHERAPY

These can be particularly helpful to deal with minor muscle strains and aches, but should be undertaken only after appropriate diagnosis from a qualified practitioner. Regular massage of the large muscles of the neck will help with neck pain and shoulder aches, as this is often the result of spasm of the powerful trapezius muscle.

Below: *An osteopath applying a longitudinal stretching technique to the spine of a patient with the aim of realigning the vertebrae correctly.*

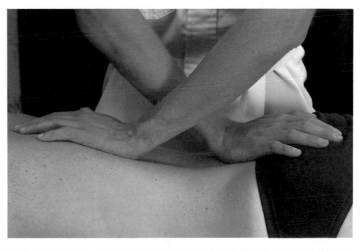

ORTHODOX TREATMENT

Increasingly doctors are working with osteopaths and chiropractors as the results of such treatment are proving so effective. Traditionally, rest and pain killers in the acute stages followed by heat, physiotherapy and ultrasound are the cornerstones of treatment. Where there is severe damage or pressure on one of the spinal nerves, then an operation is undertaken to remove the damaged disc and fuse the vertebrae. This avoids further trouble but it means that the spine remains inflexible. Surgery should be seen as a measure of last resort and an osteopathic or chiropractic assessment is particularly helpful to assist you to make a decision about such a course of action. Whichever treatment option you choose, the self-help programme outlined is essential to ensure that you do not suffer a recurrence.

SPRAINS AND STRAINS

The terms sprain and strain are not always accurately used, and occasionally (and incorrectly) they are interchanged. However, they have distinct meanings. A sprain is usually the result of an injury to a ligament (the strong, tough, inelastic bands of fibre that hold the ends of bones together around a joint); these ligaments can be sprained in an acute sports injury when the ligament is stretched, torn or ruptured, or as a result of chronic overuse or stretching, especially during pregnancy. Strains are injuries to muscles or tendons (the fibrous cords that join muscles to bones or muscles to other muscles). They can occur as a result of an acute injury, chronic overuse or poor posture.

CAUSES OF SPRAINS

Sprains involve damage to the ligaments surrounding a joint. They are caused by sudden injury or occur as a result of a period of chronic overuse.

SYMPTOMS OF SPRAINS

They will include pain, swelling, bruising and, in severe cases, the joint will become unstable. A particular form of ligament sprain affects the joints surrounding the vertebrae of the neck – the whiplash syndrome. This occurs when the head is bent forcibly backwards following a car accident. This injury may be difficult to spot and symptoms may only present a few days later (stiff neck, bruising and unstable joints). All severe sprains should be examined by a doctor and X-rays taken to exclude fractures. Chronic ligamental sprains occur mostly in the back leading to low-back pain, especially after inactivity. These are mostly the result of poor posture, lack of exercise, sleeping on soft mattresses or long car journeys.

PREVENTION AND SELF-HELP FOR SPRAINS

- Always wear appropriate sports wear.
- Never exercise from "cold" – take time to warm up slowly.
- Learn the appropriate stretching exercises.
- Gradually increase the strength and flexibility of your joints (i.e. by taking up Yoga).
- Wear protective and supportive clothing, especially around joints.
- Ensure chairs, beds, settees etc. all provide support at the lower back.
- Do not drive long distances without stopping for a stretch.
- Take long hot baths to ensure you relax your muscles.

Below: *This is an electron micrograph of skeletal muscle fibres magnified 500 times. Injuries to the tissue of a muscle are known as strains.*

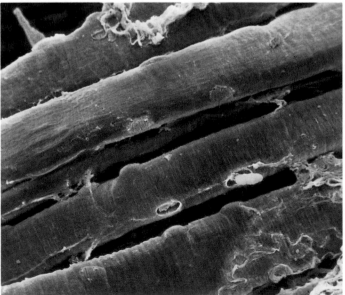

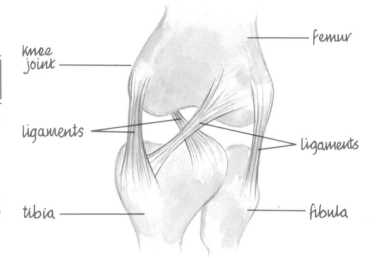

knee joint

ligaments

tibia

femur

ligaments

fibula

IMMEDIATE TREATMENT

Remember **R I C E**. This acronym stand for Rest–Ice–Compression–Elevation.
On feeling an injury, it is important to stop the activity at once, and rest the injured limb. If possible put some ice-cubes in a polythene bag or a packet of frozen vegetables, wrap a thin towel around it and place this cold compress on the injured joint. Do not prolong this for more than 20-30 minutes at a time, but it can be repeated three to four times a day. Compress the joint with a firm (but not too tight) elasticated crêpe bandage and elevate the limb, as this may slow any internal bleeding. Painkillers may be appropriate. While there is pain, the joint should be rested, but gentle movement may be attempted to ease the muscles.

MASSAGE

This will help but it requires expertise as too vigorous a massage may be harmful. However, gentle effleurage will help disperse swellings and the

Above: *Ligaments are tough bands of tissue that bind bones together around a joint, such as the knee joint. Sprains are injuries to ligaments.*

formation of adhesions (when normally unconnected parts of body tissue stick together, often as the result of inflammation). Further treatment will depend on the level of pain and gentle petrissage may be attempted.

AROMATHERAPY

Aromatherapy combined with massage is extremely helpful – apply hyssop and marjoram oils (two drops in a teaspoon of carrier oil). Only apply to the injured part if there is no skin break. A compress impregnated with the same oils can be used. Add five drops of oil to a bowl of water. Soak a towel or tablecloth in the solution and wrap it around the joint. Secure it in position, and leave on the joint for two or three hours.

HOMEOPATHY

A moist compress of *Arnica* is helpful. Add ten drops of mother

tincture of *Arnica* to 30cl (half a pint) of water. Soak a towel and place it on the injured joint. Bandage the compress in position.
Take *Arnica* 30x hourly for six doses, then *Rhus tox.* 6x, three times a day for six days. *Ruta* 6x is sometimes recommended if there is much swelling and bruising (one three times a day).

CHILDREN: Many take the same dose as adults.

ACUPUNCTURE

This can help relieve pain and stiffness but would need to be applied by an expert.

ACUPRESSURE

For ankle sprains point Urinary Bladder 60 (on the outside edge of the ankle behind the prominent bone in the depression) is recommended. Apply pressure for up to two minutes – downwards towards the sole of the foot.

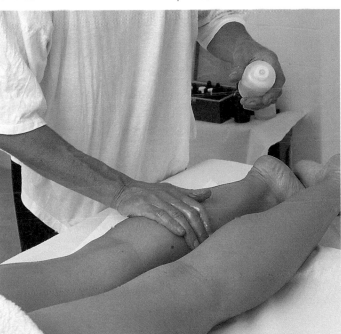

CAUSES OF STRAINS

Muscle strains may result from a direct blow in a contact sport or a tear due to over-extending the particular muscle. These often occur if the muscle is "cold" or fatigued or if there is extreme

Below: *Stimulation of the Urinary Bladder 60 acupoint is recommended for easing painful ankle sprains.*

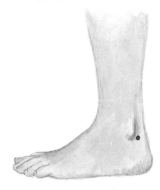

Below: *If you suffer a muscle strain in the leg, massage by a qualified practitioner has much to recommend it.*

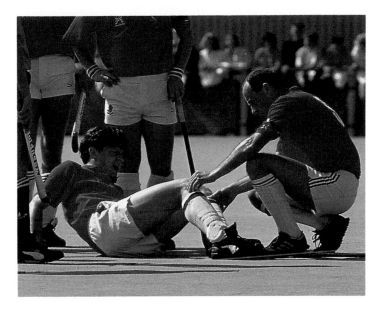

pressure to win in a competitive sport and the individual over-extends him/herself. Often there will be pain, bruising, swelling, and discoloration may follow after a few hours.
Chronic muscle strain is probably one of the most common causes of pain in the back, neck, shoulders or head. This is often the result of poor posture, tense muscles from anxiety or worry, and general unfitness. Any repetitive job that requires you to sit or stand for long periods may produce spasm in the muscles leading to stooped shoulders or back, and causing pain. Psychological tension and stress will often result in muscle spasms which may be acute, leading to a "tic" or tremor, or chronic, leading to low-level discomfort and pain. Coffee and strong tea can predispose to muscle strain as they may stimulate the muscles directly.
Strains of the tendons arise for similar reasons to muscle strains, but a particular variety known as "overuse" syndrome, or the repetitive strain injury, is caused by constant repetitive movements. This is usually associated with operating a

Above: *Sports injuries are probably the only drawback of an exercise regime. If you are injured, it is important to rest the affected limb.*

machine (typewriter, keyboard, piano) or repeating actions in sport (resulting in tennis elbow, golfer's elbow, etc.).
Shin splints are common in joggers and are the result of constant strain on the muscles along the front of the lower leg, which gives rise to pain. Occasionally overuse may lead to rupture of the tendon and occurs around the Achilles heel (the tendon at the back of the ankle).

PREVENTION AND SELF-HELP

The same advice applies for strains as for sprains. Chronic muscle strain can be relieved by a regular exercise programme, and by practising a regular relaxation routine. Frequent hot/cold baths are recommended, as well as regular rest periods and, if necessary, the wearing of support bandages or splints. All forms of alternative treatment suggested for sprains are applicable to strains.

ORTHODOX TREATMENT

Most doctors will suggest Rest-Ice-Compression-Elevation to begin with, having first excluded serious injury that may need splinting or immobilizing in plaster. Painkillers will be given and some sports physicians prescribe enzyme drugs to reduce clotting and bruising. Physiotherapy and ultrasound (which reduces pain and swelling) will also be offered. In cases of chronic strain or sprain, local injections of an anaesthetic, together with a steroid, may be suggested and this has proved very helpful for long-standing problems.

STIFF NECK

The neck contains many vital organs, other than the seven cervical vertebrae that join the skull to the thoracic vertebrae, which may be the site of disease. In front of the spine lies the gullet (oesophagus and the wind pipe). To the side lies the thyroid gland and dotted around the neck are the lymph glands that may swell and become tender during infections.

CAUSES

A serious and life-threatening cause of stiff neck associated with vomiting and headache is meningitis. Young adults are prone to glandular fever which may cause large lymph gland swellings in the neck. Most neck pain is the result of tense muscles (particularly the sternocleido-mastoid and trapezius muscles), often caused by prolonged sitting in front of a desk or VDU. Long car journeys will also cause stiff neck. In elderly people cervical spondylosis caused by degeneration of the spine and the development of osteoarthritis is relatively common. Wry neck or torticollis is another common cause of stiff neck and is often the result of an awkward movement or poor sleeping posture resulting in a "trapped nerve" leading to a stiff, painful muscle which is often in spasm. A whiplash injury when the neck is

Below: *Neck rolls can ease away pain. Roll your head slowly in a clockwise direction, inhaling as the head comes up and exhaling as it sinks down, then repeat in an anti-clockwise direction. Keep the movements loose and relaxed.*

thrown forward as a result of a car injury may leave the victim liable to repeated attacks of stiff neck.

SYMPTOMS

It is not uncommon for wry neck to present on waking up in pain and with an inability to move the neck to the centre. The head is locked in a particular position and it may be very painful to move.

PREVENTION AND SELF-HELP

Choose a good office chair that is adjustable in height and allows you to lean forward. Preferably, it should be possible to tilt it backwards to allow you to relax from time to time. Adjust the height of your seat so that your feet reach the floor and can take some of your weight. When driving long distances, try consciously to relax your neck and buy a neck support to fit onto your driving seat. In bed make sure you use enough pillows – experiment to find the right number for you. Practise exercises to avoid stiff neck such as those illustrated.

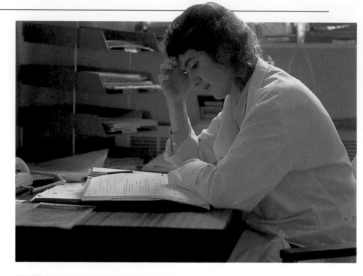

ACUPUNCTURE, OSTEOPATHY AND CHIROPRACTIC

These will all be appropriate for the treatment of neck pain, but you will need to be seen by a trained practitioner.

MASSAGE

Relief can be obtained from massage, applied either by yourself or a partner. Use lavender oils to relax the muscles and apply firm stroking

Above: *Poor posture at work and tension in the muscles of the upper body commonly cause a stiff neck.*

movements down the back. Also use the acupressure point Gall Bladder 21 in the centre of the big shoulder muscle mid-way between the shoulder and the neck (see entry on Fibrositis opposite). Electric hand-held massage vibrators can be a great help, as can warm baths containing six drops of essential oils, such as rosemary, cedarwood or benzoin.

1
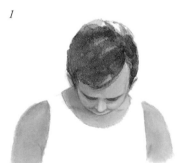

2
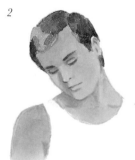

3
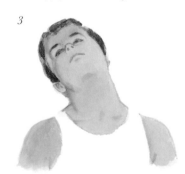

4
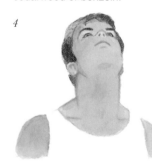

ORTHODOX TREATMENT

X-rays will be taken to exclude severe bone disease as a cause of the pain. Analgesics are prescribed together with the wearing of a neck collar. In more severe cases a course of physiotherapy or ultrasound is prescribed and very occasionally the vertebrae are fused by a surgical operation to stop them moving, so preventing them from trapping sensitive nerves. A course of neck exercises or postural retraining, such as the Alexander technique, may be very helpful in preventing further attacks.

FIBROSITIS

Fibrositis is a word in common use which is not a clearly defined medical term but which has come to mean localized pain in any part of the body – usually the back or shoulders – resulting from chronic muscular tension. In osteopathic textbooks it usually implies the sustained contraction of isolated muscle groups. The latter are often referred to as trigger points.

CAUSES

The common cause is poor posture, such as results from sitting over a desk for long periods, or poor alignment of the spine. Work that involves holding any part of the body in one position (typewriting, repetitive factory work) will introduce a state of muscular spasm Exceptionally tall people who "stoop" to reduce their height are more prone to fibrositis. Psychological causes of muscle tension such as fear, anxiety or frustration will predispose to muscle spasm. Overuse of coffee, tea, alcohol and certain foods (if you are allergic to eggs or wheat), long car journeys, lack of exercise, poor posture and a soft bed are all known factors.

SYMPTOMS

Generalized aching of muscles, with specific pain from tender spots (trigger points), are the signs of chronic muscle tension. Occasionally the pain may be felt

Below: *Here an osteopath mobilizes the neck of a patient. Tense muscles can trigger off pain around the body.*

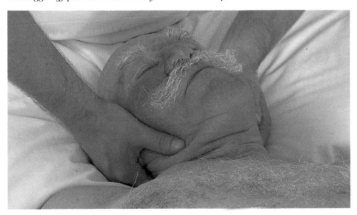

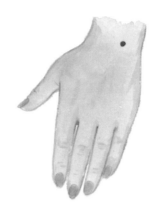

Above: *The Triple Heater 4 point is useful for allaying low back pain.*

some distance away from the tense muscles (this is known as referred pain) and the spine may "adjust' to avoid further strain. Sometimes one can actually feel "knots" of muscles. These are the contracted muscle fibres that can feel like cords – tight and taut!

PREVENTION AND SELF-HELP

◼ Regular exercise, especially Yoga, T'ai-chi, or the Alexander technique.

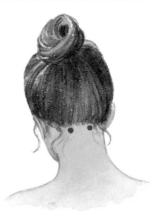

Above: *Try pressure on the Gall Bladder 20 points for neck ache.*

◼ Check your bed, chair and car seat to ensure they do not induce poor posture.
◼ Avoid spending long periods of time in one fixed position.
◼ Practise neck-rolling exercises and stretches.

MASSAGE

A general relaxation massage with long strokes along the back and the neck can provide relief from pain. Trigger points that are located especially around the neck and shoulders will be painful if pressed firmly. These areas should be massaged firmly and for sufficient time (five minutes) to allow the muscles to relax. Sometimes the neck may go into spasm and become more painful.

AROMATHERAPY

The use of aromatherapy oils, especially benzoin and cedarwood, is recommended. Apply either as a massage oil, (½ teaspoon in ½ cup of carrier oil) or three drops of essential oil may be added to a warm bath.

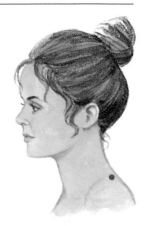

Above: *Further down the meridian are the Gall Bladder 21 acupoints.*

ACUPRESSURE

There will be several points that may be treated, depending on where the pain is located and if the muscle is in spasm. Generally pressing over the trigger point will help induce relaxation. The three main points to stimulate to relieve back pain are:
◼ Low back pain: Triple Heater 4. Run your left index finger between the knuckle of your ring and little finger to just above the wrist, where there is a little depression Press firmly for up to three minutes.
◼ Neck pain: Gall Bladder 20. These points are located at the back of the head between the bottom of the skull and neck muscles about two fingers' width either side of the midline. Apply pressure angled upwards towards the skull.
◼ Shoulder and upper back: Gall Bladder 21. Half way between the shoulder and the spine in line with the last vertebra of the neck. Apply pressure for up to three minutes, angled downwards into the shoulder muscle.

ORTHODOX TREATMENT

Doctors will usually prescribe pain killers or anti-inflammatory creams. Occasionally an injection of a local anaesthetic or cortisone will be used. Physiotherapy is suggested, together with heat and ultrasound treatment, for longstanding problems.

OSTEOPOROSIS

The term "osteoporosis" means "porous bones" and the condition results from loss of bone tissue leading to weakening of the skeleton and a consequent predisposition to fractures. It is an increasingly common disorder affecting mainly post-menopausal women, because they no longer produce oestrogen, the hormone which helps maintain bone mass. It has recently attracted a lot of publicity because of the new HRT medical treatments offered by some orthodox doctors (see below).

CAUSES

Most people mistakenly believe that this condition results from a lack of calcium. Although calcium is an important component of a healthy diet, the problem seems to lie in the inability of the bones to make use of the calcium, and that this inability is the result of the low oestrogen levels found in post-menopausal women. This explanation is still controversial, but it would be fair to say that most scientists believe there to be three contributory factors: one diet, the second exercise and the third hormonal. Osteoporosis can also occur following long-standing steroid use. It was also identified in astronauts who spent a long time in space in microgravity. Other hormones known to play a part in the causation of osteoporosis include thyroid, calcitonin and the parathyroid hormone.

SYMPTOMS

There may be none and the condition many only be discovered routinely on X-ray when a softening of bone density is noticed together with collapse of the vertebrae. Many minor falls in elderly women will lead to fractures because of their fragile bone structure. Some people will lose up to five cm (two inches) in height and develop a curvature of the spine (dowager's hump). Pain may occasionally occur but it is unusual. There is often a strong family history of osteoporosis.

PREVENTION AND SELF-HELP

Regular exercise appears to retard the development of

Below: *The pits and holes evident in the structure of this vertebra show that bone mass has been lost.*

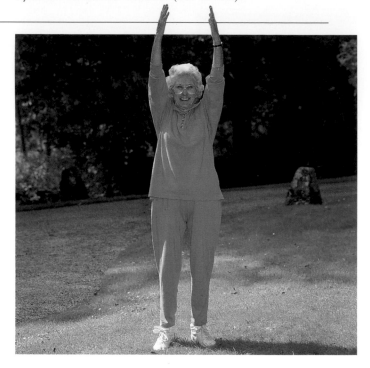

Above: *Osteoporosis commonly afflicts post-menopausal women. Regular exercise helps retard its development.*

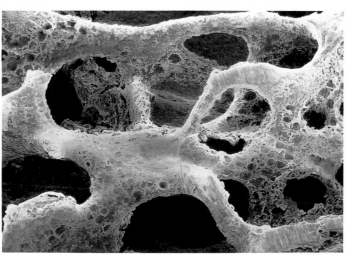

osteoporosis by holding the calcium and protein in the bone. Yoga is probably the most accessible form of exercise, but T'ai-chi, or regular walking or swimming for up to half-an-hour three times a week will also be appropriate. Dietary therapy is controversial because simply taking calcium supplements does not work, nor does drinking extra milk. Some nutritionists believe it is the combination of calcium and magnesium which is important. Avoiding excess phosphorous (found in fizzy drinks) is important and adding supplements of Vitamin C (one tablet a day), folic acid and Vitamin B_6 (one tablet a day) will help. Supplements are not required if you maintain a healthy diet with plenty of fresh fruit, green vegetables and occasional seeds (such as flax, pumpkin) and nuts (almonds). Avoid acidity in drinks and keep to herbal teas.

NATUROPATHY

Naturopaths will recommend a natural wholefood diet together with vitamin and mineral supplements. They will also encourage a regular intake of leafy green vegetables (such as spinach or kale), as well as nut oils (cashew).

ORTHODOX TREATMENT

Recently special bone densitometry tests have become available to measure more precisely the level of bone loss associated with osteoporosis. Treatment for women has included HRT (hormone replacement therapy) which provides the oestrogen that is naturally lost following the menopause. Other treatments include a combination of calcium supplements and a calcium-retaining hormone. These treatments are largely unproven and may lead to undesirable side effects, such as excessive deposits of calcium that may disturb kidney function.

REPETITIVE STRAIN INJURY (RSI)

This is a recently named condition which is not new to medicine, but which has attracted some notoriety in the media. Another name would be the "overuse syndrome" and it occurs in different parts of the body which are subject to constant and repetitive movement. Examples of RSI would include "tennis elbow", "writer's cramp" or "jogger's shin". The more recent publicity has been associated with the increase of computer keyboards leading to symptoms related to the wrists, hands and forearms.

CAUSES

Although still fiercely debated, RSI appears to be a form of chronic tenosynovitis (inflammation of the sheath around a tendon) where the tendons which attach the muscles to the bones become inflamed and develop "rough edges". Stress and psychological factors are known to exacerbate the condition and it is not uncommon in students before examinations.

PREVENTION AND SELF-HELP

Using muscles repeatedly when they have not been stretched first through passive movement and warm-up exercises is a common feature of this condition. Poor posture in

Below: *This piano student suffers from RSI. She is being taught how to modify her technique accordingly.*

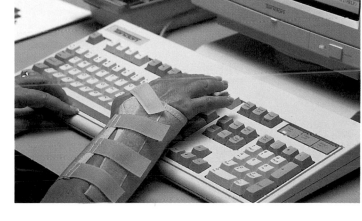

Above: *Keyboard operators appear particularly susceptible to RSI. Special wrist braces are sometimes applied to relieve the symptoms.*

writing or sitting in front of a VDU is a common cause and regular rests together with appropriate eye-guards and filters help to avoid unnecessary eye strain, which may in turn lead to a strained posture. Occasionally various types of splints and supports on the wrists and forearms have been used to help the worker.
Massage is an appropriate preventative and treatment programme.
Hydrotherapy, using ice packs, cold showers, jets, and whirlpool baths will all help. Special mud packs are available in certain health centres.

HOMEOPATHY

Homeopathic treatment includes *Arnica* and *Aconite* 6x (one tablet twice a day for three days).

Arnica cream rubbed over the affected area is a useful first aid measure. *Rhus tox.* 6x and *Ruta* 6x are prescribed for more chronic situations (one tablet three times a day for one week).

ACUPRESSURE

Acupressure points can be used to relieve pain but these will depend on the site of the problem, so the advice of a specialist may be required. The Governing Vessel meridian is often used as it has a sedative effect. Apply pressure along this meridian for two minutes.

OTHER THERAPIES

Relaxation/meditation and counselling can also be important in those conditions that remain chronic.
Acupuncture can be of great help in this condition but needs to be undertaken by an experienced practitioner.

ORTHODOX TREATMENT

It is important to seek a medical opinion if the condition does not respond to general treatments. An X-ray and general blood tests may be required to exclude other causes. Rest and painkillers, especially combined with anti-inflammatory drugs (ibuprofen or ibugel), may be prescribed. Occasionally local injections may be given directly into the joints and special splints applied. It may be necessary to immobilize the wrist and forearm in a plaster of paris cast. Physiotherapy – heat and cold treatment – will also be applied.

BUNION

DESCRIPTION

A painful swelling of the joint on the big toe which can become ulcerated and infectious. It is associated with osteoarthritis of the joint and caused almost always by tight-fitting shoes.

PREVENTION AND SELF-HELP

▪ Avoid all tight shoes and boots, especially in the case of children.
▪ Practise foot exercises daily – scrunching the toes and then spreading them out wide.
▪ Walk barefoot if possible.
▪ Massage toes and feet while having a bath.

ALTERNATIVE THERAPIES

Naturopathy Bathe feet in a mustard bath or a solution of Epsom salts (one tablespoon in a bowl of warm water). Massage around front bone of foot and avoid all tight shoes.
Herbal medicine Celery seeds are often used as an infusion (one teaspoon of seeds in one cup of warm water – take twice a

Below: Though the butt of many jokes, the bursitis known as housemaid's knee is nothing to laugh about.

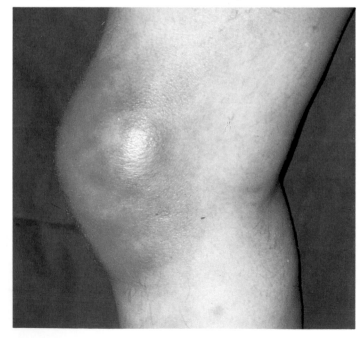

day). Local application of Biostrath Willow (a preparation made from primula and willow) will relieve pain.
Acupuncture will relieve pain.

ORTHODOX TREATMENT

Local treatment will be applied if there is any infection. Special shoes are advised and pain-killers given for arthritis. If the swelling is large, then an operation is undertaken and the excess bone removed.

BURSITIS

DESCRIPTION

A small collection of fluid in a thin sac (a bursa) provides for easy movement when a muscle or tendon moves over the bone. It lubricates and prevents friction. Bursitis is when such a sac is inflamed, injured or enlarged.

PREVENTION AND SELF-HELP

▪ Rest is important, especially if the inflammation is associated with repetitive activity, (see RSI, page 133).
▪ Bandage with crêpe bandage to give support.
▪ Taking pain-killing tablets as necessary.

▪ Apply hot/cold compresses.
▪ Use lavender and eucalyptus oils mixed in a carrier oil and massage around the painful area.

ALTERNATIVE THERAPIES

Osteopathy may help by reducing the pressure on the joint and helping with mobility.
Hydrotherapy Cold compresses (ice packs) alternating with hot towels will help.
Acupuncture will reduce pain and may improve mobility.
Homeopathy. *Apis mel.* 6x or *Rhus tox.* 6x, take one tablet three times a day until pain subsides.

ORTHODOX TREATMENT

Common sites affected by bursitis include the elbow (tennis elbow), the knee (housemaid's knee) or in the heel. Pain, redness, inflammation and swelling are common. Pain-killing tablets, anti-inflammatory pills, injections (steroids) and occasionally surgery are suggested.

CALLUS

DESCRIPTION

A thickened area of skin on the feet or hands that comes from frequent use or friction.

PREVENTION AND SELF-HELP

▪ Avoid tight shoes.
▪ Use a pumice stone in the bath to scrape off old skin.
▪ Check for poor posture, flat fleet or long protruding nails.
▪ Practice foot exercises (see Bunion above).

ALTERNATIVE THERAPIES

Naturopathy Proper attention to footwear is stressed. Soaking feet in a mustard bath and rubbing in almond oil containing essence of lavender (five drops) is also recommended.
Osteopathy will determine if there is poor posture or misalignment of the spine.

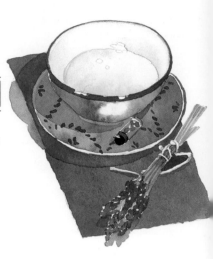

Above: *Lavender oil can soothe aching feet. Applied as part of a foot massage, it is a wonderful tonic.*

ORTHODOX. TREATMENT

This is not a serious ailment unless an underlying orthopaedic condition is involved. Advice on footwear will be provided and a chiropodist suggested who may pare off tough skin.

CARPAL TUNNEL SYDROME

DESCRIPTION

This condition is caused by compression of nerves as they pass from the wrist into the hand. It causes tingling, pain and aching of the hand and arm, occasionally causing mild paralysis.

PREVENTION AND SELF-HELP

▪ Avoid obesity.
▪ Avoid repetitive movements (typing etc.) without proper hand care – taking time to exercise and massage the wrists and forearms.

ALTERNATIVE THERAPIES

Acupuncture may help with symptoms, but if the nerves are tethered this may only be temporary.
Hydrotherapy Alternate cold and hot compresses may help to reduce discomfort.

Naturopathy Supplements of Vitamin B₆ help with nerve conduction.

ORTHODOX TREATMENT

Carpal tunnel syndrome is found commonly in middle-aged women due to a thickening of the sheath through which the nerve passes. It is made worse by obesity, fluid retention and hormone imbalance. Pain-killing drugs and local steroid injections are prescribed. On occasions, the nerves have to be released by a minor operation.

CRAMP

DESCRIPTION

A painful spasm of a muscle either in acute situations during exercise or in the form of troublesome spasms at night, especially in the elderly.

PREVENTION AND SELF-HELP

▪ Do not exercise in cold weather without first warming up.
▪ Do gentle stretching exercises at first to ease the muscles.
▪ Exercise within your limit.
▪ Relaxation exercises help to relieve tense muscles.
▪ Hot baths and proper sportswear will reduce the occurrence of cramps.

Below: *The wrist nerve affected by carpal tunnel syndrome lies under the blue and purple patches in this scan.*

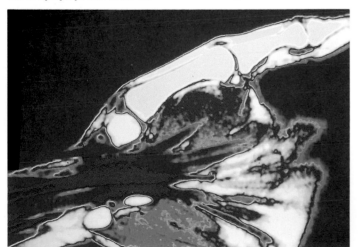

ALTERNATIVE THERAPIES

Massage, gently at first, then with chopping movements of the hands, will release the spasm.
Homeopathy *Cuprum metallicum* and *Colchicum* 6x, one tablet every hour, may help.

CHILDREN: Same dose as for adults.

Naturopathy Therapists will suggest mineral supplements obtained from seeds, nuts and green vegetables.

ORTHODOX TREATMENT

Acute cramp arises because the muscle is overstrained or overstretched and does not have enough oxygen supply. Rest is essential and manually pushing the limb to shorten the muscle will bring about relief. Quinine tablets at night help cramps in the elderly.

FLAT FEET

DESCRIPTION

An absence of or fallen arches of the feet will produce flat feet where the sole rests flat on the ground. This gives rise to pain on standing or walking.

PREVENTION AND SELF-HELP

▪ Wear appropriate footwear.
▪ Standing on the toes and then

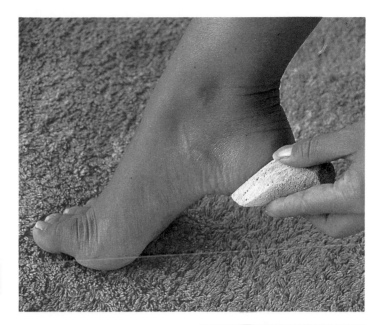

Above: *Using a pumice stone after a bath to scrape off old skin is an effective way to deal with calluses.*

rocking back onto the heels for five minutes a day will strengthen muscles.
▪ Gently massage your feet with a massage oil

ALTERNATIVE THERAPIES

Osteopathy Osteopaths will suggest proper exercises and attention to posture; realignment of the spine will help.
Massage with lavender oils will help relieve tired, aching feet.
Hydrotherapy Alternate cold and hot foot baths are recommended.

ORTHODOX TREATMENT

This is often the result of poor footwear. Foot exercises will be prescribed, and metatarsal pads placed in the shoes. Occasionally physiotherapy will help.

FROZEN SHOULDER

DESCRIPTION

Pain and inability to move the shoulder due to loss of fluid in the joint, inflammation of the tendons or bursitis (see above) can follow lack of use, especially if a wrist is fractured and arm is not moved.

PREVENTION AND SELF-HELP

▪ Be sure to rotate shoulders through all directions, especially if the arm is in a sling for any period of time.
▪ **Acupressure** Press upwards on the front top part of the humerus (upper arm bone) just as it enters the shoulder joint. Then press downwards on the point mid-way between the neck and shoulder just above the collarbone. Press firmly on each point for up to five minutes.

ALTERNATIVE THERAPIES

Osteopathy The problem may arise from misalignment of the spine and careful examination and manipulation is tried.
Homeopathy Try *Rhus tox.* 6x and *Bryonia* 6x – one tablet three times a day for one week.
Massage with warm oils of rosemary or sage can ease the joint.
Hydrotherapy Alternate hot and cold packs with gentle exercising are recommended.

ORTHODOX TREATMENT

Pain-killing drugs together with local injections of steroids are the normal measures taken. Physiotherapy and ultrasound are also used. Occasionally, physically mobilizing the joint under anaesthetic is tried.

ACNE

More than 70 percent of young people will at one time or another develop acne. It often begins around the time of puberty and for almost everyone clears up by their early twenties. It particularly affects the face but lesions may occur on the upper back and chest as well. The acne lesion arises because of a blockage of the sebaceous glands. These are small glands surrounding hair follicles that secrete sebum (an oily substance which keeps the skin moist and acts as a protective layer). If there is overproduction of sebum, which often happens during puberty, it is unable to be secreted because of a blockage, and it collects under the skin, first forming a blackhead, then, because of secondary infection, the lesions develop into infected spots and pustules which can burst causing scarring and pitting.

CAUSES

■ **Heredity** Acne is more common in certain families who appear to have an heriditary disposition towards it.

■ **Androgen hormone** This is the male hormone (secreted by both men and women at puberty) which stimulates the sebaceous glands to secrete more sebum. However, it is not the case that one individual secretes more androgen than another; it appears rather that some people's glands are particularly sensititive to it.

■ **Bacteria** Certain anaerobic bacteria (i.e. those not needing oxygen) live at the base of the hair follicle and will infect a blocked gland. These bacteria break down the fatty acids present in the sebum which then cause further damage to the skin.

■ **Diet** It is popularly believed that a high-fat diet (chocolates etc.) makes acne worse. Although many people improve when following a healthy diet, no scientific evidence has been collected to pinpoint what in the diet is the particular culprit.

SYMPTOMS

■ Small pimples and blackheads on face, back and chest.
■ The pimples become infected and turn into pustules.
■ The pustules burst leaving "pits" and "holes" which cause scarring.

PREVENTION AND SELF-HELP

■ Wash with medicated or detergent soap to remove bacteria from skin.
■ Experiment with your diet (see below), especially avoiding sugar,

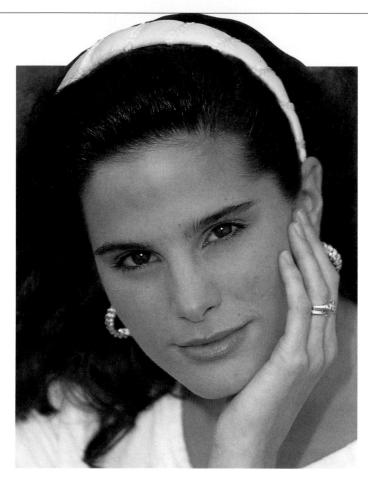

Above: *A clear complexion radiates good health. Acne, on the other hand, can result in loss of self-esteem.*

chocolate, sweets, biscuits and fried foods.

■ Try some of the several skin preparations on the market. They are of two kinds, either abrasives which remove a thin layer of skin and open up skin pores, or antiseptics which kill bacteria.

■ Do not squeeze pimples as this may cause the pus or sebum to be forced deeper in the skin causing further damage.

■ Avoid using greasy cosmetics and oil-based make-up. If you have long hair, tie it back off your face. Wash your hair regularly.

■ Visit your doctor to discuss medical treatment, but at the same time try some of the alternative treatments outlined below.

■ Remember acne is not a serious physical illness – it does go away and spots almost always seem to be worse to the self-conscious sufferer than to his/her friends.

■ If the acne is causing you difficulties with girlfriend/boyfriend, you may wish to discuss the problem with a counsellor.

NATUROPATHY

Naturopathy will emphasise many of the self-help tips and the practitioner may suggest you visit a healthfood store for some natural cosmetics. Local treatment suggested might include dabbing the spots with a garlic clove (a natural antibiotic) before cleansing or using warm lemon juice. Abrasive lotions or the action of scrubbing the face with a loofah can be replaced by using some sea-salt, rubbing it gently into the face in a circular motion and then washing it away with clear water. Diet plays an important part in prevention and care and a wholefood diet with plenty of raw vegetables will be suggested. All dairy products including cheese and eggs should be avoided, and food

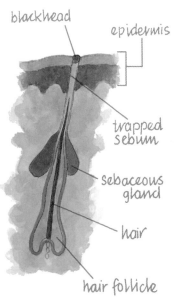

blackhead
epidermis
trapped sebum
sebaceous gland
hair
hair follicle

Above: *Sebaceous glands secrete sebum which helps to lubricate the skin. Over-production of sebum leads to blocked hair follicles and so acne.*

should be steamed or grilled, rather than fried or roasted, thus avoiding the consumption of excess fat. Vitamin A and zinc supplements are also recommended. Research suggests that people with severe acne have low levels of zinc and Vitamin A is known to be a requirement for healthy growth of skin. Vitamin A (found particularly in carrots, green vegetables and tomatoes) is not a harmless substance and its local application to the skin now used in medical treatment should be undertaken with caution. Zinc is found in most natural foods, but supplements are without risk and a daily tablet is worth trying for three months.

HERBAL MEDICINE

Many preparations are available both to nourish the skin and remove and treat infection. Calendula (one teaspoon of tincture in a warm cup of water) is useful, while a chamomile tea-bag in a cup of water can also be tried – bathe the face by dabbing it with the moist teabag. Facial steam baths are helpful to open

the pores in the skin but care must be taken not to scald or burn yourself. Sit in front of a bowl of steaming water in which you have placed some chamomile flowers or sage leaves. Place a towel over your head and allow the steam to bathe your face, but for no longer than 15 minutes. Herbal prescriptions may be given orally to help cleanse the system or balance the hormonal level. These may include burdock, clovers and dandelion.

HOMEOPATHY

Kali bichromicum and *Sulphur* (one tablet, 30c, twice a day for one week) are often prescribed for infected lesions, but practitioners will seek to identify a constitutional remedy as it is believed that acne is an indication of a "miasm" or deep-seated untreated infection. *Lycopodium* at 1m strength has been used with some partial success.

Below: *Diet plays a significant part in the prevention of acne. Avoid fatty, greasy foods and dairy products and try to eat lots of raw vegetables.*

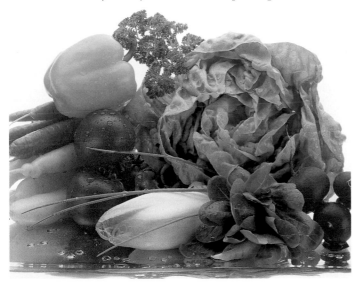

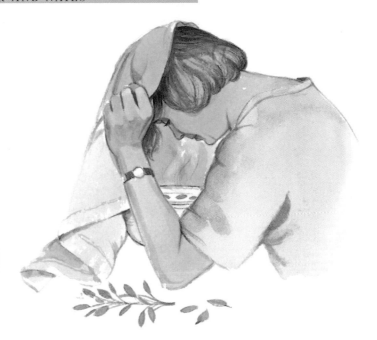

Above: *Facial steam baths are an effective way of opening the pores and cleansing the skin. Try adding some sage leaves to the hot water.*

BIOCHEMIC TISSUE SALTS

Calcarea sulph. is often prescribed: take four tablets every two hours for two days, then reduce to two tablets every four hours for two weeks.

AROMATHERAPY

Bathing the skin with distilled water in which essential oils have been added is often suggested – use two drops each of lavender, juniper and cajuput. Tea-tree oil applied directly to the spots using a cottonwool bud may help to eradicate infection.

ACUPUNCTURE

Although not particularly helpful, it can reduce the emotional stress caused by acne. Chinese practitioners believe acne is caused by wind and heat

affecting the blood and will strive to balance the energy flow in such a way as to reduce their effects. A natural wholefood diet will be suggested and herbs will be prescribed to help elimination of toxins.

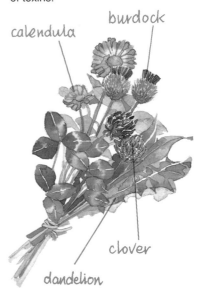

Above: *Herbal remedies prescribed to cleanse the system include calendula, clover, burdock and dandelion.*

ORTHODOX TREATMENT

Conventional doctors will suggest many of the treatments outlined above and will start by prescribing an anti-abrasive ointment. More recently, the long-term use of antibiotics has been shown to be of great help in reducing skin imperfections, but many naturopaths believe they may lead to intestinal and digestive difficulties such as candida. They nevertheless have made a great difference to many acne

sufferers and you will need to discuss the details with your doctor. Treatment needs to carry on for at least six months and some people continue for years. Vitamin A (given as a cream or tablet) is now available, but side-effects are common and medical advice must be followed. U.V. light therapy has proved effective in very severe cases, but occasionally it has been necessary to undertake skin grafting.

ECZEMA

One of the commonest skin conditions, eczema affects people of all ages and is extremely common in infants and children. Eczema or dermatitis is a response of the skin to various factors (see below), and it can run through various patterns and stages. It commences with redness of the skin due to dilation of the small blood vessels there. Thin, watery fluid then accumulates under the skin giving rise to blisters, oedema (fluid accumulation) and itching. If the blisters break down, there is weeping and wheals, which can occur from scratching. This stage is then followed by scab formation, which will heal the skin but may leave it dry, rough, thick and unsightly. On occasion scarring and disfigurement will occur. Eczema can and often does get secondarily infected, which will lead to further damage and scarring. Bleeding is not uncommon, especially where the skin is very thin (for instance, on the shins). Five types of eczema are commonly described: they are contact, atopic, seborrhoeic, varicose and discoid.

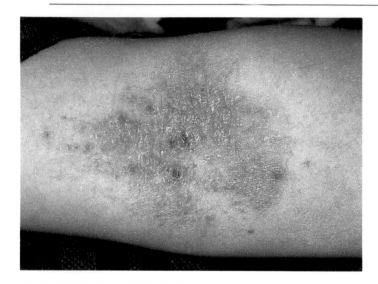

TYPES

Contact eczema As its name suggests, this is often the allergic response of the skin to an external agent that has come in contact with it. Common causes are detergents, watchstraps, perfume, anti-perspirants, deodorant, dyes of all kinds, rubber, plasters, garden plants, nickel and other metals, bracelets and occasionally powders and contraceptives (diaphragms and condoms). The eruption is usually only temporary, and will disappear once the irritant is removed. The eruption shows only on the area that has been in contact with the irritant, but occasionaly scratching may transfer the irritant to other parts of the body.

Atopic eczema This is probably the commonest form, fast appearing in young babies and infants. Usually there is a family history and the cause, although allergic, is not often the result of an external irritant. It can,

Above: *Atopic eczema, such as this, is thought to be caused by a deficiency of linoleic acid in the body.*

however, be made worse through contact. This form of eczema is commonly associated with milk protein allergy, and reaction to eggs and wheat, and an exclusion diet will be a very common approach to treatment. Infants usually get the eruption on face and hands but in older children it will spread to the elbow creases and the knees. This form of eczema presents much more with dry itchy skin than the weepy variety. It can be triggered off by infection and chickenpox is well known to cause a serious relapse. Atopic eczema is associated with later onset of hay-fever and asthma, and forms one of the major allergic conditions. It is thought to be caused by a deficiency in linoleic acid that is necessary for the proper function of the skin capillaries (linoleic acid is found in evening primrose oil).

Seborrhoeic eczema occurs where there is secretion of sebum and is common on the face, external ears, eyebrows and in young infants when it is known as cradle-cap. It causes the scaly encrustation of the eye lids known as blepharitis. Occasionally it affects the front of the chest (the breast-bone). It is not as serious or problematic as atopic eczema and usually causes only minor irritation with little skin thickening. It responds well to treatment.

Varicose eczema This is associated, as the name implies, with varicose veins although this is not always obvious. It occurs on the inside and outside of the legs just above the ankle and can be very problematic for elderly patients because of its constant soreness and weeping. The skin often breaks down into a varicose ulcer, which can be difficult to treat because of the poor blood supply found in the legs of people of an advanced age.

Discoid eczema affects young adults and appears as discs (i.e.

coin-shaped lesions) on the arms and legs, occasionally on the buttocks and lower abdomen, which itch and weep, and often become secondarily infected. This form of eczema is commonly affected by stress and tension and sometimes may be confused with insect bites or stings.

CAUSES

These are particular to each variety (see above), but all eczema is in part related to a hereditary external (contact) or internal (food) allergy which worsens at times of weather change, stress and emotional tension.

SYMPTOMS

They vary with each condition but include:
■ Dry skin which may feel rough to touch and become thickened.

Below: *Discoid eczema is characterized by the appearance of circular lesions. It is affected by stress.*

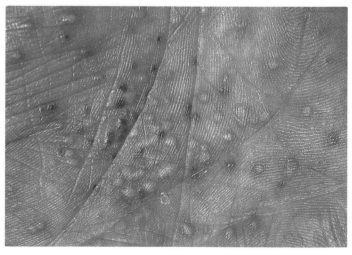

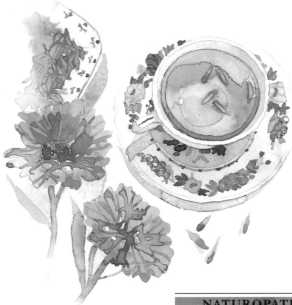

Above: *Marigold tea is one of the mainstays of herbal treatment of eczema. Take two cups a day.*

- Redness and inflammation.
- Swelling, blisters and weeping (wet eczema).
- Infection, scab formation, encrustation and weeping.

PREVENTION AND SELF-HELP

- Accurate diagnosis is important and medical care will be necessary even in mild cases.
- Avoid all material that is known to exacerbate the symptoms.
- Avoid all detergents, especially those containing biological enzymes.
- Exclusion diets, especially in atopic eczema, are well worth a try (see below).
- Try to avoid scratching, especially at night. Special gloves can be worn by small children and, if you cannot resist, rubbing is preferable to scratching.
- Contact your national eczema society as they can offer much guidance and advice.
- Learn to cope with stress and practise a relaxation and breathing exercise.

NATUROPATHY

Great emphasis will be placed on eating a suitable diet including raw fruit (properly washed) and raw vegetables. Avoid milk, eggs, cheese and wheat products, but it is best to do this under qualified supervision. A fluid fast can be tried for no more than 48 hours.

HERBAL MEDICINE

Marigold tea is a well-known treatment and it can also be bought in ointment form (calendula). Drink the tea twice a day or apply the cream three times a day. Other herbs commonly prescribed include nettle, chamomile, dandelion and burdock. A traditional remedy is to apply warm cabbage leaves over the affected areas. Bandage them on the skin overnight.

HOMEOPATHY

This is often very helpful but a precise homeopathic diagnosis is often required. First aid measures include *Sulphur* 6x or *Mercurius* 6x: one tablet every two hours for up to two days. Other remedies include *Graphites*.

CHILDREN: Same dose as for adults.

AROMATHERAPY

Lotions (12 drops of oil to 60ml [2 fl. oz.] of carrier oil) may be tried and the following are often suggested as particularly helpful for this condition: fennel, geranium, sandalwood. These can also be safely used on children.

ACUPUNCTURE

Will also be particularly helpful, especially when combined with Chinese herbs. You will need to seek the advice of a qualified therapist.

ACUPRESSURE

Pressure on the acupoint Large Intestine 4 can be beneficial. You find this by pressing your index

Below: *Eczema seems to be associated with food allergies. Naturopaths recommend raw fruit and avoidance of dairy and wheat products.*

finger and thumb together. Locate the point at the end of the crease so formed. Apply pressure with the thumb angled towards the wrist for about five minutes. This helps to relieve the itching.

Below: *Pressure on the Large Intestine 4 acupoint is particularly useful for controlling pain and itching.*

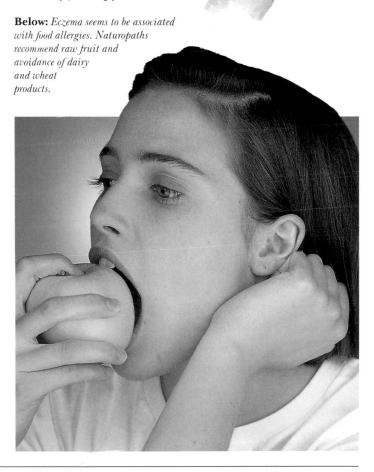

ORTHODOX TREATMENT

Doctors rely on moisturizing cream for dry skin, emulsifying ointments as a soap substitute and a different strength of hydrocortisone applications. These should not be used continuously as not only do they have a damaging effect on the skin, but there is often a rebound phenomenon once they

are stopped. Evening primrose oil is now available for treatment, both in the form of capsules and to apply directly on the lesions. Counselling and stress management are very important in the treatment of eczema, especially for children to help them to adjust to and live with their disease.

PSORIASIS

Psoriasis is a chronic skin condition affecting approximately one person in 50. It causes raised red scaly patches which affect both sides of the body. Lesions are common on the elbows and knees but can occur on all parts of the body including the scalp. Sometimes the lesions are small and circular, others will join up together to form plaques. The nails of the hands and feet are also affected leading to pitting and thickening. One in 20 sufferers will develop arthritis which is similar to rheumatoid arthritis. Psoriasis develops in fair-skinned people and is usually linked to young adults, but children can also develop psoriasis following a sore throat. When examined under a microscope, the lesions appear to affect the small blood vessels, firstly as swelling and then as rapidly growing skin cells.

CAUSES

No cause has been identified but the following factors are felt to be important:
- Heredity – it does occur in families.
- Stress is considered to be an important factor in causing relapses.
- Certain infections and drugs have been known to precipitate an attack.
- Diet is not thought to be a major factor, although alcohol does affect the condition.

SYMPTOMS

Apart from the unsightliness which may be very distressful, there are few other symptoms:
- Itchiness is not uncommon in 20 percent of sufferers.
- Scaliness of the scalp can give rise to troublesome "dandruff".
- Pitting nails do not hurt, but it can lead to permanent damage.
- Arthritis (when it occurs) can be very painful and disabling, involving all joints of the body.

PREVENTION AND SELF-HELP

As so little is known about psoriasis it is difficult to give advice, certainly regarding prevention. Once the condition has been diagnosed, those factors known to exacerbate it need to be managed and controlled. Primarily, this involves reduction in alcohol consumption and reducing stress, if this is an important factor. Certainly relaxation classes, autogenic training and what is termed tertiary prevention (reducing the impact of the disease on the individual) through counselling, have proved effective, not so much in reducing the condition, but in making it seem less of a problem for people to deal with. Alternative therapies have not proved any more successful at treating psoriasis than conventional medicine, and it is

Below: *Psoriasis causes red lesions to appear on the skin. Sometimes these are covered with scales of skin.*

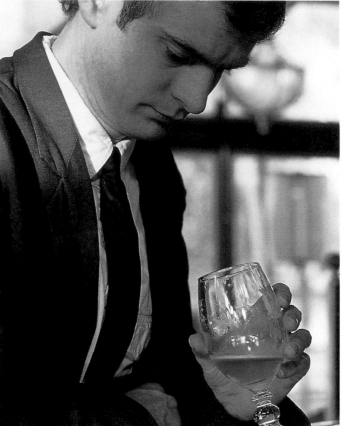

Above: *Stress and alcohol consumption are known to exacerbate psoriasis. Sufferers have to learn how to relax and must cut down on drinking.*

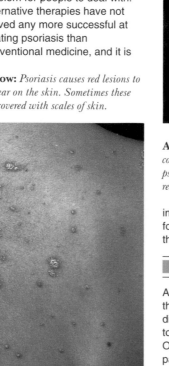

important to seek medical advice for it before embarking on any of the suggestions outlined below.

NATUROPATHY

A naturopath would emphasize the importance of a wholefood diet, together with hydrotherapy to help cleanse the skin. Occasional mud baths and mud packs have been applied, but these should not be tried if there are open lesions on the skin.

However, the general reduction in stress that comes about from visiting a natural health centre or spa may be an important factor in helping patients to improve.

HOMEOPATHY

Again, although not noted for successful treatment of psoriasis, homeopathic remedies are worth trying. *Psorinum, Graphites, Sulphur* and *Petroleum* are all prescribed depending on symptom pattern, distribution of lesions and past history of relapses. Take the 6x dose – one tablet three times a day for four days. Homeopaths will often want you to stop any hydrocortisone ointments that have been prescribed by a doctor, which may actually make the lesions worse. This worsening may also be an indication of "aggravation", a common response in several alternative therapies (the condition gets worse for a while before it gets better). This pattern of response is fairly common in homeopathy and it is important to consult an expert practitioner and follow his or her advice.

HERBAL MEDICINE

Contrary to medical opinion, herbalists believe that diet does play an important part in psoriasis and you may be asked to change to a raw food diet and cut out dairy products as well as meat and fried food. In addition, vitamin supplements (Vitamin B complex – one tablet twice a day) might be prescribed. Specific herbal remedies used include burdock, dandelion, Oregon grape, chamomile and echinacea. The

Below: *Hydrotherapy has proved effective in controlling some cases of psoriasis. The general air of calmness associated with a spa also helps to reduce stress levels.*

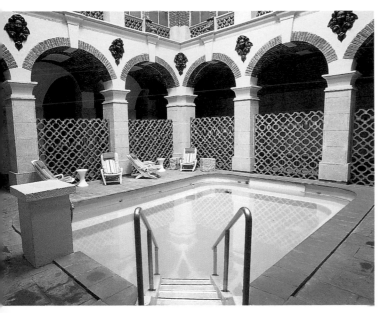

latter increases resistance to infection, a factor felt to be important by alternative practitioners in the causation of psoriasis. Herbal skin lotions would also be prescribed. Again, it is important to consult a qualified practitioner who will make a detailed assessment of the condition.

ACUPUNCTURE

It would not hold out a cure for psoriasis but may improve the general health and wellbeing of the individual sufferer. Chinese medicine sees the skin as being closely linked to the lungs, and treatment would focus on strengthening the flow of Chi between lungs and skin. Infection is thought to block this flow, so that any source of infection, like the tonsils, would be treated separately.

AROMATHERAPY

A white lotion base is suggested when psoriasis is quiescent, and the use of essential oils in the bath help to soothe and heal skin lesions – try three drops of bergamot and lavender oil added to your bath water.

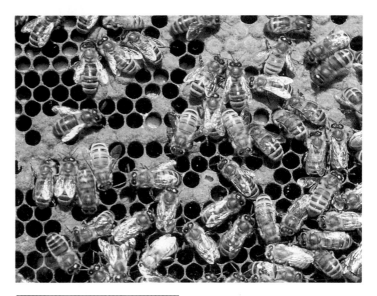

Above: *Bee larvae destined to become queens are fed with Royal Jelly. A folk remedy for psoriasis recommends Royal Jelly in capsule form.*

FOLK REMEDY

A traditional remedy for psoriasis worth trying is Royal Jelly, which can be taken in capsule form. Sunlight or exposure to an ultraviolet lamp can help dry the lesions, but care must be taken not to overexpose the skin to the Sun, as prolonged exposure carries a danger of skin cancer.

CONVENTIONAL MEDICINE

While not being able to cure psoriasis, medical treatments can have a very effective role in making the condition quiescent and removing the symptoms, especially itching. Hair shampoos have been very good at removing scaly lesions and allowing normal hair growth. Local treatments are of three kinds.

Coal tar applications, in the form of pastes, lotions, and scalp application shampoos have been the long-standing treatment for psoriasis. They are effective, but messy and smelly. They also stain clothes and for this reason they are not very popular with the "client".

Dithranol or Lassers paste is a sulphur-containing compound which does not have the cosmetic problems of coal tar, but which

can sting and burn the skin. It comes in various strengths and it is usual to build up gradually.

Steroid applications are by far the commonest and most widely used treatments and there is no doubt they are effective. Steroid-based shampoos can almost keep psoriasis of the scalp at bay. Long-term use of these compounds is not a good idea and in certain cases a rebound effect can occur. The condition gets much worse when the treatment is stopped. Advice and careful monitoring for side-effects is important if one is on steroid treatments.

In severe cases individuals may need to be admitted to hospital and two further treatments are now available.

P.U.V.A. Psoralen-Ultraviolet A light treatment involves taking the substance psoralen and having ultraviolet light exposure. Although very successful, cancer is a more common occurrence after this treatment.

Cytotoxic drugs (which kill body cells) are also effective in severe cases, but can have serious and long-term side-effects.

ORTHODOX TREATMENT

None of the treatments outlined above cures the condition and because psoriasis is characterized by relapses and remissions, many clinicians now believe that it is more useful to help patients adjust to their disease. Those individuals with psoriasis who accept counselling or psychotherapy have three times fewer relapses than those who do not.

RINGWORM AND ATHLETE'S FOOT

These are both examples of fungal infections which affect the superficial layer of the skin and can be very infectious. They are not caused by "worms" but by a type of fungus called tinea. It can infect various parts of the body and the different varieties are found on the scalp (tinea capitis), on the trunk (tinea corporis), and on the groin (tinea cruris). Similar fungal infections affect the space between the toes (athlete's foot) and the vagina (thrush). The fungus lives on the dead horny part of the skin, usually in moist warm areas, and it can also affect the nails leaving them pitted and scarred.

CAUSES AND SYMPTOMS

Tinea capitis Ringworm of the scalp is common in children and is often caught from pets. Usually it causes itching and redness of the scalp followed by hair loss and rings of baldness. The patches may grow and join up leaving the head with a moth-eaten appearance. It is particularly infectious.
Tinea corporis affects the trunk of both adults and children and presents the classic ringworm appearance of a ring of red (sometimes raised) inflamed skin with a pale centre. It may itch, scale and occasionally bleed. One form called pityriasis versicolor affects the skin overlying the rib-cage which can become depigmented so that it

Below: *This is the classic appearance of ringworm. In fact the lesion is caused by a fungus, not a worm.*

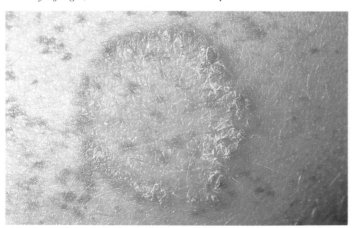

leaves pale areas of skin, which nevertheless recover in sunlight.
Tinea cruris affects the groin area and is common in sportsmen and people who sweat a lot and wear tight underwear. It is often caught in swimming pools.
Athlete's Foot (tinea pedis), like tinea cruris, is commonly caught in swimming pools, is very common and can be difficult to eradicate. It causes itchiness, and scaly white patches of skin between the toes, often because they are not dried well. The fungus causing this is from the family known as Trichophyton, but the treatment for all fungal infections is similar.

PREVENTION AND SELF-HELP

■ Use your own towel especially in swimming areas, dry very carefully between the toes and use talcum powder or a homeopathic calendula ointment.

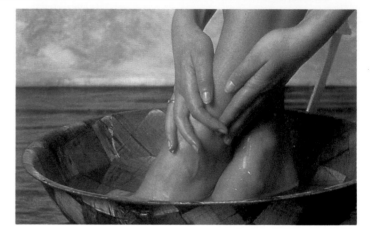

Above: *A footbath containing tagetes will help eradicate the fungal infection that causes athlete's foot.*

■ When possible avoid socks and heavy shoes, and wear sandals to keep the feet dry and well ventilated.
■ Boots and shoes can themselves become infected with the fungus and may need sterilizing or changing if necessary. Socks should be boiled.
■ Avoid tight jockey shorts and wear loose-fitting cotton underwear. Women need to avoid tights and close-fitting jeans if they develop thrush.
■ Apply Vitamin E oil directly on affected areas of the skin, making sure they are dry first

NATUROPATHY

In recurrent infections the diet may need to be examined and all white bread, sugar and

carbohydrates excluded. Calendula ointment is often prescribed and garlic capsules three times a day will help.

AROMATHERAPY

Tea tree essential oil applied directly to the skin lesion on the end of a cotton bud for no more than two seconds will help, as will a special form of marigold known as tagetes (two drops diluted in a bowl of warm water, applied three times a day).

CHILDREN: These remedies should **not** be used on children.

HERBAL MEDICINE

Ready-prepared mixtures with which you can make a herbal footbath can be obtained from healthfood stores or herbalists. Useful herbs to counter this affliction are mustard seed, ginger, aloe, myrrh and rosemary.

ORTHODOX TREATMENT

Fungal infections respond well to treatment with proprietary products in the form of shampoos, lotions, powders or creams. If the fungus is in the nail, a special paint can be applied, or in a severe case an anti-fungal tablet, which has to be taken for at least six weeks, is often prescribed.

BALDNESS

A common and non-serious problem, baldness can nevertheless cause much psychological distress, especially in women. Most male baldness is an hereditary condition which can appear relatively early in a man's life and start with loss over the temples. It results from new hair not growing fast enough to replace natural hair loss. Stress also plays a large part in accelerating hair loss and can be sudden in onset. Often the loss occurs a few days or weeks following the stressful period and may be associated with anaemia and hormonal changes, especially of the thyroid gland. Some women will lose hair during pregnancy, but this is usually only temporary. Scalp and skin conditions such as fungal infections and psoriasis may cause hair loss, and a condition known as alopecia may produce small patches of hair loss, which if extensive can affect the eyebrows and eyelashes as well. The most common cause of alopecia is stress.

PREVENTION AND SELF-HELP

Sensible hair care, avoiding chemical dyes, excessively hot rollers or frequently used dryers is important. Permanent waving works by destroying the hairs' natural keratin, which is a fibrous protein that protects the hair, and should not be used if the hair is thinning. There are now many "natural" hair products sold commercially and these are to be preferred.

Below: *Baldness is often an hereditary condition, mostly affecting men. Stress can also cause hair loss.*

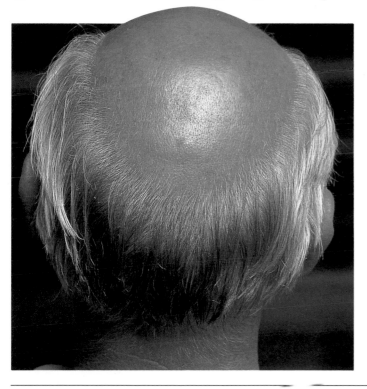

MASSAGE

Massaging the scalp with warm almond oil will not only feel good but reduce tension in the scalp muscles and improve the condition of the hair. This oil can be washed out after massage.

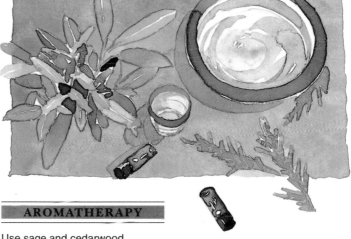

AROMATHERAPY

Use sage and cedarwood essential oils to rub gently into the scalp and move the skin over the bone (prepare this lotion with five drops of essential oil in 30 ml/1½ fl. oz. of surgical spirit). Another way of stimulating the scalp is to use a plum blossom hammer (seven small needle tips mounted on a special instrument) – it is available from acupuncture retailers. Gently tap the scalp with the hammer for a few minutes, repeating several times daily.

HOMEOPATHY

Homeopaths will suggest *Lycopodium* 6x (one tablet twice a day for a month). Baldness associated with pregnancy is often treated with *Sepia* 6x (one tablet twice a day for a week).

Above: *A sage and cedarwood oil scalp rub is not guaranteed to cause new hair growth, but it will feel good!*

DIET

Although not helpful in preventing hereditary baldness, a healthy diet with a plentiful supply of Vitamin A, Vitamin B and zinc is known to ensure healthy shiny hair. These vitamins are found in fish, seaweed, green leafy vegetables, carrots and pumpkin seeds. Avoiding smoking and caffeine will also help with reducing hair loss. Specific causes such as anaemia and thyroid disease all need appropriate treatment.

ORTHODOX TREATMENT

Usually little can be done to prevent baldness unless a specific cause is identified. Local hydrocortisone injections in areas of alopecia have helped to stimulate regrowth. Wigs are often suggested especially for women who lose their hair as a result of chemotherapy while undergoing treatment for cancer. Hair transplants have proved successful and popular for those who are very distressed as a result of premature hair loss.

CHICKENPOX AND SHINGLES

Chickenpox is one of the common childhood infectious diseases caused by a virus (varicella zoster). The same virus will cause shingles in adults (herpes zoster). It is highly contagious, usually occurs in epidemics every two or three years, but for children is not particularly serious, although complications can occur. One attack provides immunity, but the virus can remain dormant in the body, usually on nerve tissue, and can at a later date cause shingles.

SYMPTOMS

Chickenpox After an incubation period of 14-21 days, the child will notice the appearance of small red spots (papules) which usually start on the body and spread to hands, legs and face. Within three to four days the spots become blisters (vesicles) and may burst to form sores which develop a scab. The child remains infectious for about five to seven days after the last spot has appeared, i.e. until all the scabs have formed. Occasionally lesions will occur in the mouth, conjuctiva (the membrane that lines the eyelid), vagina, and, rarely, in the lungs giving rise to pneumonia. They may become secondarily infected and lead to scarring. Chickenpox in a child with eczema, or an adult, can be a much more serious condition and occasionally hospitalization is necessary.

Shingles Usually affects the over-65s and presents occasionally with pain only along one nerve route, across the chest, down the leg, into the face. This may be confused with pleurisy, sciatica or neuralgia, but a few days after the pain, the spots and papules will appear as in chickenpox and may be associated with a temperature.

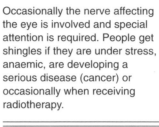

Below: *A mother dabs calamine lotion on her son's chickenpox rash. This helps soothe the itching while the body gradually overcomes the virus.*

Occasionally the nerve affecting the eye is involved and special attention is required. People get shingles if they are under stress, anaemic, are developing a serious disease (cancer) or occasionally when receiving radiotherapy.

PREVENTION AND SELF-HELP

There is no immunization against chickenpox or shingles so avoidance is the only measure that can be taken. Once you have developed the infection, you yourself will be infectious for up to 21 days, or seven days after the last spot has appeared. Chickenpox does not affect an unborn child but the child can be born with chickenpox if a mother in late pregnancy is in contact with it or has not had it herself. Self-help measures include
- Painkillers.
- Rest.
- Cold showers.
- Do not pick the spots.
- Apply calamine lotion to soothe the itchiness.
- Do not cover the spots and keep them dry.

NATUROPATHY

A diet of raw fruit and vegetable juices would be recommended. Honey drinks or orange and lemon juice sweetened with honey are also considered beneficial. A supervised fast for 24-36 hours is another option that might be considered, to stimulate the body's immune system.

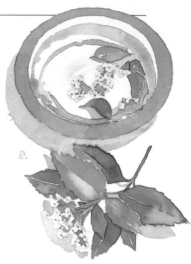

Above: *An herbal palliative: an infusion of elderflower applied to the spots helps to take away the pain.*

HERBAL MEDICINE

Soothe inflammation with an infusion of elderflower dabbed on the spots. Take garlic capsules three times a day and try herbal teas of yarrow, and lime blossom (one cup every two hours).

CHILDREN: For children under 12 and over two, use half the adult dose.

HOMEOPATHY

Rhus tox. 6x will soothe restlessness and irritation. *Antimonium tart.* 6x will help with healing of blisters. In each case, take one tablet every four hours for three days.

CHILDREN: Can take the same dose as adults.

ORTHODOX TREATMENT

Chickenpox is usually a mild condition requiring symptomatic treatment only (calamine, antihistamine). Recently an anti-viral medication has been introduced that can be taken early in the disease process. This helps to reduce the length of the period of the infection and the number of skin lesions that develop.

MEASLES AND GERMAN MEASLES

Measles is one of the most common of childhood infections and is still a major cause of death in developing countries. It has become much rarer in Western Europe and the USA as a result of the mass immunization campaign that began some years ago. It does still sometimes occur but not in the epidemic form it once did. German measles (or rubella) is a less serious viral disease that takes a mild form in children and adults. It is dangerous, however, in the case of pregnant women as it can affect the foetus.

CAUSES

Measles is caused by a small virus particle and the infection is spread by direct contact and by air which contains millions of infectious particles being breathed in. It is a mild disease in most well nourished children, and recovery is swift. It can, however, give rise to complications, such as pneumonia, encephalitis, otitis media (ear infection), but immunization will protect against this eventuality.

SYMPTOMS

▪ High temperature and respiratory symptoms – runny nose, dry cough.
▪ A rash appears on the fourth day as red/purple raised spots which begin behind the ears, spread to the full trunk and eventually cover the whole body. The rash can be felt as well as seen. In the case of German measles, the rash cannot be felt.

▪ Red eyes and conjunctivitis are not uncommon, and occasionally an infection of the middle ear occurs.
▪ Lymph glands may be swollen.
▪ Before the rash appears on the body, it is possible to see spots on the inner side of the cheeks (Koplik's spots).
▪ The incubation period is anything up to twelve days, although it is usually eight. The child is infectious for up to seven days after the rash has first appeared.

PREVENTION AND SELF-HELP

Immunization provides up to 95 percent protection and is usually undertaken routinely at eighteen months. Complications can occur but these are much less than the complications of measles itself. If

Below: *The faint pink rash that is characteristic of German measles. The infection is usually quite mild.*

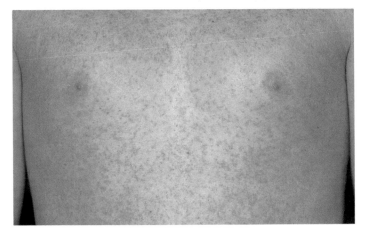

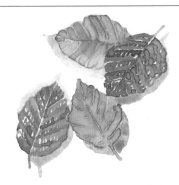

Above: *Witch hazel and water helps soothe itchiness of the skin.*

a child develops the disease, rest, fluids, and temperature-reducing medication are usually all that are required.

HOMEOPATHY

Apis mel. for high temperature.
Euphrasia for red eyes.
Pulsatilla for cough.

CHILDREN: Give a child two drops of the appropriate remedy every two hours for two days.

NATUROPATHY

Vitamin A and C supplementation and fasting when the fever is high are the recommendations here.

HERBAL MEDICINE

To reduce temperature, take an infusion of yarrow and elderflower, one cup twice a day; children half the adult dose. To help itching, dab the skin with a cool infusion of lavender or a teaspoon of distilled witch hazel added to 60cl (one pint) of water.

GERMAN MEASLES

A very mild but infectious disease of children and occasionally adults. It is caused by a virus but may often only present as a "cold" with no evident rash. The importance of German measles is that it can cause genetic deformities in a foetus under 12-14 weeks if the pregnant mother is in contact with a child who has it and has not herself developed immunity to the condition. All pregnant mothers are now tested to see whether they are immune to German measles, and any pregnant mother in doubt about her immunity who comes into contact with someone with the disease should seek advice from her doctor.

SYMPTOMS

German measles presents – normally in children between the ages of six and ten – as a mild respiratory infection followed (usually the same day) by a faint pink rash which may join together to form an area of redness. Occasionally there is some swelling of the glands. The condition is very mild and recovery normally takes place within two to three days. The incubation period is about 14 days and the condition is infectious from five days before the onset of the temperature and rash to five days after. No specific treatment is required because of the mildness of the condition and complications are extremely rare. Immunization is now routine at eighteen months and gives 80 percent protection.

ORTHODOX TREATMENT

Treatment for measles is usually symptomatic. Temperature is reduced with aspirin or paracetamol and antibiotics are given only if there are signs of a secondary infection (usually in the ears or lungs). For German measles, other than general symptomatic treatment (fluid and rest), no specific medical treatment is required or given.

DANDRUFF

Dandruff is a form of seborrhoeic dermatitis which affects the scalp, eyebrows, occasionally the breastbone and outer ears. It arises where sebum is secreted from around hair follicles in the skin and causes the flaky patches of dead skin that appear on the shoulders or clothes. Recently a fungal infection has been isolated from the scalp, and this has revolutionized treatment. One of the factors causing dandruff seems to be the over-production of superficial skin cells. The many local treatments that can be bought over the counter are keratolytics, i.e. drugs that help dissolve and remove excess skin.

CAUSES

For many years it was thought that diet played a part in the causation of dandruff, and since the isolation of the fungus, this theory has been confirmed in that fungal infections are found in people on high carbohydrate diets (i.e. eating a lot of sweets, fried foods). The fungus is known

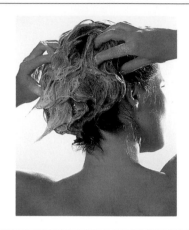

Right: *Why not try one of the many herbal preparations that can be used to improve the condition of your hair?*

as *Pityrosporum ovale* and is a form of yeast.

PREVENTION AND SELF-HELP

Keep to a healthy diet, avoiding sugar and fried foods. Additional Vitamin B, zinc, selenium and Vitamin E will help restore hair growth. Take one multivitamin tablet a day. Natural herbal shampoos include infusions of rosemary or lavender; alternatively, boil 15g (half an ounce) of sage leaves in one litre (one-and-three-quarter pints) of water for five minutes. Leave to infuse for five minutes. Strain, allow to cool and rub the mixture into scalp. Other approaches include using live yoghurt as a hair conditioner. Leave it on for ten minutes, then rinse it away with an infusion of thyme to which two tablespoons of vinegar have been added. Many other rinses can be used, including parsley, chamomile tea and lemon juice or apple cider vinegar in water.

ORTHODOX TREATMENT
Orthodox medicine now prescribes an anti-fungal shampoo and cream which has proved very effective in not only curing the dandruff but also in preventing its reappearance.

HEAD LICE

Head lice are a species of small insect parasite which live on the head sucking blood and causing inflammation and itchiness. Other varieties live on the body and pubic area. Lice are small pinhead-sized insects which are only rarely seen themselves. They lay their eggs which are pearl drop-like in character on the side of the hair shaft. These are known as nits.

CAUSES AND SYMPTOMS

Other than an itching head, lice cause few symptoms. They are very infectious, so whole schools and families can be affected. Lice are caught from close personal contact (sexual, where pubic lice are concerned) but can also be caught from infested bedding, mattresses and towels. Good hygiene practices and keeping to your own personal towels will avoid cross infection.

TREATMENT

Treatment is very effective with anti-lice shampoos which need to be left on for a few hours and then the hair combed with a steel comb to remove all the eggs. Natural product shampoos are not as effective as those obtained from your doctor or chemist, although they will help to reduce inflammation and infection. Washing hair in cider vinegar or rubbing lemon juice on the scalp have been used for adults and

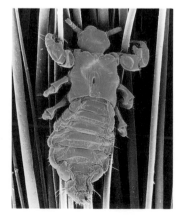

children. However, these actions may not kill all the lice and then re-infection can occur. Any of the shampoos suggested for the treatment of dandruff can help, especially those containing vinegar. The bitter herb, common wormwood, can also be used to kill lice and fleas – it should be scattered among clothes, linen cupboards and in bedlinen.

Left: *This fierce-looking creature is in fact a head louse, magnified 25 times, clinging to shafts of hair.*

ORTHODOX TREATMENT
Head lice are best treated by the orthodox means outlined above. Proprietary anti-louse shampoos are available at local chemists everywhere. They are best left on overnight, and the hair washed and rinsed in the morning.

ITCHING

Itching is a common symptom in many skin disorders, but can also occur as a result of generalized disease. It is important to ascertain the cause, especially in long-standing situations, so that the appropriate treatment can be given. Generalized itching or pruritis can result from allergies, or intolerances to drugs and foods. It can be caused by soap powders, and is a common complaint in severe jaundice, prickly heat and pregnancy (due to hormone changes or other causes). It is not uncommon in the elderly. Stress is another causative factor, leading to neurodermatitis.

CAUSES

Some of the causes of generalized itching are discussed above. However, probably the most common cause is stress, resulting in what has been called neurodermatitis which can occur on most parts of the body, but is often found only where the hand can reach – the back of the neck, forearm etc.

Skin causes include eczema, occasional psoriasis and a condition called lichen planus, which particularly affects the middle-aged Infestation with lice, scabies and other parasites will cause intense itching, as will urticaria (hives or nettle rash) arising from bites, stings and other allergic responses.

Itching of the anus is common, irritating and unpleasant. In children it is often the result of threadworms, and in adults is generally caused by haemorrhoids or other local skin conditions. However, it is often psychological in cause.

Itching of the vagina is most commonly caused by thrush infection or by the use of an inappropriate deodorant or perfume. Skin conditions affecting the vulva cause a marked form of irritation (leukoplakia) but, as with other areas of the body, it can also be a symptom of stress and tension.

PREVENTION AND SELF-HELP

Itching of whatever variety is often made worse by bathing in warm water, and by changes in the pollen count or temperature. Cold baths do help to relieve the problem and are often used as a first aid remedy, especially in the case of stings and bites. It is important to identify the cause of itching but other self-help measures may include:
 ▪ Local application of chickweed, either in the form of an infusion, oil or ointment.

Below: *This angry rash is called urticaria or hives. It is caused by an allergic reaction in the skin cells.*

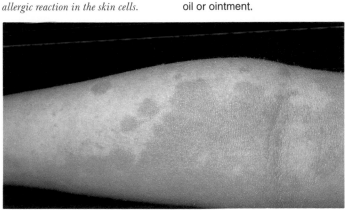

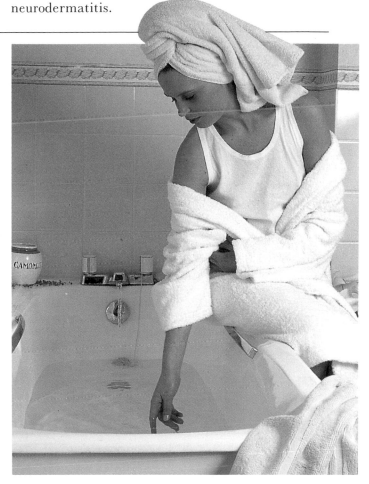

Above: *The agony of itching can be reduced by taking baths in cold water. Avoid getting into warm or hot baths, though; that could make matters worse.*

 ▪ Calendula ointment made from marigold flowers.
 ▪ The oils from sweet almond, avocado or wheatgerm massaged gently into the skin will help prevent the skin from drying out.
 ▪ Aloe vera juice or gel can have a soothing effect.

HOMEOPATHY

Useful remedies include *Apis mel.*, *Sulphur* and *Pulsatilla*. Take one tablet twice a day for three days, 6x potency in all cases. Same dose for children. Specific treatment for skin conditions will depend on accurate diagnosis and if you have to wait to see a homeopathic practitioner, it can be helpful to put yourself on a fluid fast.

ORTHODOX TREATMENT

After a diagnosis, antihistamine creams and tablets are usually the first line of treatment. These may cause drowsiness. Local steroid applications to the anus or vagina are often prescribed to relieve soreness but should not be used long term unless under supervision. Stress management, counselling, relaxation techniques and biofeedback may all help to reduce the psychological element which is often the major factor in chronic itching.

RASHES AND SPOTS

Rashes are both symptoms and signs of disease. They vary tremendously in importance and severity and may be the result of a chronic long-standing condition, e.g. psoriasis, or an acute allergic response, e.g. urticaria. Rashes represent the body's physical response to either infection, allergy or chronic disease. They may or may not be infectious and treatment must always depend on an accurate diagnosis. The appearance of rashes varies; they can be macular (discoloured but not raised), papular (raised), bullous (containing liquid as in chickenpox), pustular (filled with pus as in acne), or scaly as in psoriasis. Rashes may cause loss of pigmentation, and can be itchy or not.

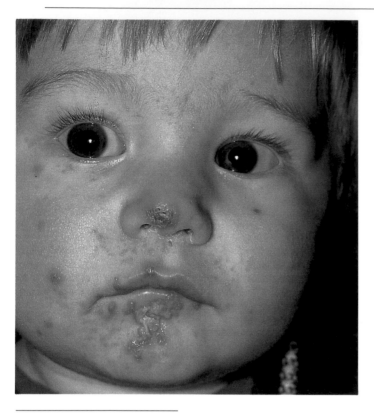

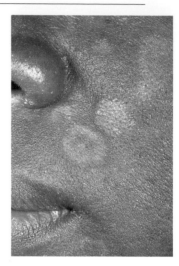

Above: *These discoloured patches of skin are caused by a fungal infection known as pityriasis versicolor. It is not contagious.*

PREVENTION AND SELF-HELP

It is not possible to provide a general guideline to the management of rashes as they vary enormously and a proper medical diagnosis is always necessary to determine appropriate treatment. However, the following precautions are helpful:

▪ Avoid all powerful detergents, especially biological agents for washing children's clothes.
▪ Avoid sunburn which can cause a heat rash, and wear loose clothing in hot weather.
▪ Avoid allergic food if there is a history of allergies.
▪ Reduce or omit dairy products (under guidance) in children with eczema.
▪ Ensure a wholesome and balanced diet.

▪ Consult a doctor if the rash lasts for more than a day and if it is accompanied by temperature or other general symptoms of illness.

Below: *Some rashes affect the whole body and are associated with fever; this is one, a scarlet fever rash.*

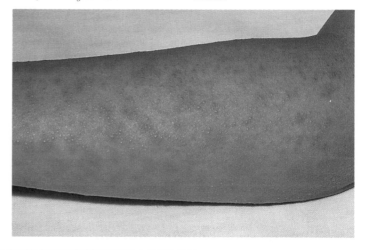

TYPES OF RASH

It is possible to separate rashes into three groups:
Those that affect the whole body and are associated with fever or general disease
These are usually related to infection, e.g. measles, German measles, chickenpox, scarlet fever, glandular fever.
Those that affect the whole body but without general symptoms Sometimes these rashes are further subdivided into those that are itchy, usually due to allergy (food, soaps, detergents, nettle rash, drug

Above: *This poor child has impetigo – a contagious rash on the skin caused by a bacterial infection.*

reaction), eczema, scabies or psoriasis. Less common rashes occur, and they are usually not itchy. Examples of these are pityriasis and ichthyosis.
Those that are localized to one part of the body These may or may not be infectious, e.g. cold sores, impetigo, thrush (all infectious), acne, acne rosacea, contact dermatitis (not infectious). Hot weather can bring up a harmless heat rash, particularly in babies and obese adults.

ORTHODOX TREATMENT

The causes of skin rashes are so varied that it is not possible to give a broad summary of how doctors will treat them here. Specific treatment will depend on an accurate diagnosis, and the reader is directed to the related entries in this book for more detailed information.

NAPPY RASH

This is a fairly common condition in young babies resulting from the skin being in contact with urine. The normal bacteria on the skin will react with the urine to produce ammonia which causes irritation and chafing of the skin. The rash is often around the "line" mark of the nappy, encircling the waist, thighs and buttocks and can be limited to a few red, raised spots. Sometimes the irritation will cause a form of eczema which will make the skin blister and weep. The common complication is infection with thrush (a fungus commonly living in the vagina and intestine). This infection is transmitted from the mother who herself may have symptoms of a vaginal discharge and itching.

CAUSES

It is important not to leave babies for too long in wet nappies, and many of the new disposable variety have the added virtue of being able to protect the skin from urine soaking through. Any infection in the mother should be treated at the same time,

Below: *Nappy rash occurs because bacteria present on the skin react with the baby's urine to produce ammonia which irritates the skin.*

otherwise re-infection is common. Thrush can sometimes be present in the baby's mouth and be caused by unsterilized teats and bottles.

PREVENTION AND SELF-HELP

Frequent changing and the use of nappy liners are to be recommended. Try not using plastic pants as this not only keeps the nappy wet but increases the likelihood of the

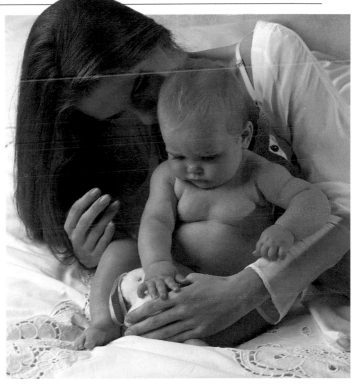

Above: *Frequent changes of nappy and the use of barrier creams are the keys to keeping a baby dry and contented.*

baby sweating and developing a heat rash. One change of nappy during the night is also helpful in ensuring the baby keeps dry. Sometimes changing the type of nappies will help, i.e. change to disposable or vice-versa depending on what you normally use. Leaving the baby without a nappy will help avoid the chafing against the skin, and so allow the skin to recover.
Barrier creams to protect the skin are now easily available and the commonest in use are zinc and castor oil or cod liver oil.

Careful washing and drying of the skin is essential. An old remedy is to use dilute vinegar (half a teaspoon in a cup of water) to wash the affected areas.
Nappies Disposable nappies are almost always used these days for convenience and some of the new varieties contain a layer of cellulose fibre to increase the absorption of urine and avoid any wet contact with the skin. Fabric nappies are made of a natural cotton or muslin and, although offering a more natural alternative, do not have the convenience factor. However, disposable nappies can be more costly, so there are pros and cons on both sides.

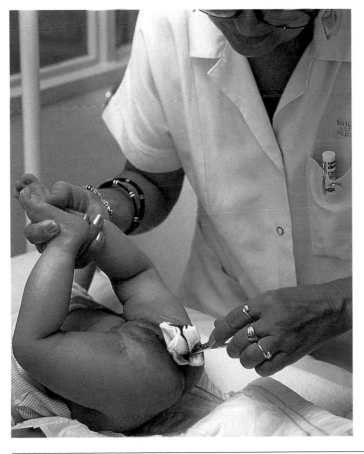

ORTHODOX TREATMENT

This will include most of the above advice but the doctor may prescribe an anti-fungal cream if he thinks there is a thrush infection present.

ABNORMAL MOLES

DESCRIPTION

Moles are coloured, flat or raised swellings on the skin. They are common in fair-skinned people and increase in occurrence with age and exposure to the Sun. Greater frequency now is apparent because of the destruction of the ozone layer above the Earth which allows harmful UV radiation through to damage the skin and predispose to skin cancer.

PREVENTION AND SELF-HELP

▪ Avoid exposure to the sun if fair-skinned.
▪ Wear protective clothing.
▪ Use sun tan preparation. Remember you can still burn under cloudy skies.
▪ Limit exposure to 30 minutes on the first day of a holiday and 30-60 minutes daily thereafter.

ALTERNATIVE THERAPIES

Alternative therapists will refer to a doctor if there is evidence of a change in the appearance of a mole, as this may be a symptom of developing skin cancer.

ORTHODOX TREATMENT

Seek advice from a doctor if a mole:
▪ Changes size.
▪ Changes in colour.
▪ Bleeds.

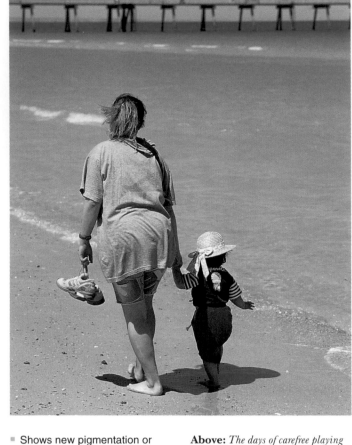

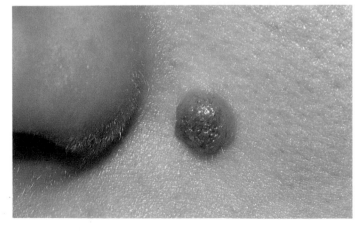

▪ Shows new pigmentation or goes dark in colour.
A doctor will send for biopsy for definite confirmation of diagnosis.

BLISTER

DESCRIPTION

A blister is a clear vesicle or pocket of skin containing clear

Below: This is how an ordinary skin mole looks; any abnormalities should be reported to a doctor.

Above: *The days of carefree playing on a sunny beach are sadly no more. Parents and children must cover up to protect their skins from UV radiation.*

fluid (serum) usually as a result of friction or a burn. Similar vesicles occur in chickenpox and shingles.

PREVENTION AND SELF-HELP

▪ Avoid badly fitting shoes. "Break in" new shoes. Wear thick socks.
▪ Wear gloves for unaccustomed long periods of manual work.
▪ Use protective creams in the Sun.

ALTERNATIVE THERAPIES

Biochemic tissue salts Take four tablets of *Nat. mur.* every 30 minutes until pain goes away.
Aromatherapy Dab lavender oil on blisters.

ORTHODOX TREATMENT

Keep the blister clean with antiseptic and a dressing. Do not lance.

BOIL

DESCRIPTION

An inflamed area of the skin which collects pus and develops into a swelling usually round the base of a hair follicle or in places of skin friction (thighs or buttocks). Can be a sign of poor nutrition or diabetes. If untreated it may lead to a carbuncle.

PREVENTION AND SELF-HELP

▪ A good diet with plenty of raw vegetables and fruit, good personal hygiene and skincare should prevent the appearance of boils.

ALTERNATIVE THERAPIES

Naturopathy Apply poultices of crushed fenugreek seeds or a softly boiled onion which can bring the boil to a head. Lightly bandage a thin slice of juicy lemon over the boil to encourage a head to form.
Biochemic tissue salts *Ferr. phos.* and *Kali mur.*, one tablet alternately every four hours are recommended.
Homeopathy *Hepar sulph.* 6x, one tablet every two hours.

CHILDREN: One tablet every four hours for children.

ORTHODOX TREATMENT

Local treatment with a Mag. sulph. dressing or poultice is the normal procedure. If large, the boil may require lancing and antibiotics may be prescribed to deal with the bacteria.

CORNS

DESCRIPTION

A corn is a thickening of the outer horny layer of the skin usually over a bone, mostly found on the feet and toes. Corns can be painful and become infected. They have a tendency to recur, particularly if footwear is too tight.

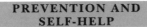

PREVENTION AND SELF-HELP

- Wear properly fitting shoes.
- Protect the feet with socks. If appropriate wear sandals.
- Corns will wear away if pressure on the toes and feet is removed.

ALTERNATIVE THERAPIES

Naturopathy Wash feet regularly. Remove rough skin with a pumice stone or bathe feet in a tub of warm water containing a tablespoon of Epsom Salts.
Herbal medicine Paint corns with fresh lemon juice or crushed garlic juice.

ORTHODOX TREATMENT

Corn plasters and salicylic acid will encourage corns to peel. Paring skin after softening in a warm bath with a sharp sterile steel blade can help. You may be referred to a chiropodist.

HANGNAIL

DESCRIPTION

A split at the side of the nail bed which may develop into an infection and produce a boil or whitlow. They are common among people who immerse their hands in water for long periods.

Below: *Corns such as this classically occur on the toes; tight or ill-fitting shoes are often to blame.*

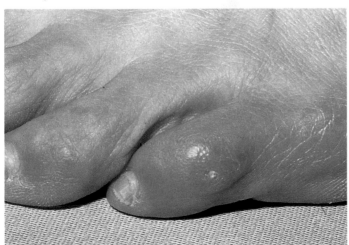

PREVENTION AND SELF-HELP

- Use rubber gloves during washing up.
- Use protective hand cream.
- Use antiseptic soap.

ALTERNATIVE THERAPIES

Treatment as in Boils (above).

ORTHODOX TREATMENT

Treatment as in Boils (above).

WARTS

DESCRIPTION

Warts are small solid growths appearing on hands, feet (verruca), mouth and lips (cold sores) and on genital areas. They are caused by viruses and are contagious. They may become quite large, unsightly and

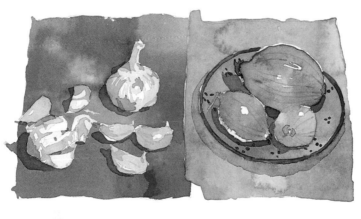

infected. They are not pre-cancerous and if left alone will disappear. This may take up to two years, however, so treatment is often required.

PREVENTION AND SELF-HELP

- Do not scratch warts or they will spread.
- Wear footwear in gyms and around swimming pools.
- Use proprietary creams carefully.
- Do not try to cut away yourself.
- Do not attempt any self-medication if elderly or diabetic.

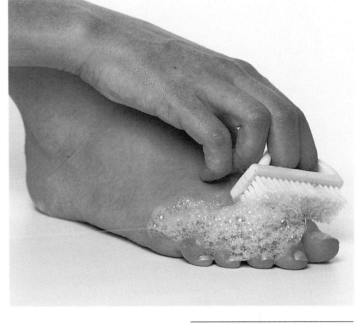

Above: *Regular washing of the feet is one of several measures that are advised to prevent corns from forming*

Below: *Onion and garlic, either in the form of oils or applied as a poultice, are well-tried remedies for warts.*

ALTERNATIVE THERAPIES

Acupuncture Some points, particularly on the Lung and Large Intestine meridians, have proved effective.
Hypnosis Occasionally works through the power of auto-suggestion while the patient is in a trance.
Laying on of hands This is a traditional treatment based on faith healing. It can work.
Aromatherapy Onion and garlic oils applied six times a day, for children twice a day, are recommended. Chopped onion and garlic bandaged on the wart overnight can also be effective.
Homeopathy Treatment can work but is a bit hit-and-miss. Try *Calc. carb.* and *Kali mur.* 6x – one tablet twice a day for seven days.

CHILDREN: For children under four, try four to six drops of the preparations mentioned above taken twice a day.

ORTHODOX TREATMENT

Proprietary paints of salicylic acid or podophyllin will destroy the exposed area of the wart. Normal skin needs to be protected with petroleum jelly before applying these. They can also be removed by means of surgery, burnt off (cauterization) or frozen off (cryotherapy).

HEADACHES

Headaches are a common and usually not serious symptom that most people experience from time to time. They form part of the symptom picture of many minor complaints (colds, 'flu, allergies), but can be a symptom of a specific condition (such as sinus problems or migraine). The commonly held view that headaches are related to high blood pressure is very rarely the case, but occasionally a headache can accompany a serious disorder (such as meningitis, or a brain tumour). It is because of this rare link with serious conditions that it is wise to seek medical advice if a headache persists for longer than a few days. Such headaches, however, are probably the result of the commonest cause: anxiety and tension.

CAUSES

Allergies Wheat products, alcohol, chocolate, and cheese. Coffee is sometimes taken to relieve a headache, and if you are a heavy drinker of coffee and then stop you may experience a headache while your body gets used to the absence of caffeine circulating in the system.

Brain tumours Both by compressing the brain and producing extra fluid, the tumour signals its presence with a chronic persistent headache which may be associated with vomiting, loss of vision and drowsiness. This can also occur following a head injury, which clearly will give rise to a headache, but which after settling, may recur because of a haemorrhage or clot pressing on the skull.

Infections Particularly meningitis, but any respiratory infection or virus infection may give rise to a headache. The pain occurring with meningitis is often accompanied by a stiff neck and severe vomiting.

Blocked sinus Chronic catarrh and sinusitis, which cause blockage and infection of these cavities in the skull, will be a major cause of headache (see pages 66-67).

Migraine and cluster headaches These are caused by changes in the blood vessels affecting the brain and will cause the one-sided, throbbing headache typical of this condition (see pages 154-155).

Muscle tension Probably the commonest cause of headache occurring in the back of the head or behind the forehead. This is related to tension in (and at times spasm of) the large muscles of the shoulders and neck (sternocleidomastoid and trapezius) which are partly attached to horny structures of the skull. The tension produces pain signals to be transmitted to the brain. If persistent, the headaches may not go away while the tension persists. Trigger points in neck and shoulder often refer pain to the head.

Below: The sternocleidomastoid and trapezius are large muscles in the shoulders and neck that attach to the skull. Tension in these muscles often gives rise to headaches.

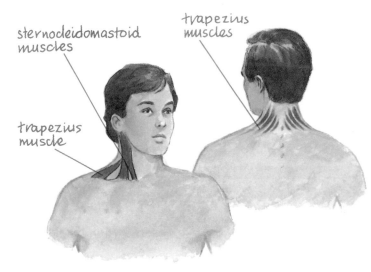

sternocleidomastoid muscles

trapezius muscles

trapezius muscle

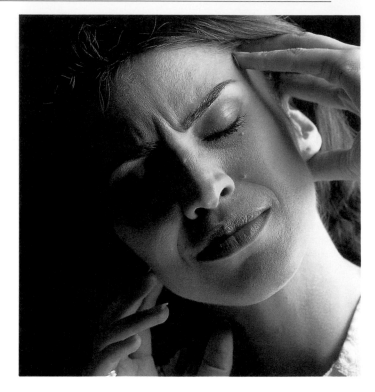

Above: We can all sympathize with this woman. Headaches are one of the most common sources of everyday pain.

Neck problems Cervical spondylitis (arthritis in the neck vertebrae), and malignant and postural abnormality are very common causes of headaches, sometimes by the direct trapping of the spinal nerves supplying the muscles of the scalp and forehead.

Eye problems Eye-strain and eye infections can give rise to a persistent pain behind both eyes which can be made worse by eye movement.

SYMPTOMS

They will depend on the cause of the headache but it is helpful both for yourself and your practitioner if you keep a diary of the frequency, site, and quality of the pain, using a scale "0" (no headache) to "10" (severe headache). Write down any associated symptoms, such as nausea, vomiting, worse in the light, left or right side, made worse by movement, coughing or sneezing, etc. Try to get familiar with the state of muscle tension in the back of your neck and shoulders, and use this as a guide to indicate whether this may be the cause. "Common things commonly occur", so do not think every headache is a signal of a brain tumour or meningitis, but seek help if your own self-help approach has not produced results within three to seven days.

PREVENTION AND SELF-HELP

Everyone will have their own particular favourite remedy for

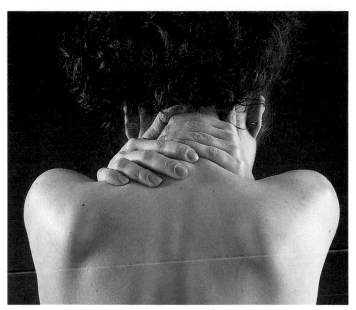

Above: *Self-massage of the neck is a useful preventative measure to combat the onset of a headache. It helps ease away tension in the muscles of the neck and upper shoulders.*

headaches, but the commonest one is rest and pain-killers. Try to avoid using "distracting therapies", i.e. drinking more coffee or more alcohol to suppress the pain signals.
▪ Fresh air, exercise and ionizers may help.
▪ Exclude dietary causes and particular allergies.
▪ Fast for 24-48 hours, taking fresh fruit and raw vegetables and liquids.
▪ A hot water bottle or warm pad applied to the site of the pain may help.
▪ Self-massage or by using a hand-held instrument will relieve tension in the neck and shoulders.
▪ Yoga exercises, deep-breathing, the corpse posture and progressive muscular relaxation all help to relax tense muscles.
▪ Reduce the glare on VDUs, and avoid staring at a screen for long periods. Take a few minutes' rest regularly when using a computer to let your eyes relax.

MASSAGE AND AROMATHERAPY

Both will help to remove most common muscle-tension headaches but they will return if the primary cause is not addressed. Specialized soft tissue techniques can remove trigger points (see the illustrations on this page for useful massage treatments).

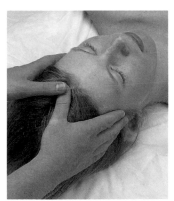

Above: *Massage along the vertex, the front-back central line of the skull, can help with headaches. Put one thumb on the other and massage a point on the vertex by rotating the thumbs gently in circles. Then move them a little and massage the next point.*

OSTEOPATHY/ CHIROPRACTIC

It is helpful to have a consultation if you are subject to recurrent headaches, as malignant and poor posture can be corrected by spinal manipulation. Be careful if you are over 50. It is wise to have an X-ray first to rule out severe osteoarthritis of the neck that may make some forms of active manipulation contra-indicated. Cranial osteopathy is very useful.

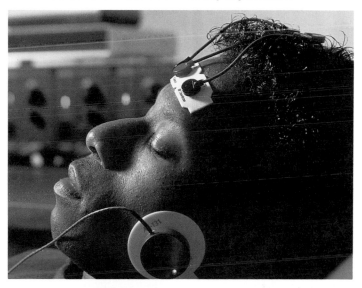

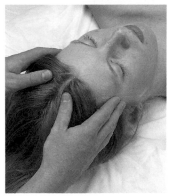

Above: *Eye-temple massage also alleviates headaches. Stroke with your fingers from the outer edges of the eyebrows to the bony mounds on the temples, and rotate the fingertips here for a few seconds. Press gently but firmly, and then repeat.*

HERBAL MEDICINE

A change of diet and hydrotherapy, e.g. taking a hot mustard foot bath will be advised, and several of the herbal teas available will help to soothe and release muscle tension. Try chamomile, rosemary, thyme and lemon balm.

Below: *Biofeedback enables people to monitor their brain waves and so learn techniques of relaxation.*

ACUPRESSURE

This can be of immense help, both in the acute states of the headache as well as in preventing recurrence. You can learn the various acupressure points that will serve as a self-help measure (see migraine pages 154-155, neuralgia page 159, and stress pages 102-103).

BIOFEEDBACK

This technique has been used to reduce the frequency of headaches as a result of migraine and muscle tension by allowing the patient to monitor his or her physical responses and to learn relaxation and meditation techniques.

ORTHODOX TREATMENT

Most doctors will treat persistent headaches as a sign of anxiety or tension and you may be asked to see a counsellor. However, a full physical examination will be done first to exclude any serious causes. Blood tests and X-rays will be undertaken if necessary, and you may be sent to see a specialist to have a sinus examination. In situations where headaches are recurrent and no obvious cause is identified, a brain-scan may be undertaken.

MIGRAINE

Migraine is a form of recurrent headache which affects both sexes. It has been estimated that up to five percent of the population suffer from it. There are various different types. Classical migraine usually affects one side of the head, is preceded by an aura, and is characterized by throbbing, nausea, occasionally vomiting and photophobia (the pain is worse in the light). There is usually a family history and people with migraine are, characteristically, hard-working and obsessional. Attacks can be triggered off by overwork or emotional tension. Migraine appears to be a disease of the blood vessels of the brain. In the initial stages (the aura), the blood vessels constrict, restricting the blood flow to the brain, and then dilate, causing the throbbing pain and eye symptoms. The headaches may last a few hours, but in a variant called cluster migraine the headache may occur daily for up to three months and is often associated with watery red eyes. Common migraine is not so severe as the two previous types and is often confused with a simple headache. Abdominal migraine is rarer but occurs relatively frequently, especially in children. It presents with stomach pain, nausea and occasionally vomiting.

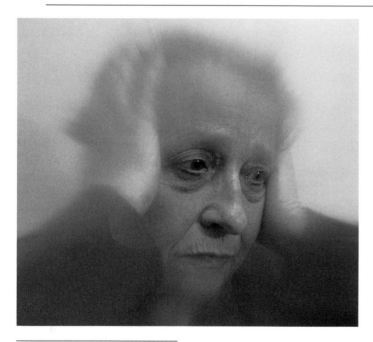

- Review your diet and cut out known causes of migraine, such as chocolate, wine or cheese. Other "danger" foods include eggs, dairy and wheat products.
- Put yourself on a short, three-day, purifying fast (eating only raw fruit and vegetables).
- Cut out coffee and strong tea.
- Start exercising and take up a relaxation technique.
- Once you have developed a headache, lie down in a dark room and practise deep-breathing and relaxation exercises.
- Visit your doctor and make sure the diagnosis is right.

Below: *For migraine sufferers these are "danger" foods. Chocolate and alcohol are other known causes of an allergic migraine.*

NATUROPATHY

Treatment may include an osteopathic assessment to ensure that there is no cervical-disc misalignment causing the headaches. Fasting and diet will be emphasized together with hydrotherapy. Massage is very helpful especially if the shoulder muscles are very tense.

ACUPUNCTURE

This is particularly helpful, both in the acute stage, as well as being a way of preventing and reducing the frequency of attacks. Chinese practitioners view migraine as a blockage of Chi in the Yang channels and will treat accordingly.

CAUSES

- Hereditary predisposition.
- Personality characteristics.
- Stress and emotional tension.
- Allergy to certain foods, i.e. chocolate, alcohol, cheese, and possibly others.
- Taking the contraceptive pill can bring on migraine.
- It may affect women at the time of their menstrual period.

SYMPTOMS

- Aura – a feeling that the attack is going to occur, possibly with disturbances of vision (flashing bright lights), funny smells or nausea.
- Nauseousness and tingling of the face and both hands, which may become very cold.

Above: *An image that captures the misery of migraine. An attack is often preceded by an aura that may cause disturbances of vision and nausea.*

- Confusion and dizziness with poor concentration.
- Headaches at the front of the head over the eye on one or both sides, or at the back of the head and neck. The headache is throbbing.
- Vomiting and photophobia (aversion from light).

PREVENTION AND SELF-HELP

- Keep a diary of your headaches and try to identify their frequency and any trigger factors, including food, menstrual period, or stressful situations.

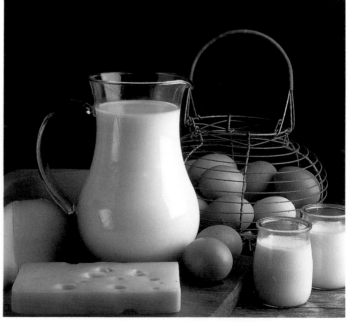

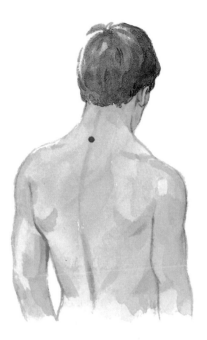

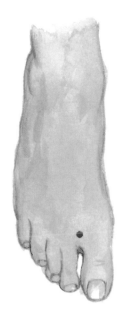

Above: *Two points to stimulate to alleviate the pain of migraine are Governing Vessel 14 at the top of the spine, and Liver 2 between the toes.*

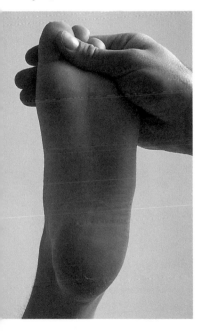

Above: *Reflexologists maintain that pressure on the tip of the big toe can relieve the pain of a migraine attack.*

ACUPRESSURE

A self-help technique should be learned to try and avert an acute attack. Three points may be stimulated to help alleviate the pain.
- At the end of the crease between the first finger and thumb, press in towards the first finger for up to two minutes.
- Behind the head at the base of the neck, press between the two prominent vertebrae for up to three minutes.
- In the well between the big toe and first toe press inwards and towards the centre of the foot for up to two minutes.

HOMEOPATHY

Many remedies exist for migraine and a proper consultation is necessary to identify the right one. As a first aid measure try
Arnica – for constant pain.
Nat. mur. – for a throbbing burning headache.
Nux vomica – for nausea and vomiting.
Iris ver. – for watery painful eyes.

Sanguinaria – right-sided headache.
Spigelia – left-sided headache. In all cases, take one tablet, 6x potency, twice a day for three days.

CHILDREN: Same dosage as for adults.

REFLEXOLOGY AND MASSAGE

Will help both in the acute stages, as well as in prevention. The toes represent the head and neck in reflexology and pressure on the tip of the big toe is particularly helpful in relieving migraine headaches.

BIOFEEDBACK

This became very popular as a way of controlling migraine and for a while many machines were used in the home as part of a relaxation technique. Most people, however, found this both difficult and time-consuming, and such machines are no longer used very widely.

Below: *Acupuncture has proved a very effective remedy for migraine. The therapist aims to balance the flow of Chi in the Yang meridians.*

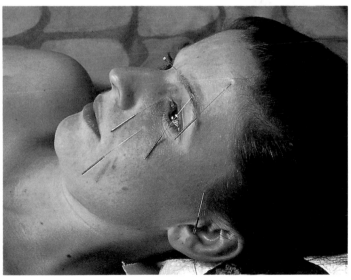

HERBAL MEDICINE

Feverfew is the classic herb considered to be effective in preventing migraine, and other recommendations are rosemary and chamomile. Each can be taken as a tea or infusion, one cup twice a day.

Below: *Teas made from feverfew, rosemary and chamomile are the classic herbal preventative remedies.*

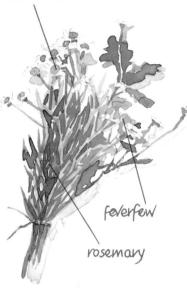

chamomile

feverfew

rosemary

ORTHODOX TREATMENT

A full examination and blood tests, and occasionally X-rays, would be taken to ensure the correct diagnosis, while treatment would consist of specific medication. The classic treatment is ergotamine tablets which help to reduce dilation of the blood vessels, and so stave off the throbbing headache associated with the visual disturbance phase of an attack. Other tablets include beta-blockers and certain new drugs that appear to prevent the onset of migraine. During an attack, rest in a darkened room and painkillers are generally advised.

DIZZINESS

Dizziness can be both a very minor and not uncommon symptom, or, if persisting, it may be the harbinger of serious disease. It is, therefore, important to have a proper medical examination if the symptoms persist. The spinning sensation and feeling of faintness may be accompanied by nausea and actual vomiting. If there is a loss of balance and staggering (vertigo), it is important to seek medical help. Occasionally dizziness may be accompanied by ringing in the ears (tinnitus).

CAUSES

▪ Anything as simple as rising too quickly from a chair or bed, to being frightened or having a shock will cause dizziness.
▪ Acute food poisoning which is often associated with nausea (alcohol abuse, or over-intoxication is probably the most common form of acute food poisoning).
▪ Anaemia and poor circulation to the brain (transient Ischaemic attacks).
▪ Dizziness may be associated with motion sickness while

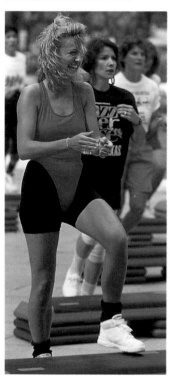

Above: *Fainting is caused by reduced blood flow and lack of oxygen supply to the brain. Happily, people who keep fit are unlikely to faint.*

travelling in cars, boats, aeroplanes etc.
▪ Very hot climates and high altitudes will produce fainting attacks in the vulnerable.

PREVENTION AND SELF-HELP

▪ During an attack, sit or lie down on the floor or bed and untie and loosen tight clothing. Open windows to reduce the temperature.
▪ If the attacks are simple fainting attacks, check you level of stress and introduce a relaxation exercise, especially diaphragmatic breathing, into your daily routine.
▪ Make sure you are not hyperventilating as this can cause dizziness and fainting just on its own.
▪ Check your level of fitness and join a Yoga or aerobics club – very few people who are physically fit faint.
▪ If there are any auditory symptoms (tinnitus or vertigo) seek medical help.
▪ Persistent dizziness and fainting should always be properly investigaged.
▪ The use of a "hot drink", brandy or smelling salts immediately after an attack is not particularly helpful. Lying down should suffice to alleviate the symptoms.
▪ Many alternative practitioners believe that dizziness can be a sign of low blood pressure and low blood sugar. Neither of these conditions is thought to exist by American and UK-based conventional doctors, although low blood pressure is considered a condition to be treated in Europe, and low blood sugar is recognized by naturopaths.

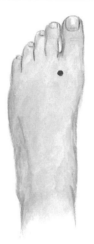

Above: *The Liver 3 acupoint is found on the top of the foot. Massage of it can help with an attack of dizziness.*

NATUROPATHY

Naturopaths will examine the diet thoroughly and suggest a reduction in the sugar content together with an increase in complex carbohydrates (oats, wholewheat, brown rice). High fibre from green leafy vegetables will also be recommended. Chicory and endives help liver metabolism of sugar.

HERBAL MEDICINE

An infusion of broom will raise blood pressure if it is considered too low and other herbs such as oats, gentian and wormwood may be given to improve circulation.

OSTEOPATHY AND CHIROPRACTIC

A not uncommon cause of dizziness, especially in the elderly, is a malalignment of the

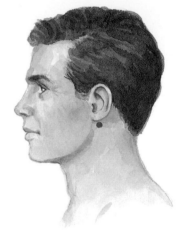

Above: *Triple Heater 17 is another useful point to stimulate in the event that you start to feel faint.*

vertebral joints, especially if there is poor circulation. Often dizziness occurs on looking up or moving the neck. It is important *not* to have manipulative treatment in such an instance: instead seek advice from a qualified doctor.

ACUPRESSURE

Stimulation of two acupoints – Liver 3 on the foot and Triple Heater 17 on the neck – can help during an attack of dizziness.
▪ *Liver 3* is found between the big and second toes, about three fingers' width above the angle where the two toes meet. Press hard with the thumb for about three to five minutes, massaging in a circular movement. Repeat six times as day.
▪ *Triple Heater 17* is found just behind the ear lobe. Massage it in the same way with your index finger.

ORTHODOX TREATMENT

Simple faints and dizziness do not require treatment, other than general advice about lifestyle.
Further treatment will depend on an accurate diagnosis but very commonly no specific cause is found.

EPILEPSY

Epilepsy is a condition of the central nervous system affecting the brain which leads to recurrent "fits" or seizures that are associated with loss of consciousness. The nerve cells in the brain send messages to one another through small electric impulses that can be picked up by an EEG machine that produces an electro-encephalogram. In epilepsy, disturbances of electrical discharge occur both during and between attacks. Epilepsy does not affect the mental state and although there may be some psychological disturbance as a result of long-standing disease, sufferers feel quite normal between attacks.

TYPES

Grand Mal This is characterized by a few seconds warning or "aura", which may be a noise or visual disturbance, followed by loss of consciousness, falling to the ground, and the fit which can affect both sides of the body. It involves stiffening and rhythmic clenching of the hands and shaking of the body. The tongue may be bitten during an attack and saliva may dribble from the mouth. Following an attack, the patient usually falls asleep and may appear confused and drowsy when woken up. Often there is loss of memory.

Petit Mal This occurs in children and during adolescence. It is not accompanied by seizures but presents with momentary loss of consciousness, which can be confused with day-dreaming. Occasionally the eyelids may blink and flutter.

Temporal lobe epilepsy There may be an aura as in Grand Mal but usually there is no major fit. The subject experiences feelings of unreality or *déjà-vu*. He may act strangely, not know where he is, complain of sounds and smells and not be able to recognize people. He rarely loses consciousness or falls to the ground.

Jacksonian fit This is what is called a "local fit" and affects one part of the body only, usually the hands or face. There is no loss of consciousness. This sort of fit is usually caused by an injury or infection of the brain that stimulates an abnormal electrical discharge.

CAUSES

In most cases of epilepsy, no specific cause is found. It does have a hereditary tendency, and may occur following a head injury or brain tumour. In all cases it is associated with an abnormal electrical discharge that can spread throughout the brain. Epilepsy may occur as the result of a birth injury, drug abuse or excessive alcohol intake, or stress and emotional tension.

PREVENTION AND SELF-HELP

▪ If you have epilepsy, always carry a card stating this, and ensure you take your medication regularly. Avoid taking stimulant drugs, excessive amounts of alcohol and caffeine.

▪ If you observe someone having a fit, lie them down on their side – loosen clothing around the neck – remove objects that can be broken (such as spectacles), and make sure there is enough space to allow them to stretch without harming themselves. Keep the airway free. Put a pillow under the head. **Do not** open the mouth, remove false teeth or try to give a drink. Once the fit is over, allow them to sleep and cover with a blanket.

▪ Living with the disease means accepting it, not denying it, but do not let it control your life.

▪ Avoid working with machinery or on tall buildings, bridges etc.

▪ Avoid rooms with flickering fluorescent lights or VDU screens, and strobe lights in night clubs as they may trigger an attack.

▪ All people with epilepsy are not allowed to drive a car unless the fits are well-controlled (no fits for two years), and they pass a special driving test.

▪ Sport is not prohibited, but avoid solitary mountain sports.

Below: *A brain scan showing the blood flow of someone who has just had an epileptic attack. The vivid colours indicate abnormal brain activity.*

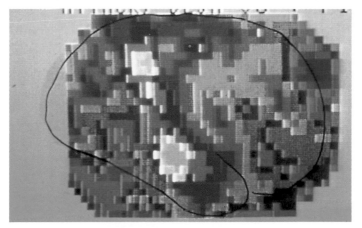

Swimming is permissible, but it is best to ensure you swim when someone else is present.

▪ Join your national epilepsy association.

HELPFUL THERAPIES

Alternative treatments have little to offer as a cure or means to control the epileptic fit and it is important that you seek medical advice and take all the medication prescribed. However, certain therapies are helpful in reducing the frequency of attacks and some have been known to help control the severity of the attack.

▪ Follow a wholefood diet and avoid stimulants.

▪ Develop a relaxation programme and learn how to meditate.

▪ Avoid trigger factors and take chamomile tea at night to help relaxation.

▪ Cranial osteopathy has had some success in helping people with epilepsy. Pressure point GV26 (on channel of upper lip just below the nose) is extremely efficacious in children and can be used during a fit. Apply steady pressure for up to two minutes.

AROMATHERAPY

As relaxation is important in staving off epilepsy attacks, aromatherapists recommend taking essence of Roman chamomile for its sedative effects. Put three drops on a half a spoonful of brown sugar, and take three times a day, between meals.

ORTHODOX TREATMENT

The mainstay of treatment is the regular use of medication which will vary according to which type of epilepsy is present. Some medication can have long-term side-effects and it is important to have regular checks which can include making sure the blood level of the drug is high enough to prevent seizures.

MULTIPLE SCLEROSIS

Multiple sclerosis is a disabling and distressing illness of the central nervous system that affects young people and is characterized by remissions and relapses. Lesions develop in the fatty protective covering of the nerves (the nerve sheath) that is made from myelin. The damage results in loss of nerve conduction (the ability of nerves to carry nervous impulses), more in the sensory part of the nervous system than in the motor part, i.e. it affects the nerves carrying sensation rather than the nerves that carry movement messages. MS can affect all nerves but is most common in the nerves supplying the hands and legs. Other vulnerable nerves include the optic nerve and the vestibular nerve (affecting balance).

CAUSES

The precise cause of MS is not known. It seems to be more common in temperate climes and women are affected twice as often as men. There is a suggestion that it occurs more frequently in families. The two factors that are now felt to be the most likely causes are the effects of a "slow virus" (a virus that lives in the body for a long time) and diet. There is some evidence that diet (lack of certain essential fatty acids that make up the myelin) may be a cause.

SYMPTOMS

These vary enormously and it can take two or three episodes of MS before the diagnosis is certain. They include
- Pins and needles.
- Manual clumsiness – i.e. dropping drinks or cigarettes.
- Loss of balance and vertigo.
- Loss of vision, blurring or dimmed sight.
- Weakness and loss of control of the limbs.
- Bladder disturbances, especially sudden incontinence.

PREVENTION AND SELF-HELP

A proper diagnosis is essential and you should visit your doctor if you have any symptoms or are concerned. Blood tests, and possibly a lumbar puncture and a scan of the spinal cord will help

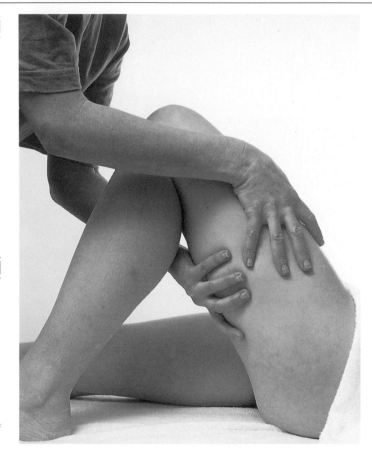

Above: *As there is no cure for MS, treatment must centre on controlling the symptoms. A massage helps maintain body mobility and muscle tone.*

confirm the diagnosis one way or another.
Foods to eat Fruits and vegetables, fructose and honey, oats, brown rice, wholewheat flour, low-fat milk, pulses, fish.

Foods to avoid Alcohol, coffee, animal fats, full-cream milk, meat, peanuts, white flour products.
- Take up a gentle exercise routine, which helps with posture and awareness, such as Yoga, or the Alexander Technique.
- Learn a relaxation and breathing exercise; try meditation.
- Massage and reflexology will help.

NATUROPATHY

A naturopathic approach will involve
- Hydrotherapy to keep joints and muscles loose and exercised.
- Relaxation exercises to relieve stress.
- Dietary guidance – eat fresh fruit, vegetables, low fat meats, white fish such as cod and haddock, sprouted seeds such as bean sprouts and cress, and pulses.
- Dietary supplements – take Vitamin B_{12}, one 50mcg tablet three times a day, and evening primrose oil, one tablet three times a day.

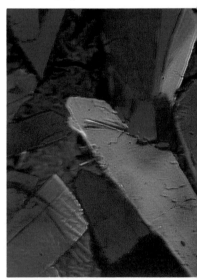

Above: *A highly magnified view of molecules of Vitamin B_{12}. Naturopaths recommend B_{12} supplements for MS.*

ORTHODOX TREATMENT

Like alternative therapies, orthodox medicine cannot offer a cure for multiple sclerosis and management of the illness will concentrate on controlling the symptoms. In the acute phase of an attack, cortisone treatment can restore function, especially if the eyes are affected. Rest and physiotherapy are encouraged. Hydrotherapy can be particularly useful to exercise muscles and maintain mobility in the knee joints. Infections are treated if they occur in the bladder and kidney, and walking and occupational aids may also be necessary.

NEURALGIA

Neuralgia is a term for pain arising from a nerve that is being irritated or "trapped", usually between bones (sciatica is a form of neuralgia). The pain may be felt all along the course of the nerve and not just at the point under pressure. The pain may be constant, or intermittent as in trigeminal neuralgia affecting the trigeminal nerve of the face. As neuralgia is a symptom, there are many different causes.

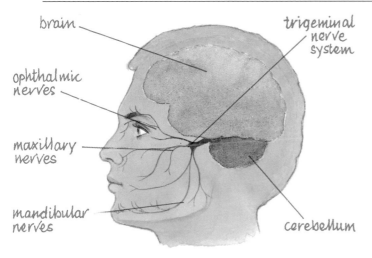

brain
ophthalmic nerves
maxillary nerves
mandibular nerves
trigeminal nerve system
cerebellum

CAUSES

Post-herpetic neuralgia is the pain that follows an attack of shingles where the nerve has been irritated and inflamed by the herpes zoster virus. It can be of a very distressing kind but usually lasts only a few weeks. The pain is felt along the course of the nerve affected.
Trigeminal neuralgia is a condition affecting the trigeminal nerve and produces a lancing, severe pain in the face and over the eye. It is often triggered by eating, smoking or a cold wind.
Bony neuralgia arises from a trapped nerve, either as a result of an old fracture that has not healed or a collapsed vertebra in the lumbar region of the spine or in the neck.

PREVENTION AND SELF-HELP

It is important to obtain a correct diagnosis and a visit to a doctor or osteopath/chiropractor who will carry out a full examination with X-rays, if necessary, is essential.

Above: *The trigeminal nerves split into several branches across the face. They can be affected by neuralgia.*

■ Home treatments include painkillers, and using hot water bottles on the affected area to relieve pain.
■ Reducing muscle tension through breathing and relaxation exercises will also help.

ACUPRESSURE

For trigeminal neuralgia, press inwards at the inner end of the eyebrow on the affected side, or you can press downwards at points just next to the corners of the mouth. Apply light pressure for at least two minutes. Other pressure points will depend on where the neuralgia is situated.

ACUPUNCTURE

It can be very useful in removing troublesome neuralgia both because it reduces muscle tension and restores nervous function. Electro acupuncture is sometimes used, as well as a small machine that performs what is known as transcutaneous nerve stimulation. The TNS machine emits small electrical impulses which can be used at home to stimulate the nerve and so reduce the pain. However, people with heart pacemakers should **not** use a TNS machine.

OSTEOPATHY AND CHIROPRACTIC

A therapist will help to restore bony alignment if possible, and remove pressure from the nerve. Cranial manipulation is a gentle and effective way of easing pressure or tension on the affected nerve.

AROMATHERAPHY

Add two drops of clove oil, one of basil and one of eucalyptus to a tablespoon of carrier oil and rub it over the affected area.

Below: *Cranial osteopathy is an option to help relieve the excruciating pain associated with facial neuralgia.*

SPIRITUAL HEALING

This is one condition where laying on of hands has helped several individuals with chronic pain and certain "pain clinics" now make use of a healer to help with the most difficult cases.

Below: *TNS pads are electrical devices that aim to relieve pain by using an electrical current to block pain signals along a nerve.*

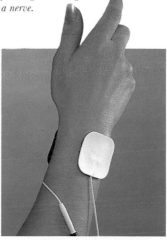

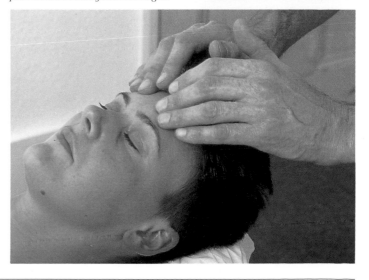

ORTHODOX TREATMENT

Conventional analgesics will first be tried. Trigeminal neuralgia responds well to a nerve drug and occasionally, for chronic pain, a small dose of anti-depressant is given. The nerves can be injected, frozen and occasionally removed if the problem has overwhelmed the patient.

STROKE

A stroke is the result of a cerebrosvascular accident – damage to blood vessels in the brain – commonly as a result of an embolus (clot) or haemorrhage. It results in a sudden loss of movement on one side of the body affecting the face, arm or leg, or all three. It is a condition affecting the elderly and it is unusual before the age of 50. Strokes can be fatal but usually leave the individual paralysed. Depending on which side the stroke occurs will determine whether speech is affected. Recovery of both speech and movement can happen for anything up to one year after the stroke.

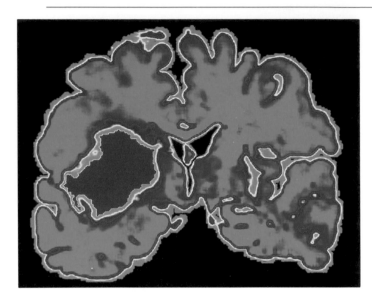

Above: *This scan shows a slice of a brain which has suffered a haemorrhage (red), one of the causes of a stroke.*

exists, it is important to ensure that medication is taken regularly. Alternative therapies do have a place in aiding recovery and helping the individual live with the disability. The focus of treatment is on proper rehabilitation, and under expert supervision, massage, aromatherapy, hydrotherapy, Yoga and postural re-education help. A diet to help reduce weight is important if you are overweight and herbs and vitamins may help to restore a sense of wellbeing. It is not uncommon, and understandably so, that people often get depressed following a stroke, and much help can be given by sensitive support, advice and counselling. Some people whose speech is badly affected will learn to paint or play a musical instrument to help with self-expression. Massage with gentle aromatherapy oils (lavender, almond oil) will soothe and relieve discomfort in the paralysed side.

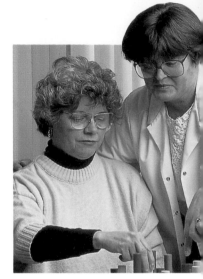

Above: *A stroke victim undergoes occupational therapy to help improve co-ordination and muscle control.*

Below: *Massage with aromatherapy oils can relieve some of the discomfort of paralysis and promote relaxation.*

CAUSES

An embolus or clot occurs as a result of atherosclerosis (see page 91) when it is dislodged, and travels to the brain causing blockage of the blood supply which leads to death of the brain tissue. A thrombosis may also build up on the walls of a cerebral artery, so blocking blood supply to part of the brain.

Haemorrhage (the rupture of blood vessels in the brain) often occurs in younger people and is accompanied by severe headaches. Occasionally the haemorrhage is due to malformation of the walls of the blood vessels – high blood pressure is a common associated factor.

Transient ischaemic attacks, or "stuttering strokes", are minor episodes of dizziness and vertigo where the blood supply to the brain is briefly interrupted. If paralysis occurs, it is usually only temporary.

SYMPTOMS

■ Dizziness, confusion, loss of consciousness and memory.
■ Paralysis of one side of the body.
■ Loss of control of bladder and occasionally the bowels.
■ Loss of speech or the ability to put the right name to objects.

TREATMENT

Treatment should be by a doctor and will almost always require the patient to be sent to hospital. **Do not attempt to treat the patient yourself.** If high blood pressure

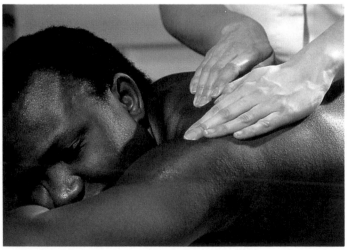

ORTHODOX TREATMENT

Medical treatment consists of care of the body, physiotherapy and active rehabilitation. Sometimes X-rays are taken to explore the degree of atheroma in the arteries of the neck and by-pass operations can be performed to prevent further recurrences. In strokes caused by haemorrhage, occasionally the blood clot is removed by surgery.

PARALYSIS

Paralysis is a symptom that arises as a result of many different conditions, particularly affecting the nervous and muscular systems. The causes of paralysis are diverse, as is explained below.

CAUSES

Injury Often the result of road-traffic accidents, sporting injuries or war wounds where the spinal cord is compressed or severed, leading usually to total loss of movement below the site of the injury, which may include loss of control of the bladder, bowels and sexual function. There is usually a phase of "shock" to the system after which partial recovery can occur. Muscle wasting and contractures (tightening of the ligaments) will occur if proper attention is not given.

Birth injuries Cerebral palsy is often the result of lack of oxygen to the brain at the time of delivery and may lead to loss of movement and co-ordination of the muscles, with involuntary writhing movements of arm and face. Mental function is not affected and with proper care and rehabilitation, people can be helped to live a creative and fulfilled life.

Below: *This man broke his neck and is paralysed in all four limbs. His rehabilitation includes physiotherapy.*

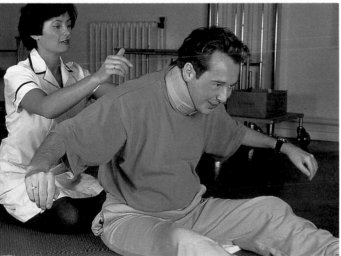

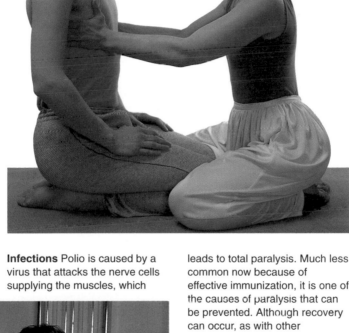

Below: *Yoga is one of the alternative therapies that can help victims of paralysis improve their muscle tone.*

Infections Polio is caused by a virus that attacks the nerve cells supplying the muscles, which leads to total paralysis. Much less common now because of effective immunization, it is one of the causes of paralysis that can be prevented. Although recovery can occur, as with other conditions the focus of treatment is on rehabilitation and recovery. A transient paralysis can occur following a virus infection (Guillain-Barré syndrome) which often affects young people, usually in the lower limbs. Recovery is almost always complete but can take weeks.

Nervous disorders Strokes and multiple sclerosis (see page 158) will also cause paralysis which can be transient or permanent. Hysterical paralysis (loss of the use of one limb or voice) is not uncommon and can occur after attacks of hyperventilation. There is usually a major element of stress or emotional tension present.

Muscular disorders These include the muscular dystrophies and motor-neurone disease which have a hereditary predisposition and which affect the muscles of the body causing them to waste and lose their power. The muscles involved in swallowing and respiration are also affected which leads to severe distress and eventual death.

USEFUL THERAPIES

All forms of paralysis should be seen by a doctor but much good work can be achieved through alternative therapies.

Acupressure and acupuncture Help to reduce physical pain.

Yoga, T'ai-chi Improve muscle power and co-ordination.

Massage, breathing and relaxation exercises Decrease muscle tension and induce relaxation.

Wholefood diet, vitamin and mineral supplements Improve diet and increase overall level of well-being.

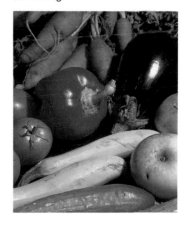

Above: *A good diet induces a sense of well-being. It is obviously not a cure for paralysis, but it does help.*

ORTHODOX TREATMENT

The primary approach that orthodox medicine offers is an individual rehabilitation programme to include physiotherapy, speech therapy, and hydrotherapy. Research has been carried out in using drugs to prevent the condition deteriorating but these have not been very successful.

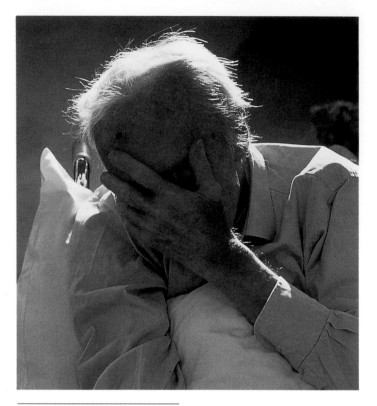

ALZHEIMER'S DISEASE

DESCRIPTION

Loss of mental faculties (memory, concentration and intellect) as a result of death of brain cells. This condition is similar to senile dementia but affects a younger age group. No clear cause has been identified although one suggestion links it to high levels of aluminium in the body. There may also be a genetic factor that predisposes to Alzheimer's.

PREVENTION AND SELF-HELP

▪ If the cause is related to high aluminium levels (not proven), then cooking in stainless steel pots is a sensible precaution.
▪ Counselling, especially for the relatives, may help with this distressing condition.

ALTERNATIVE THERAPIES

Herbal medicine Rosemary tea helps circulation, especially of the nervous system. Ginkgo biloba (maidenhair tree) is a herb often used for memory loss.

Above: *The mental degeneration caused by Alzheimer's is very distressing for family members to witness.*

Acupuncture helps to reduce stress and improve learning.

ORTHODOX TREATMENT

Diagnosis is often confirmed with an M.R.I. (magnetic resonance imaging) scan which reveals loss of the "normal" pattern of the brain surface. There is no known cure but treatment is given to relieve and reduce symptoms.

ENCEPHALITIS

DESCRIPTION

Inflammation of the brain following a serious viral infection or a brain abcess.

PREVENTION AND SELF-HELP

Not applicable.

ALTERNATIVE THERAPIES

No known alternative therapy helps.

ORTHODOX TREATMENT

Usually causes a coma and can lead to permanent brain damage. Treatment with antiviral drugs can be successful if the cause is identified soon enough.

FEBRILE CONVULSIONS (FEVER FITS)

DESCRIPTION

These are fits or seizures which occur in young children as a result of a high temperature. The child may lose concentration, go vacant and twitch. They may last up to five minutes. After the fit, the child may want to sleep.

PREVENTION AND SELF-HELP

▪ Do not allow a small child's temperature to rise unobserved.
▪ Do not wrap him or her up.
▪ Loosen clothing.
▪ Cool the body down with tepid sponging or a tepid bath. If temperature rises, open windows.
▪ If a fit occurs, summon medical help. Lie the child on its side; do not try to open the mouth.

ALTERNATIVE THERAPIES

Alternative practitioners do not necessarily feel a temperature should be treated if it is not too high.
Naturopaths would suggest fasting with plenty of fluid, and cold compresses.
Homeopathy *Aconite* 6x, *Belladonna* 6x, *Byronia* 6x and *Nux vomica* 6x are all remedies useful for a small child. Make the child take one tablet every two hours until the temperature subsides.
Herbal medicine Willow bark tea, which contains the same ingredients as aspirin, reduces fever. A cup may be sipped regularly, up to three cups daily.

Below: *The two large orange patches on the left of this brain are lesions caused by viral encephalitis affecting the cerebral hemisphere.*

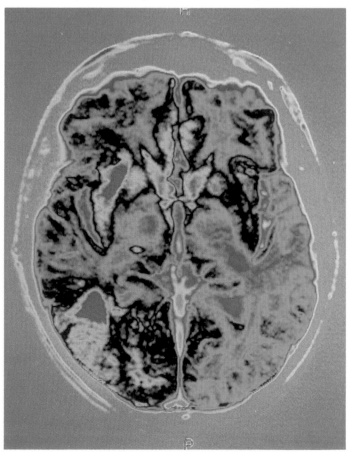

ORTHODOX TREATMENT

This is not a very common condition of childhood, which is more frightening than serious. It may accompany measles, chickenpox, or viral infection. A doctor will advise cooling the child down and anti-convulsants may be prescribed. A lumbar puncture may be performed to exclude meningitis.

MENINGITIS

DESCRIPTION

An inflammation of the meninges (the lining of the brain) caused by virus or bacteria. It can be of rapid onset and can be fatal if not detected early on. It is more common in children.

PREVENTION AND SELF-HELP

- There is now a vaccine available that will protect against some forms of meningitis.
- If there has been any contact (at school or in playgroups) then preventative antibiotics are given.

ALTERNATIVE THERAPIES

Treatment should not be attempted by alternative therapists for this is a serious and potentially fatal disease.

ORTHODOX TREATMENT

Meningitis is diagnosed from the symptoms of a headache, vomiting, neck stiffness and photophobia (light hurting the eyes). A lumbar puncture (a needle in the spine) will draw out fluid for accurate diagnosis. Treatment will include antibiotics and occasionally steroids.

NERVOUS TIC

DESCRIPTION

An involuntary twitch of the muscles which may become a nervous habit. It can affect any muscle, but often the eyelid or facial muscle is involved. Occasionally it may be the sign of a muscle disorder.

PREVENTION AND SELF-HELP

- Exercise, especially aerobic, to clear any lactic acid will help.
- Relaxation and meditation may help to reduce underlying tension.

ALTERNATIVE THERAPIES

Acupuncture will help to relieve general stress levels, as will **hydrotherapy**, **massage** and **reflexology**.
Naturopathy A diet with added Vitamin B_6 and zinc is recommended.
Homeopaths may suggest *Aconite* 6x – one tablet three times a day for one week.

CHILDREN: Same dose as for adults.

Behaviour therapy is also of help.

ORTHODOX TREATMENT

Often underlying stress/anxiety or fear will produce a tic, especially in children who cannot easily talk about their concerns. Usually reassurance and support is suggested. Very occasionally, tranquillizers or hypnosis may be recommended.

NEUROPATHY

DESCRIPTION

A disturbance in the peripheral nerves of the hands or feet leading to pins and needles, weakness and muscle wasting. It can be caused by a variety of conditions such as vitamin deficiency, alcoholism, diabetes, carpal tunnel syndrome and anaemia.

PREVENTION AND SELF-HELP

- A proper balanced diet and added supplements may be required if you are a strict vegan.

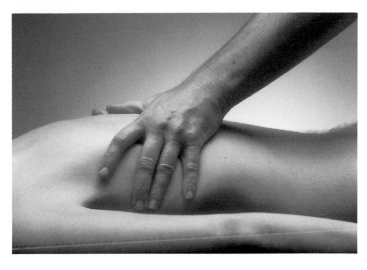

- Yoga and stretching exercises will reduce muscle tension and help to restore balance.
- Early diagnosis of the cause will help to plan a self-help programme.

ALTERNATIVE THERAPIES

Naturopathy A proper medical diagnosis is necessary first, but supportive therapy through diet, vitamin supplements, and minerals can help if appropriate.
Herbal medicine Lemon balm and rosemary herbal teas are often used as nerve tonics.
Biochemic tissue salts *Kali phos.* and *Mag. phos.* may help restore function. Take one tablet a day for a month.

ORTHODOX TREATMENT

A proper diagnosis is arrived through examination, blood tests and nerve-conduction tests and treatment will depend on the cause and will include medication as well as surgery. Splints are sometimes used to prevent permanent damage to muscles as a result of contractions and muscle wasting.

PARKINSON'S DISEASE

DESCRIPTION

A degenerative condition of the nervous system which causes muscle stiffness, tremor and loss of facial expression. It occurs

Above: *As there is no known cure for Parkinson's disease, treatment must concentrate on relieving the symptoms. Massage is particularly effective.*

mostly in people aged over 50 and is more common in men than women.

PREVENTION AND SELF-HELP

- A relaxation exercise especially if accompanied with deep breathing can help with the symptoms.
- Yoga has been used effectively to improve confidence and co-ordination.
- Counselling is often helpful to address the accompanying psychological issues.

ALTERNATIVE THERAPIES

There is no effective treatment but alternative approaches may help sufferers cope with the symptoms of the disease.
Acupuncture may help to relax muscle stiffness.
Aromatherapy has been suggested to reduce trembling. Four drops of lavender essence on a sugar cube may be taken three times a day.

ORTHODOX TREATMENT

Parkinson's disease may be the result of a viral disease but its cause is not known. Treatment is with drugs and occasionally surgery. Recently implanting new cells into the brain has been tried, without much success.

BREAST DISORDERS

The breasts are part of the endocrine system responding to hormonal changes occurring at puberty, menstrual periods and the menopause, and producing milk following the giving of birth. They are also the most obvious of sexual characteristics of women. Having healthy, well-shaped breasts is important for most women and psychological distress is not an uncommon consequence of mis-shaped, too small or too large breasts. Almost every women's magazine will give tips for developing well-shaped breasts and millions of pounds are spent each year on breast enlargement or breast reduction. The breasts are made of glandular tissue supported by fibrous bands and interspersed with fatty cells which swell and are sometimes visible during pregnancy and periods. The nipple is made of erectile tissues similar to that found on the lips or vagina, which respond to sexual stimulation. There are a number of disorders that can affect the breasts, and the most common are described below.

CAUSES

Mastalgia, or painful breasts, is a fairly common occurrence of many women and is the result of the raised oestrogen levels found at times during the menstrual cycle and pregnancy. A high circulating level of oestrogen and sodium will trap more water in the breasts so that they swell and become tender and painful. If this occurs regularly during each monthly cycle, the condition is called fibrocystic disease and can lead to "lumpy" breasts: the lumps are benign and do not lead on to cancer.

Benign breast lumps are not uncommon in women and may be single cysts or multiple cysts, often associated with fibrocystic diseases.

Mastitis is another painful condition of the breasts resulting from an infection, usually occurring during breast feeding because of a cracked nipple.

Breast cancer will affect around one in 12 women in the Western world and is associated with certain well-known risk factors:

■ Race: More common in white races.
■ Menstrual history: Early onset of periods and late menopause.
■ Age: Over 50.
■ Family history: Increased risk if your mother or sister has had cancer.
■ Marital history: Never having married or been pregnant increases the risk.
■ Hormonal drugs: HRT for women over 50 is thought by some authorities to increase breast cancer. The contraceptive pill is thought to protect against breast cancer.
■ Diet: A high saturated fat diet (high in dairy products, red meat, and fatty foods) increases the risk.
■ Emotions: This is still controversial but there is some evidence that the way women respond to stress may affect their chances of getting breast cancer.

Below: *Taking evening primrose oil can be effective in reducing the pain associated with mastalgia.*

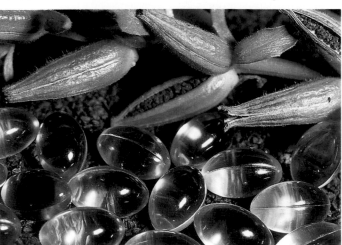

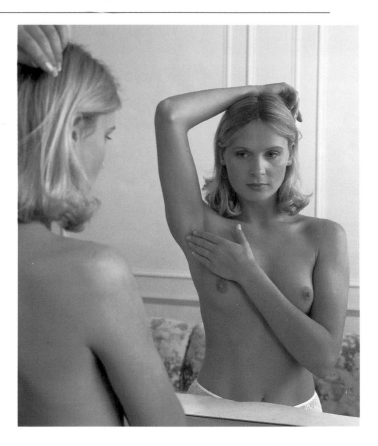

Those who do not express their emotions and have a sense of hopelessness and helplessness seem at greater risk.
■ Previous breast cancer: Women who develop breast cancer in one breast are six times more likely to develop breast cancer in the other.

SYMPTOMS

■ Pain and swollen, engorged breasts are a common feature of hormonal changes and affect both breasts.
■ Pain in one breast may be the result of mastitis.
■ A painless lump is the most common presentation for breast cancer; painful lumps are not usually malignant.
■ Discharge from the nipple – clear, milky or blood-stained – may accompany infection or a lump.
■ A change in skin texture (for instance, a rough and "dimpled" feel, like the surface of an orange) may indicate a malignant growth.
■ Different sizes of breast are not uncommon and do not necessarily indicate disease.

Above: *Women should develop the habit of carrying out a breast self-examination regularly every month.*

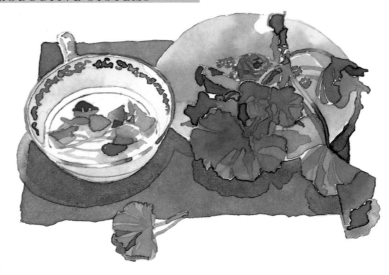

PREVENTION AND SELF-HELP

Breast self-examination is easy to learn and you should get into the habit of examining your breasts once during your monthly cycle. Regular medical examinations if you are on oral contraceptive pills or hormone replacement therapy is an important part of a preventative programme.

Diet is an important factor in preventing breast disease. You should aim to reduce the fatty content of your diet, together with your salt intake. Eat plenty of fresh fruit and salads. The fatty acid gamma linolenic acid (GLA) is known to reduce the pain of mastalgia and is found in evening primrose oil. Supplements of Vitamin B_6 (pyridoxine) (one tablet twice a day for two weeks before the period) will help with the symptoms associated with pre-menstrual tension and has been used as a treatment for this condition.

Exercise Many exercises are to be found in women's magazines that are claimed to improve breast-size, but as the breast itself contains no muscle tissue, the effect of exercise is only on the pectoral muscles beneath the breast. Strengthening these muscles may improve breast "lift" but a good supporting bra and ensuring you are not overweight are equally helpful measures. Breast sagging is more often the result of poor posture and the Alexander technique may help with this condition.

NATUROPATHY

Naturopaths will suggest a diet including plenty of green vegetables, including cress, and cabbage (vegetable juice may be a more convenient way of obtaining the ingredients known to improve healthy tissues).

Below: *This woman is undergoing mammography. Regular medical breast check-ups are a sensible precaution.*

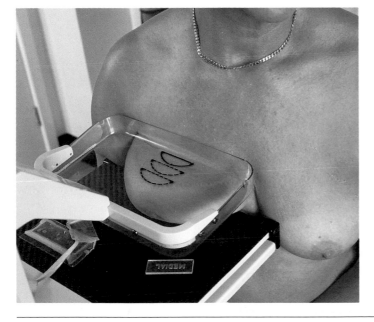

Additional vitamins are sometimes prescribed in fibrocystic disease or in breast cancer: zinc (5mg, one tablet per day), selenium (10mg, one tablet twice a day), Vitamin A and Vitamin B_6 (one tablet daily is sufficient). Splashing or spraying the breasts with cold water on a regular basis will help to keep them healthy and firm.

ACUPRESSURE

For mastalgia, pressure between the third and fourth rib above the nipple will help to relieve breast tenderness and improve lactation.

AROMATHERAPY

Add a few (three or four) drops of essence of geranium to a bowl of warm water, and bathe both breasts in the solution. This will reduce engorged and tender breasts. Massage with oil of chamomile will help cracked nipples.

HOMEOPATHY

Cal. phos. and *Calc. ostrearum* (6x, one tablet three times a day) may help painful breasts.

Above: *Swollen or tender breasts can be relieved by bathing them in warm water containing essence of geranium.*

OTHER HELPFUL THERAPIES

Visualization/meditation/relaxation exercises will help to improve the sense of general well-being and have been shown to alleviate the level of depression found in women who have developed breast cancer.

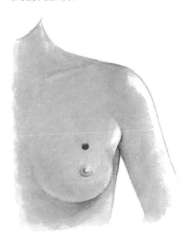

Above: *This acupoint can be used if you are troubled by breast pain, particularly that caused by mastalgia.*

ORTHODOX TREATMENT

Hormonal and cyclical changes affecting the breast are often treated with a variety of hormonal combinations which alter the balance of progesterone and oestrogen. Painful cysts will be "aspirated" (having the fluid drawn off) using a fine needle, and most lumps in the breast will be subjected to careful examination including mammography (special X-ray of the breast). In almost all cases, a biopsy will be taken to reveal whether the lump is malignant. Surgery is now confined to removing the lump (lumpectomy) or removing some or all of the breast (mastectomy). Radiotherapy and chemotherapy will be utilized if thought appropriate, and currently a scientific trial of the drug tamoxifen is being conducted to establish whether it prevents subsequent breast cancer developing in women who are at high risk of developing this condition. Many of the complementary therapies are now much more readily available and several centres are happy to combine orthodox and complementary therapies in the management of breast cancer.

CYSTITIS

Cystitis is an inflammation of the lining of the bladder and urethra – a tube leading out of the bladder – that gives rise to a burning sensation on passing water, increased frequency of urination, and low abdominal pain. It predominantly affects women, although occasionally men do get it. It can occur in young girls but it is usually a condition of sexually active women. It can come on very suddenly and start with lower abdominal pain; often the individual suffers severe attacks and it can lead to kidney infection. Children occasionally get cystitis and this should be treated by an orthodox doctor.

CAUSES

The infection is commonly due to a bacterium called E.coli which normally lives in the bowel and gets transmitted to the bladder, either through poor hygiene or during sexual intercourse. The symptoms of cystitis need not necessarily mean there is an infection, as they can also occur as a result of the bruising that may arise during intercourse or after childbirth. Cystitis also arises if there is a vaginal infection – thrush and more seriously gonorrhoea. It can occur through irritation caused by vaginal deodorants, and because of diabetes. Diet does play a part in predisposing to attacks of cystitis, as does the wearing of tight jeans and underwear.

SYMPTOMS

■ Burning sensation and pain on passing urine.

Below: *This X-ray image shows the bladder (red oval) and the ureters that connect it to the kidneys.*

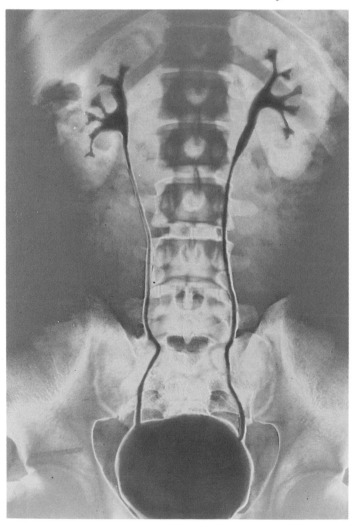

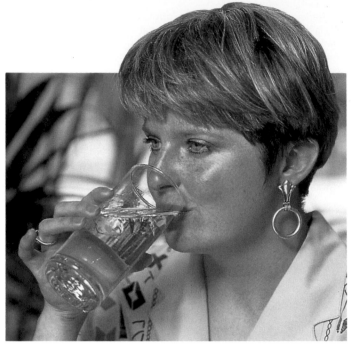

■ Frequent urination and pain just at the end of passing urine.
■ Low abdominal pain and occasionally low-back pain.
■ Temperature and shivering fits.
■ Cloudy, smelly urine with occasional blood.

PREVENTION AND SELF-HELP

During an attack
■ Drink a large glass of water or a cup of mild chamomile tea, three or four times a day.
■ Pass urine in a warm bath if very painful.
■ Stop consuming alcohol, coffee and tobacco.
■ Use hot water bottles to alleviate lower abdominal pain.
■ Change the acidity of your urine by adding a teaspoon of bicarbonate of soda to a glass of water and drinking the solution three or four times a day.
■ Apply live yoghurt to the vagina. This helps to relieve distress as well as to recolonize

Above: *If you develop cystitis, cut out alcohol, acidic fruit juices and coffee and make sure that you drink plenty of water during the day.*

the vagina with the "right" bacteria.
■ Avoid citrus juices and acid fruits.
■ Drink cranberry powder dissolved in water frequently (one teaspoon in a cup of water).
Between attacks
■ Change your underwear if it is too tight and avoid tights.
■ Maintain a high standard of hygiene after using the lavatory.
■ Always empty your bladder before and after intercourse.
■ Change from tampons to sanitary towels.
■ Always go to the lavatory if you feel the need to pass urine – do not hold back.
■ Use a lubricating jelly during intercourse if the vagina is very dry, and experiment with different positions as the pressure on the bladder and vulva will vary.

NATUROPATHY

Attention will be paid to diet, especially to the reduction of acid content, sugar and white flour products. Irrigating the vaginal area with warm water after going to the lavatory or having intercourse is recommended – you should take care to wipe the area from the vagina to the anus, and not vice versa. Drink vegetable juices – carrot and raw apple mixed are particularly good. Take propolis tablets – one tablet three times a day. Allergy tests may be done to exclude specific items, and candida may sometimes cause this problem.

Below: *Chamomile tea bags and the flowers from which they are made. The tea helps in cases of cystitis.*

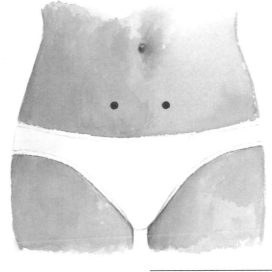

Above: *During an attack, gentle stimulation of the two Stomach 28 acupoints can relieve the pain.*

HOMEOPATHY

First aid treatment during an attack includes *Cantheris* 6x (one tablet every two hours). Others are *Staphisagria* for cystitis following intercourse, and *Sarsparilla* for pain on urinating, (dosage as above). A more long-term remedy would require a homeopathic consultation.

BIOCHEMIC TISSUE SALTS

Remedies include *Ferr. phos.* in the early stages followed by *Kali phos.* (one tablet twice a day for three days).

AROMATHERAPY

Recommendations here are juniper and eucalyptus oils (one to two drops in a cup of warm water). Drink two cups a day. Adding essential oils to a bath (ten drops) will help the soreness and aid recovery. Oils to try in this case include benzoin, bergamot and sandalwood.

ACUPRESSURE

Massage to the acupressure point Stomach 28 can help relieve the pain of an attack. This point is found three fingers' width on either side of the midline of the abdomen, and four fingers' width below the navel. Apply pressure gently on both sides angled downwards for one to two minutes.

OTHER THERAPIES

Massage, reflexology and hydrotherapy can all be of great help in the acute stages to relieve the tension and pain that is often associated with this condition.

Below: *Barley water is a traditional remedy to soothe the urinary tract. It can be made by boiling a heaped teaspoon of barley in a litre (1¾ pints) of water for half an hour and then straining off the liquid.*

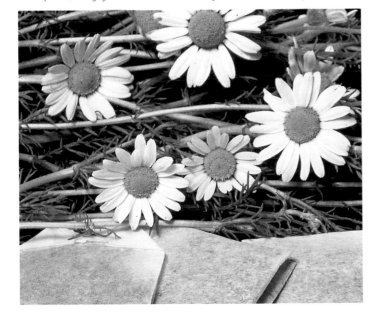

HERBAL MEDICINE

Much the same advice would be given. Specific herbal remedies include couch-grass, which aids the excretion of urine and heals the lining of bladder, and buchu which acts as an antiseptic and restores the damaged lining.

Echinacea is a good herb to restore resistance to infection, especially in the pelvic area. In an acute attack, drinking large amounts of yarrow infusion will help, and barley water (obtainable from food stores) is a traditional remedy for its soothing diuretic effect.

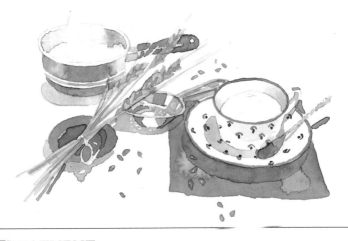

ORTHODOX TREATMENT

Cystitis is not in itself a serious condition and the occasional attack is not uncommon. Urine tests are taken to exclude infection and antibiotics prescribed if appropriate. If the attacks are frequent, it may be necessary to have a gynaecological examination, and an X-ray of the kidneys will reveal any problems. A cystoscopy involves looking into the bladder itself with a special instrument to rule out any polyps or other growths. The stretching of the urethra itself when this is done may help to reduce the frequency of the condition. Prevention is much the best policy and doctors will advise many of the self-help tips outlined above. If the problem is clearly associated with intercourse, taking one dose of antibiotics after intercourse can sometimes ensure the problem does not arise.

SEXUAL PROBLEMS

The freedom and willingness to discuss openly sexual activity that has become apparent over the last thirty years unfortunately does not seem to have reduced significantly the frequency and type of problems that men and women experience during sexual intercourse. More recent studies of sexual activity have identified certain patterns and types of "normal sexual cycle" and it is now common to discuss problems of desire (lack of sex drive), problems of excitement and arousal, and problems associated with orgasm and climax. Notwithstanding the physical nature of the sexual act and the importance of the appropriate "technique", the major causes of difficulties are still largely psychological, educational and emotional. It has also been important to separate the need for intimate physical contact from the sexual act itself. Many couples have found that to be liberated from the need to have a "technically" good sexual life has allowed them to enjoy the intimate physical and emotional closeness that can be achieved by the sensitive use of touch and sharing.

MALE PROBLEMS

Physical difficulties usually refer to impotence and premature ejaculation, both of which are largely caused by anxiety and psychological tension related to the sexual act. Impotence is the failure to achieve an erection which enables penetration. It can be caused by drugs, surgery, alcohol or fatigue and by certain medical conditions (diabetes, prostate disease etc.). Most men will experience impotence at least once in their lives as a result of "performance anxiety". The next occasion intercourse is attempted, the fear of impotence itself can produce impotence and a vicious circle is established. Sensitive and sympathetic response from the partner is often all that is required for this problem to right itself and sexual abstinence usually allows for the natural sex

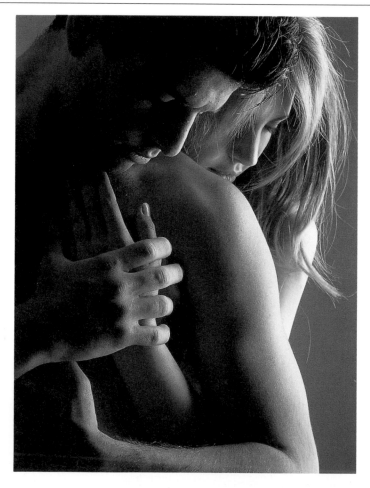

Above: *Tenderness and loving touch all play a part in a sexual relationship. When things go wrong, the causes can be mental just as much as physical.*

drive to return. Aphrodisiacs from oysters to ginseng or rhinoceros horn have been much used as a traditional folk cure. Little evidence suggests that these stimulants work in any other way than psychologically. Fatigue and stress are important to address

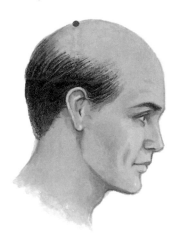

Above: *This point, called Governing Vessel 20, is specifically recommended for dealing with impotence.*

and massage, especially of an overtly sensual variety, will help.

ACUPRESSURE

The point specifically used to help impotence is called Governing Vessel 20. This is found on top of the head midway along a line joining the tops of the ears. Apply pressure perpendicularly downwards using the middle or index fingertip for two minutes.

HERBAL MEDICINE

Herbal practitioners will suggest a review of your diet and recommend the exclusion of coffee, alcohol, and saturated fat. Smoking will also be discouraged.

PREMATURE EJACULATION

This is the condition in which the man reaches his climax too rapidly – either before or immediately after penetration. This pattern of sexual activity causes distress both to himself and his partner. Again, anxiety and stress are felt to be the major factors and relaxation methods using deep breathing exercises actually during intercourse will help to reduce the level of excitement. Other natural methods have involved having more frequent intercourse, using a condom to decrease sensitivity of the penis and desensitizing the aspect of penetrative sex by encouraging touch and massage without proceeding to sex itself. The squeeze technique – whereby the partner squeezes gently behind the glans or head of the penis for about three to four seconds to reduce sensitivity and erection – has helped many couples with this problem.

ACUPRESSURE

Stimulation of acupressure point Kidney 3 is said to help. It is found on the inside of the ankle. Just before intercourse apply pressure with the tip of the index finger slightly downwards and towards the heel, for about two minutes.

WOMEN'S PROBLEMS

Dyspareunia or painful intercourse may be related to a lack of lubrication, either because the woman does not feel aroused by her partner or because there has not been sufficient attention to foreplay. The vagina contains mucus-secreting glands which will normally lubricate the vagina if the clitoris or vulva is stimulated. Other causes of dyspareunia may be physical in nature (especially likely if the pain is deeply felt) and can be caused by infection or cysts. It is important to seek the advice of a doctor if this is the case. A particular type of painful intercourse is called **vaginismus** where there is a painful spasm of the vaginal muscles. This will occur where intercourse is not acceptable to the woman or because of some previous frightening or painful experience (such as rape, surgical operation, labour). Penetration may be impossible in vaginismus and should not be attempted. It is important for a woman to feel confident of her ability to control the sexual act and treatment often involves suggestions that the woman should feel her own vagina in the bath and allow her fingers to enter gradually, recovering her confidence of

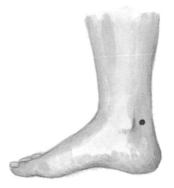

Above: *Stimulation of the Kidney 3 acupoint is thought to overcome difficulty with premature ejaculation.*

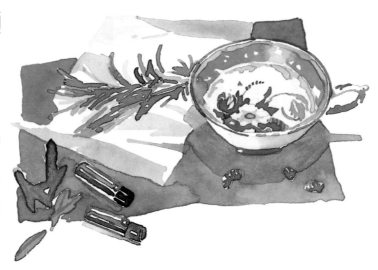

Above: *Tension is the enemy of good sex. A massage or bath using these oils will help you unwind.*

being penetrated. As in all sexual problems, good communication and a sensitive partner will ensure many of the problems can be dealt with without seeking professional help. Touch, massage and the use of aromatherapy are the key to overcoming many of these sexual difficulties. Oils such as cedarwood, sandalwood, myrrh and rosemary have been used both to relieve tension as well as stimulate sexual desire. Add three drops of the essential oil to a warm bath, or make up a massage lotion by adding half a teaspoon of oil to half a cup of a carrier oil and apply as part of a sensual full body massage. If vaginismus persists then expert help from a trained sexual counsellor will be required.

FAILURE TO ACHIEVE ORGASM

This is a subjective problem and many women do not always want to have an orgasm every time they have sex. Worry about failure to achieve orgasm can be the result of a masculine wish to indicate his sexual powers.

Usually this is indicative of problems in the relationship which are psychological rather than physical. Proper "technique" to achieve orgasm involves an appropriate level of foreplay, and gentle stimulation of all erogenous zones including the clitoris. Many women can achieve orgasm when the clitoris is manually stimulated, either by masturbation or by their partner. Scientific studies suggest that women can achieve a different form of orgasm (vaginal) by penetrative sex, but that a clitoral orgasm occurs only when that organ is directly stimulated.

LACK OF SEX DRIVE

This can occur in both sexes and it is important to remember that human beings are different when it comes to the frequency with which they want to have sex. Good communication is essential between the couple and general measures to relieve stress, fatigue and depression are as important as good sexual technique. Variety is well known to awaken sex drive and willingness to experiment with atmosphere, positions, time of day, the use of incense etc. may all help to address this particular problem. Many herbal folk remedies exist to help with sexual problems, ginseng being the best known, but it is really more important to talk and communicate effectively with your partner, than to rely on some external aid which almost always acts as a psychological prop.

Below: *If you can communicate with and understand your partner, love and desire may last a lifetime.*

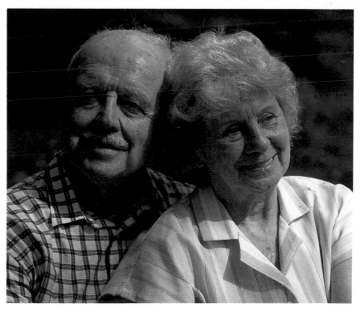

ORTHODOX TREATMENT

Much of the advice given above will be very similar to that you will encounter when visiting a doctor to deal with a sexual problem. Attention may be given to the male menopause and certain doctors are using testosterone for male sexual difficulties. Occasionally, injections into the penis will enable erection to take place and prosthetic appliances and surgical operations will be used in specific circumstances.

PERIOD PROBLEMS

Menstruation usually commences in young girls between the ages of 12 and 14 and often coincides with the development of secondary sexual characteristics (breast enlargement and pubic hair growth). Two hormones, oestrogen and progesterone, control the course of the menstrual cycle which allows the lining of the womb (uterus) to thicken in preparation for the egg (if fertilized) to be embedded and then nurtured during pregnancy. The egg is released between day 10 and day 14 of the cycle and if fertilized by the sperm will travel down through the fallopian tube and reach the cavity of the uterus. If the egg is not fertilized, then the lining of the womb sloughs and the period or menstrual flow occurs. It usually lasts anything from three to seven days. Disorders of menstruation are not uncommon and about three percent of all visits to general practitioners relate to a menstrual problem. These can be amenorrhoea (lack of periods), dysmenorrhoea (painful periods), menorrhagia (excessive or too frequent bleeding) and pre-menstrual tension (PMT – excessive or abnormal response to hormonal changes). Other concerns may include irregular bleeding, spotting between periods or post-menopausal bleeding (intermittent bleeding following the menopause).

CAUSES

Amenorrhoea The most common cause is pregnancy and this has to be excluded in all cases. This may also occur while taking the oral contraceptive pill or when the pill is discontinued. A common cause is breast-feeding; this is a normal occurrence. Severe illness, frequent travel and severe dieting may also cause the periods to stop. Stress is another major factor and it is not uncommon before academic examinations.

Dysmenorrhoea A certain amount of pain is a normal consequence of menstrual bleeding. Periods with no pain usually suggest that the egg has not been released, a frequent condition at the beginning of a woman's reproductive life. Severe pain (low back, abdominal or pelvic) can accompany a condition called endometriosis, where a small piece of the lining of the womb may lie outside the womb itself, or chronic pelvic infections.

Menorrhagia and dysfunctional uterine bleeding These conditions are commonly caused by hormonal imbalance but may indicate pelvic infection or the presence of fibroids (small "gristly growths" in the wall of the uterus). Heavy bleeding may also be caused by a late and missed abortion.

Pre-menstrual tension (PMT) This is probably the most common period problem and is usually the result of hormonal changes affecting the body metabolism leading to fluid retention. It can be an hereditary condition but is also affected by stress and psychological disorders.

SYMPTOMS

Amenorrhoea Absence or stoppage of periods usually for up to three months. Occasionally very slight and scanty periods.

Dysmenorrhoea This may be spasmodic in type and be of very severe intensity for one or two days at the beginning of the period. It may cause severe distress, loss of work. The more common kind lasts through the period, is often associated with low back pain and is less severe. Sometimes the pain may cause vomiting and fainting.

Menorrhagia Heavy periods with clots requiring several tampons or pads throughout the day. Occasional "flooding" which is not controlled by pads. This may be accompanied by tiredness and anaemia.

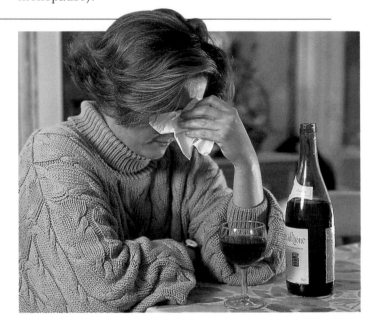

Above: *If you suffer from PMT it makes sense to cut out alcohol, as drinking may simply exacerbate the feelings of depression and moodiness.*

Below: *The beautiful fragrance of rose otto helps to disperse headaches and lift feelings of gloom.*

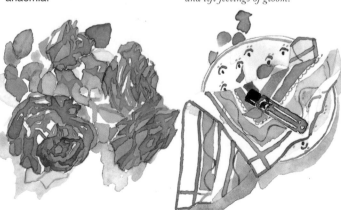

Pre-menstrual tension syndrome Moodiness, irritability, depression, low self-esteem, headaches, painful enlarged breasts, gain in weight, swollen ankles, headaches, changes in appetite, loss of libido, increase in arguments and bizarre behaviour (shop-lifting, car accidents and violent outbursts) have all been associated with PMT, and are most commonly experienced three to seven days before the period is due. Symptoms usually disappear once the period starts.

SELF-HELP FOR PMT

PMT, although a harmless condition, can be a major problem for many women and needs to be taken seriously and treated sympathetically.

■ Keep a chart of your periods

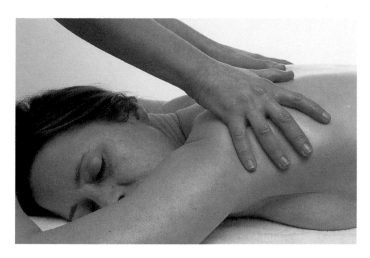

together with a list of your symptoms

■ Check your diet – avoid or stop consuming sugar-containing food, caffeine, alcohol, salt, and eat lots of fresh fruit and salads. Some naturopaths suggest a fluid-only fast (herbal teas, dilute juices, natural water) for two days before your symptoms of PMT are due to start.

■ Supplements have been found to help some women, especially Vitamin B_6 (10mg three times a day for seven days), Vitamin C (500mg daily), zinc (5mg daily) and magnesium (one tablet a day). If these are taken for one week before the period starts, they may help.

■ Evening primrose oil can also be helpful. Take two 500mg capsules twice daily for two days (2.2.2) before the symptoms are likely to commence.

■ Regular exercise, cold showers and relaxation techniques will all help to reduce the symptoms. If you have skin symptoms associated with PMT (greasy skin, spots), a Vitamin E supplement (one tablet a day for eight weeks) will also help.

Aromatherapy As well as a cold shower, soaking in a warm bath containing three drops of essential oils (one of these: lavender, sage, geranium) before sleeping will help. Headaches

Above: *A soothing body massage with aromatherapy oils is a fine way to pamper yourself and relieve PMT.*

moodiness) and *Nat. mur.* (sadness and fluid retention).

Herbal treatment may involve a strong diuretic (couch grass), but drinking a cup of chamomile tea three times a day, for up to one week, will also help.

Acupuncture is of great help in all menstrual problems but advice and treatment should be sought from a trained practitioner.

Acupressure on the point Bladder 23 may help. It is found on the waist line, two fingers' width from the midline at the level of the second lumbar vertebra. Apply pressure for two minutes.

Below: *The positions of acupoints Bladder 23 (on the waist line) and Bladder 32 are shown here.*

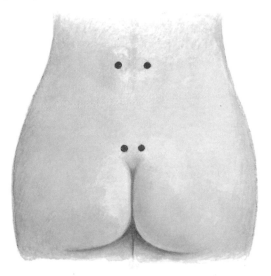

and irritability can be helped by inhaling the scent of a drop of essential oil (Roman camomile, rose otto) in the palm of your hand. A full body massage will relieve some of the tension and reduce fluid retention.

Homeopathy should be started 24 hours before the symptoms start, taking the following remedies 30x potency, one tablet four times a day, for up to one week: *Pulsatilla* (breast engorgement and fluid retention), *Sepia* (depression and

Reflexology and massage help with reducing muscle tension and the acupressure point Bladder 23, suggested above, will reduce pain. Herbalists recommend an infusion of ginger to reduce period pain; acupuncture can be of great help as well. Bach remedies include crab apple, and the biochemic tissue salt *Mag. phos.* (one tablet twice a day) will also help.

SELF-HELP FOR IRREGULAR AND HEAVY PERIODS

It is important to obtain a medical opinion first regarding these symptoms because they may signal an underlying gynaecological disorder that would require specific treatment. However, if the condition is related to hormonal imbalance, many of the general measures outlined above will help.

Aromatherapists recommend three drops of essential oil on a sugar cube three times a day.

Acupressure on the acupressure points Bladder 23 and Bladder 32 will help to regulate and reduce menstrual flow. For scanty periods, pressure on the Large Intestine 4 point is helpful. This is located between the thumb and index finger on the triangle made when fingers are outstretched.

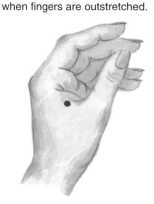

Above: *The Large Intestine 4 point can be stimulated to help deal with scanty or irregular periods.*

SELF-HELP FOR DYSMENORRHOEA

Many of the general measures suggested above should be followed, but for severe pain aromatherapists recommend the following oils: marjoram, aniseed, cypress, rubbed gently into the abdomen and lower back. The oils need to be diluted in carrier oil, 1/2 teaspoon in 1/2 cup. Homeopathic remedies include *Viburnum* 30x and *Belladonna* 30x – one tablet four times a day,

ORTHODOX TREATMENT

Most doctors will want to conduct a gynaecological examination which will include an internal with a cervical smear, vaginal swab and ultrasound to exclude a physical cause for period problems. Hormonal treatment may be prescribed for menstrual irregularity and occasionally a D & C (dilation and curettage whereby part of the lining of the

uterus is scraped away) will be undertaken to treat heavy menstrual blood loss. In severe PMT, diuretic tablets may be prescribed or a series of hormone tablets to regulate the cycle. Painful periods may respond to simple analgesics but occasional specific medicines (such as mefenamic acid) will provide relief for spasmodic dysmenorrhoea.

THE MENOPAUSE

Technically this is the cessation of periods and usually occurs for most women around the age of 50, but can occur as early as 35. There is no set pattern – the periods can stop suddenly, or there can be a gradual decrease in blood loss, or gradually more infrequent periods. Women who have had their ovaries removed will experience early menopause. Most of the descriptions of menopause concentrate on the physical symptoms, but it is also a time of emotional change for most women which may result in profound psychological symptoms. It can be a time for women to take stock of their lives, femininity and career paths. It has been common to describe the menopause as a time when women will feel less womanly and develop unpleasant physical symptoms (tiredness, hot flushes, irritability, mood swings). For many it is the reverse, however. It is important to remember that it is a normal event in a woman's life and is not necessarily associated with unpleasant symptoms. For many women throughout the world, the idea of treating the menopause as if it were a "disease" would be unthinkable.

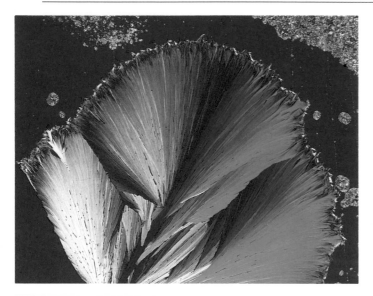

PREVENTION AND SELF-HELP

Anticipating the onset of the menopause can help in adjusting to the physical and psychological effects that may be experienced, and many women have found self-help groups and information leaflets of value in helping them prepare for the "change". Openly discussing the onset of menopause with your partner will also ensure that anxiety about loss of sexual attraction is addressed. Symptoms are often made worse by overwork and stress; paying attention to the routine habits in your life (exercise, good diet, relaxation) will be important at this time. Specific symptoms can be helped by many of the alternative therapies. However, it is important to keep reminding yourself that this is a normal occurrence during every woman's life and it should not be seen as a disease which immediately requires treatment, whether it be complementary or orthodox.

Below: *The menopause is a time of change, but it does not have to be unwelcome. Try to find time for yourself, and plan some relaxation.*

CAUSES

The menopause occurs because the ovaries reduce their production of the hormone oestrogen, which causes the cessation of menstruation and ovulation. It signals the end of fertility, although it has been known for women to become pregnant up to one year following cessation of periods.

SYMPTOMS

As mentioned above, for the majority of women the menopause is a significant state and indeed it may coincide with a feeling of liberation and increased energy. For others, the reduction in oestrogen will produce unwelcome local symptoms (dry vagina, painful intercourse, dry wrinkled skin) and other more general symptoms that are also undesirable: typically hot flushes, night sweats, decreased sexual

Above: *A magnified view of crystals of oestradiol, one of the naturally occurring oestrogen hormones.*

interest and libido, tiredness, depression and irritability. Headaches can also occur and at times it can be difficult to separate the physical causes from the psychological ones. It is often important to explore the marital, social and economic context in which the menopause occurs. It is regrettably true that for up to 25 percent of women, menopausal symptoms can be fairly distressing and may require treatment. Most menopausal symptoms run their course (if untreated) within a year or eighteen months. The more serious effects of a lower oestrogen level include development of osteoporosis and the increased risks of developing heart disease (oestrogen protects against the development of arteriosclerosis).

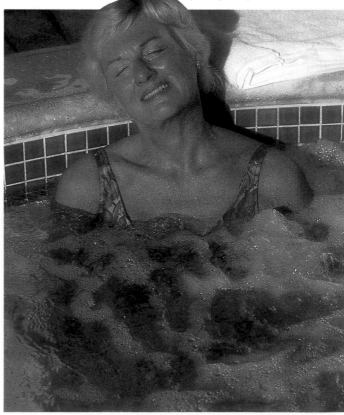

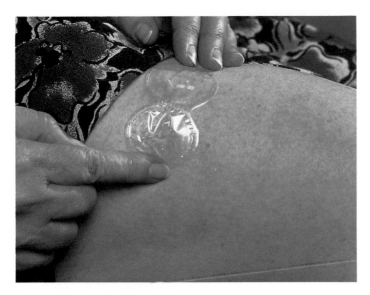

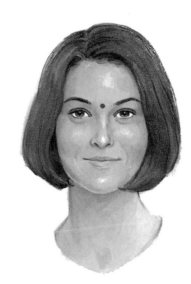

HERBAL MEDICINE

Herbal teas including chamomile and lime blossom will aid with fluid retention. A traditional remedy for night sweats involves honey (one teaspoon) and three drops of sage oil in a cup of hot water. Drink before going to bed.

NATUROPATHY

A wholefood diet eliminating sugar, tea, coffee and cold drinks will help with general symptoms. Small meals of raw food, salads, nuts and cereals together with the following supplements have been recommended by naturopaths:

HOMEOPATHY

Treatment will often be geared to your specific personality and may require a proper consultation. *Lachesis* 30x and *Glonoinum* 30x (one tablet four times a day for three days) will help with hot flushes and *Pulsatilla* 6x (one tablet twice a day) Is a good remedy for irritability and mood swings that accompany the change.

Above: *Hormone replacement therapy. The patch releases oestradiol into the skin, which helps to relieve menopausal symptoms.*

Below: *Night sweats are unpleasant; try inhaling oils of sage, cypress and geranium from a muslin handkerchief to relieve such symptoms.*

Above: *Gentle massage of the Yintang point between the eyebrows is recommended for dealing with problems associated with hormonal changes.*

- Six to ten brewer's yeast tablets daily.
- Two kelp tablets daily.
- One multivitamin/mineral tablet daily.
- Two garlic capsules daily.

Hot flushes may respond to Vitamin E, in tablet form, taken twice daily together with Vitamin C (1g daily).

MASSAGE AND AROMATHERAPY

These are good general treatments for recapturing a level of well-being and reducing stress. Oils of sage, cypress and geranium either used in a warm bath (six drops) or taken as an inhalation (one drop on a muslin handkerchief) will help night sweats.

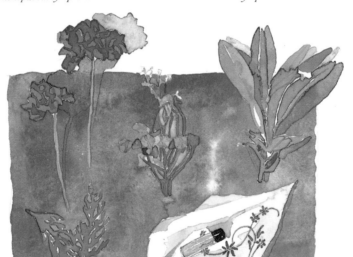

ACUPRESSURE

Apply gentle pressure for two minutes to the Yintang acupressure point which is found on the forehead, above the bridge of the nose halfway between the inner edge of each eyebrow. This will help with troublesome symptoms.

ORTHODOX TREATMENT

Orthodox treatments have been revolutionized in recent years with the introduction of hormone replacement therapy (HRT). This treatment has attracted much publicity. For some doctors the menopause is viewed as a hormone deficiency condition which requires treatment, while others consider it to be a normal physiological occurrence which requires no treatment. Oestrogen can be used as a local treatment in the form of vaginal pessaries or vaginal cream. HRT can be given as an oestrogen-only pill or as a combination of oestrogen and progesterone. It can be taken orally, as a skin patch or as a "depot" deep muscle injection which can last for up to six months. More recently some gynaecologists have used testosterone as well in the injectable implants, as it is the lack of this particular

hormone that can lead to the feelings of profound tiredness and loss of energy. The dangers of using HRT include the possibility of increased cancer of the womb and/or breasts although many experts still dispute this. The greatest benefit of taking HRT (other than reducing the menopausal symptoms) is in the prevention of osteoporosis (see page 130). The inconvenience of using HRT is the continuation of monthly bleeding. Before prescribing HRT your doctor will want to conduct an internal examination, may take blood tests to determine your hormone levels and conduct a breast examination. You will need regular medical check-ups. Many women have praised the results of HRT but it is important to remember long term studies have not been undertaken and so the long term risks are still unknown.

VAGINAL DISCHARGE

A small amount of vaginal discharge is a normal part of the physiological response of a woman to hormonal changes and is usually of a clear mucous colour. However, excessive or unpleasant vaginal discharge can be a sign of the presence of thrush – a bacterial infection – or one of a number of sexually transmitted diseases. Absence of vaginal discharge, which may occur during stress or after the menopause, may give rise to painful intercourse and require specific treatment.

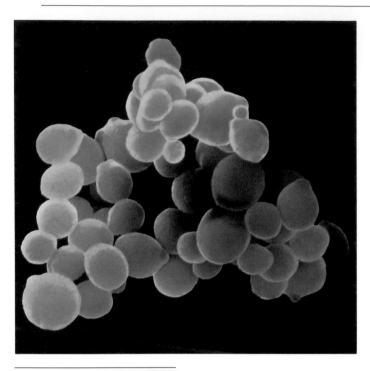

PREVENTION AND SELF-HELP

■ Avoid tight-fitting clothes and synthetic underwear. Tight jeans and wearing tights rather than stockings can all increase the dampness and temperature that will encourage thrush to grown in the vagina.
■ Maintain good personal hygiene, ensuring you use toilet paper from front to back to ensure you do not infect yourself by transferring matter from the anus to the vagina. Avoid constipation and take regular baths, ensuring you dry yourself carefully.
■ Review your diet and reduce all sugar-containing foods, high fat foods and reduce your intake of carbohydrates. Avoid eating mushrooms and any other yeast-containing foods.
■ Eat plenty of fresh fruit and

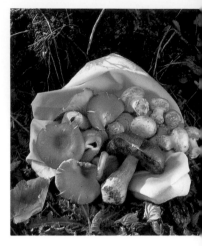

Above: *If you are prone to thrush, mould-containing foods like mushrooms should be excluded from your diet.*

Below: *This tiny organism, here magnified more than 6,000 times, causes trichomoniasis.*

CAUSES

Most causes of vaginal discharge are as a result of infection: the commonest is thrush. This is caused by the fungus candida albicans which itself is a normal constituent of both the large bowel and the vagina. Normally it gives rise to no symptoms, but under specific conditions it will cause a thick creamy white discharge, which may cause staining on the underwear. Thrush occurs for a number of reasons. It may be triggered by hormonal changes (the use of an oral contraceptive, pregnancy), poor diet (high carbohydrate, sugar and white flour intake) as well as poor hygiene. Thrush is also caused by antibiotics and steroid medication and can be transmitted during sexual intercourse. Vaginal deodorants and diabetes mellitus will also predispose to the development of thrush. Other causes of vaginal discharge are most commonly related to sexually transmitted

Above: *This unwelcome guest is the fungus* Candida albicans, *which gives rise on occasions to thrush, the commonest vaginal infection.*

diseases, such as gonorrhoea, trichomoniasis and chlamydia. The discharge is of a different nature – yellow, watery – and is often offensive. Another cause is the use of a tampon which has been forgotten, the use of vaginal pads that are not changed frequently enough, and sensitivity to perfumed vaginal deodorants.

SYMPTOMS

Vaginal discharge (yellow, white, clear, milky) together with itchiness and soreness. Your partner may have similar symptoms or itchiness of the penis. Difficulty with or pain during intercourse is not unusual and the infection may spread to the vulva and skin folds. Pain on passing urine may accompany the vaginal infection and suggest cystitis and bladder infection.

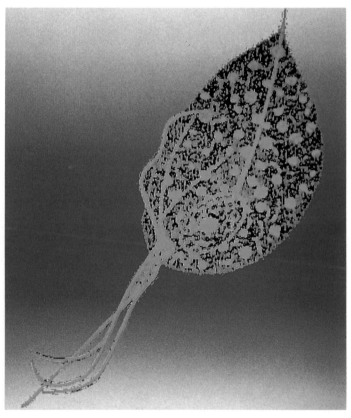

salads, and supplement your diet with Vitamin B complex. Lactobacillus acidophilus is a normal ingredient of the gut that keeps the candida under control. Take one tablet twice a day while you have the thrush infection and for at least two weeks after that. It is also helpful to eat natural live yoghurt which helps to restore the intestinal flora with beneficial bacteria.

■ Take short baths adding either a tablespoon of salt or wine vinegar to the water.

■ Do not use any medicated vaginal deodorants. Do not use biological powders to wash your underwear as the fungus can live through the lower temperature of a washing cycle that uses biological powder. Occasionally you may need to buy a completely new set of underwear or use disposable panties.

■ Avoid taking unnecessary antibiotics and if you are prone to thrush, mention this to your doctor who may prescribe some pessaries to use at the same time as you are taking the antibiotics.

■ Review your choice of contraceptive as the pill affects vaginal secretions and sugar levels, making it easier for the fungus to grow. Sequential contraceptive pills are less prone to causing thrush than combined pills. If you use a cap, make sure it is properly cleaned after use and if necessary obtain a new one. Ask your partner if he has any symptoms as you may be re-infecting one another. He may need treatment as well as you if the infection is persistent and difficult to shake off.

■ You can treat yourself by dabbing a pad of cotton wool soaked in a weak solution of wine vinegar, lemon juice or salt water directly on the external genitalia.

Below: A good diet and good health are closely related. Eat plenty of salads and fresh fruit if you get thrush; cut down on sugar and fat.

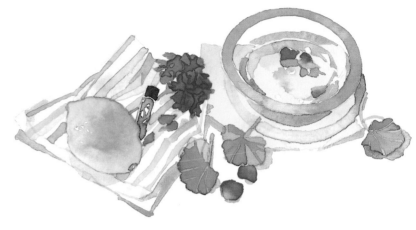

HERBAL MEDICINE

Herbalists suggest an infusion of the herb arbor vitae. Add 30g (1oz) of the leaves of the plant to half a litre (¾ of a pint) of boiling water. Leave it to infuse for one hour, strain the liquid, check the temperature and apply the infusion to the external genitalia three to four times a day.

BIOCHEMIC TISSUE SALTS

Particularly recommended is *Nat. mur.* 6x, one tablet to be taken four times a day. If the thrush is particularly troublesome it is important to seek the advice of your doctor. Any discharge that does not clear up quickly should be examined to exclude other causes of infection.

AROMATHERAPY

Essential oils can be used to prevent re-infection. Six drops of essential oils of lemon, sage and geranium may be added to a carrier oil and the body massaged with this preparation. This can help build up resistance to thrush. If the vulva is sore, a soothing

Above: Aromatherapists maintain that massage with oils of lemon, sage and geranium builds resistance to thrush.

mixture of diluted essential oils of sandalwood and peppermint can help. Two or three drops in an egg cup full of carrier oil and applied locally will help to treat the infection, as will live yoghurt placed directly in the vagina and around the external genitalia.

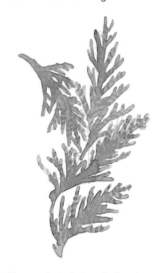

Above: An infusion of arbor vitae, obtained from the Thuja tree, makes a solution for soothing the vulva.

ORTHODOX TREATMENT

A gynaecological examination is normally undertaken and vaginal swabs will reveal the cause of the infection. Anti-fungal pessaries are often prescribed and are inserted in the vagina using an applicator provided. If there is external soreness, a cream or anti-fungal ointment will clear the infection quickly. Occasionally it may be necessary to take a short course of anti-fungal tablets (such as nystatin) to clear up the excess fungal overgrowth in the large bowel. This is often the result of prolonged use of antibiotics or inadequate diet. Other causes of vaginal discharge will be revealed following examination of the vaginal swab and specific treatment will be prescribed (metronidazole or penicillin). It is important that these infections are treated early and properly, as they may lead to wider pelvic infections which may result in fertility problems at a later date due to blocked tubes. Stress is a common cause of recurrent thrush and you will be advised to examine your lifestyle and practise some relaxation routine or take part in regular exercise.

CONTRACEPTION

Planning your family is one of the most important choices you will have to make in your life, and it is now possible to choose from a variety of contraceptive methods, each having advantages and disadvantages. The ovum or egg is usually released between the 10th and 14th day of the menstrual cycle (the time between periods) and remains capable of being fertilized for about 24 hours after it is released. However, the male sperm can survive in the genital tract for much longer and have been found alive and kicking up to seven days after intercourse has taken place. Contraceptive methods include: hormonal (the pill, deep muscular injections), barrier methods (condom, cap, pessaries, contraceptive creams), inter-uterine devices (the coil) and more natural methods. If it is impossible for you to proceed with a pregnancy, then you may wish to consider a form of oral contraception as the most foolproof. If intercourse is infrequent, one of the barrier methods – if properly used – may be perfectly acceptable.

NATURAL METHODS

Other than often lurid "folk" methods of avoiding pregnancy, the three most common methods are withdrawal, calculating your infertile days and breast feeding.
Withdrawal This is probably the most commonly used natural method and has certainly been used since biblical times. It is sometimes known as coitus interruptus, and is a method acceptable to the Roman Catholic Church. It depends on a man withdrawing his penis before he ejaculates and ensuring that no pre-ejaculate leaks into the vagina before or during penetration. For obvious reasons this is neither a safe nor a satisfactory method of contraception. Mistakes are all

Below: *The moment of conception – an egg (pink sphere) is fertilized by a male sperm (yellow tail at top).*

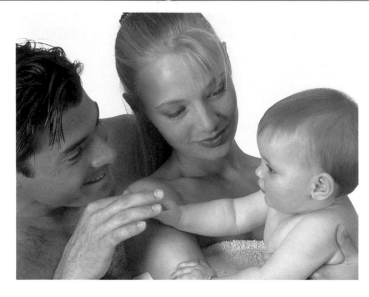

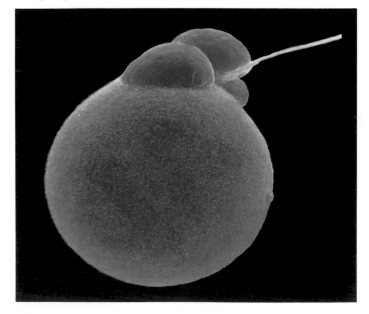

too common and the failure rate appears to be as much as 10 percent. It is, however, cheap, it is always available and there are no adverse side effects – unless you get pregnant.

Above: *Contraception allows a couple to plan when they will embark on a family. Unforeseen pregnancy can impose strain on a relationship.*

Calculating your fertile period
Because it is not always possible to be accurate as to the time of ovulation and because as mentioned earlier, sperm can live in the genital tract for some time, the safest time for intercourse is after you have ovulated and before your next period. Calculating when you ovulate can be achieved by a number of methods:
▪ *The calendar method* Keep a diary of your periods for at least six, or preferably twelve months. Calculate your longest cycle, taking the first day of your period as day one. Subtract 11 from this figure which will give you the beginning of your infertile period. For instance, if your longest cycle is 30 days, 30 minus 11 equals 19, so your infertile period starts on the 20th day of your cycle.

Then calculate your shortest cycle and subtract 19 from this; e.g. 25 days – 19 = 6. This figure indicates when you are likely to be fertile again in your next cycle. So, in this example your **unsafe** days would be from day 6 to day 20 in each cycle.
▪ *The temperature method* This is a little more accurate but again requires you to take your temperature every day (under the tongue) before your early morning cup of tea. You can obtain easy-to-read thermometers and charts from your local family planning clinic. This method relies on the fact that there is a slight rise in the basal temperature of 1° Fahrenheit (0.5°C) immediately following ovulation until the next period. The fertile period is calculated from the fourth day before to three or four days after the rise in temperature. Intercourse should be avoided during this time.
▪ *Cervical changes* Some women are able to detect when they ovulate because the neck of the womb softens and rises slightly in the vagina. The external opening (os) is slightly larger. This physical evidence again indicates unsafe days for intercourse.
▪ *Mucus changes* Changes in the mucus produced by the cervix also occur before and after ovulation and some women are able to detect the point of ovulation by examining the mucus. For about three days preceding ovulation the mucus becomes copious and watery, while following ovulation it becomes sticky and minimal. The infertile period is calculated as beginning four days after the most copious secretion.

Breast feeding This is probably the most natural of birth control methods and is nature's way of protecting a mother from another immediate pregnancy. Ovulation usually restarts within three months of delivery, but breast feeding (due to the sucking) can switch off this process and mothers who are able to breast feed can delay the recurrence of ovulation for up to two years. Like all natural methods it is not entirely reliable and it is important to take other precautions if a pregnancy is not wanted.

If practised effectively natural methods can provide a satisfactory protection against pregnancy. A failure rate of only about one to three percent has been recorded in well motivated couples. Figures above 10 percent are, however, the average as most couples do not or are unable to maintain the disciplines that these methods require.

BARRIER METHODS

The condom is an acceptable and safe method of contraception which is now more frequently used as it protects against sexually transmitted disease and AIDS. Although not "natural" it is without side effects and if used with a spermicide can produce over 98 percent reliable protection.

Below: This diagram shows how a woman can work out her infertile days by temperature change or calculation based on her monthly cycle.

The cap or diaphragm will suit some women especially those who have had a child and who are in a stable relationship. It needs to be fitted by a doctor or a nurse at a family planning centre, and because it can be inserted some time before intercourse takes place does not interfere with the spontaneous act the way that a condom does. Caps are of two kinds – diaphragm and suction caps which fit over the cervix. Recently a "female condom" has been developed which is rather like a plastic disposable lining which is inserted into the vagina before intercourse takes place.

Spermicides are special preparations that kill sperm. Their use is really essential when using a condom or cap for they increase the safety rate by at least 10 percent. These come as soluble pessaries, or gels, or aerosol foams. The contraceptive sponge is another option; it is made of polyurethane and impregnated with spermicide. It is, however, not entirely reliable.

THE PILL

The pill is the most common artificial form of contraception used and has revolutionized the management of conception. Many women have found that the convenience and ease of taking one pill a day has freed them from the fear of pregnancy. The pill is a combination of the hormones oestrogen and

progesterone and prevents the release of the egg, thus avoiding the risk of fertilization. It can both regulate the menstrual cycle as well as prevent ovulation. With the "low-dose" pills now available, the side effects are minimal and long-term risks have been much reduced. Nevertheless you will need to be seen by a doctor to

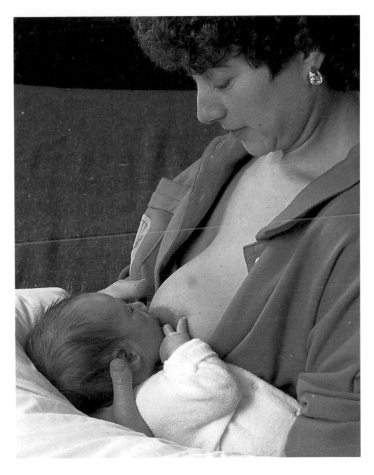

Above: Breast feeding a baby delays the restart of ovulation; it is nature's way of controlling pregnancy.

check your blood pressure, weight, breasts (the pill may increase the risk of breast cancer in some cases) and have a gynaecological examination before starting on the pill.

The temperature method

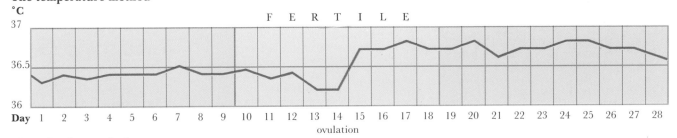

The calendar method

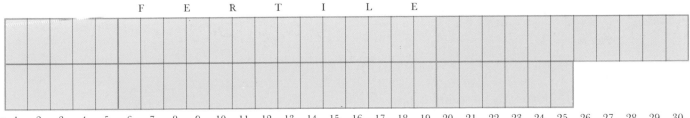

BEDWETTING

By the age of two and a half, two out of every three children are dry by day and half also by night. After five years of age only ten percent of children are still wet by night, but this condition may continue until the age of 15 in two percent of cases. Enuresis (or bedwetting) is of two types: it is found in children who have never been dry and those who have been and then start wetting the bed again.

CAUSES

Nervous control of the bladder in childhood is variable and there may be no specific abnormality other than delayed control. Often the difficulty occurs if the parents react with punishment, and the child becomes frightened and/or guilty because he or she has wet the bed. Certainly, anxiety and loss of security can make a child wet the bed and it can be a sign of childhood depression. Another major set of causes are related to bladder infection, bladder control and occasionally kidney disease. All these causes can be eliminated simply by examining the urine.

Below: *What goes in must come out! Try to discourage children from drinking at night if bedwetting is a problem.*

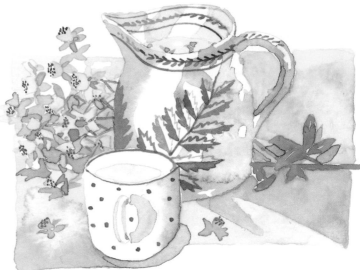

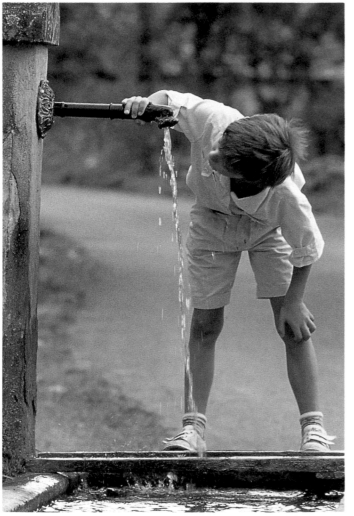

SYMPTOMS

These are usually self-apparent and it is important the child is not made to feel ashamed. Some children will sleep right through the night and still wet the bed while asleep; others will wake up and then wet the bed. Any specific symptoms such as pain or general fatigue should be reported.

PREVENTION AND SELF-HELP

The commonest form of bedwetting is because of delayed bladder control and the child should not be admonished or punished when accidents occur. A simple explanation should be given and measures such as reducing the child's fluid intake before going to bed, or waking the child up to pass urine once in the night could be all that is required. If persistent, urinary infections should be excluded

Above: *A few sips of an infusion of St. John's wort taken before bedtime promotes peaceful sleep.*

through consulting your doctor who may, if the test is positive, wish to send you to see a specialist. Placing a rubber sheet over the mattress and using a buzzer apparatus to wake the child is the next method to try. Any dampness or urine activates the buzzer which wakes the child. Massaging the child before sleeping will help as well, as it will help relax the child and allow him or her to sleep peacefully.

HERBAL MEDICINE

Herbalists may prescribe an infusion of St. John's wort to reduce anxiety and produce a level or relaxation. Add a handful of dried flowers to one litre (1¾ pints) of hot water. Allow the mixture to stand for one hour, strain, and give the child half a cup before bed.

ORTHODOX TREATMENT

Orthodox medical measures will include all of the above, but the doctor may also suggest counselling if it appears that either the child or the parents are particularly anxious about this symptom. Recently a mild anti-depressant in the form of a syrup has been found to be helpful.

PROSTATE PROBLEMS

The prostate is a small, walnut-shaped gland that lies at the neck of a man's bladder encircling the urethra (the tube through which the urine flows) at the base of the penis. It produces a lubricating fluid in which the sperm are carried during ejaculation. The prostate can become infected (prostatitis), usually as a result of a sexually transmitted disease, or it can enlarge, usually after the age of 50, causing disturbance in passing urine. The enlargement of the prostate is fairly common and can lead to cancer of the prostate, which is the third most common cancer afflicting men.

CAUSES

The cause of overgrowth of the prostate gland is unknown but approximately 80 percent of men over the age of 80 will develop it. It is considered to be caused by a hormonal change, although more recently a dietary factor has been identified.

SYMPTOMS

Infection of the prostate gland will lead to pain in the lower abdomen or on sitting down. There may be a temperature and a general feeling of fatigue and unwellness. In severe cases it will cause difficulty in passing urine together with a urethral discharge. An enlarged prostate gland will

Below: *A section through the tissue of a healthy prostate gland, here seen magnified 75 times.*

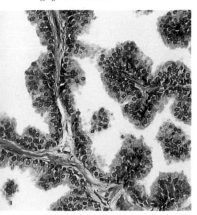

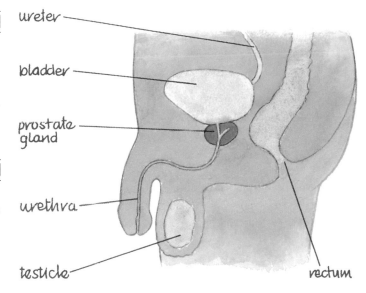

ureter
bladder
prostate gland
urethra
testicle
rectum

Above: *The prostate gland is situated under the bladder. It produces fluid to carry sperm during ejaculation.*

initially not produce any symptoms other than a mild reduction in the flow of urine. Most troublesome symptoms include high frequency of urination (having to get up at night), dribbling and incontinence, often accompanied by urine infections.

PREVENTION AND SELF-HELP

Recently it has been discovered that the prostate contains ten times more zinc than any other organ in the body and regular zinc is now prescribed (one tablet a day). Eating more of the zinc-containing foods (such as

brewer's yeast, wheatgerm, pumpkin seeds, powdered mustard) is also recommended. Herbalists may prescribe a diuretic such as chamomile or couch grass. Traditional remedies include a course of propolis and pollen (one tablespoon a day).

NATUROPATHY

Naturopaths will suggest a regime of hot and cold compresses applied on the perineum, the area between the scrotum and anus, or sitz baths (alternate hot and cold baths with salt powder added). Reduction of tea, coffee and alcohol will also be recommended.

BIOCHEMIC TISSUE SALTS

Nat. sulph. one twice a day or *Mag. phos.* (same dosage) may reduce the need to micturate.

ACUPRESSURE

Stimulating point Spleen 6 will help to improve urinary control. It is found on the inside of the leg above the ankle, four fingers' width above the tip of the ankle bone. Apply the pressure slightly upwards towards the knee for two minutes.

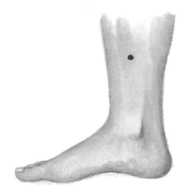

Above: *Distressing symptoms such as incontinence and dribbling can be relieved by stimulating the Spleen 6 acupoint on the inner leg.*

ORTHODOX TREATMENT

Most men with prostate enlargement will remain symptomless and require no treatment. If symptoms occur, then the doctor will examine the prostate gland by doing a rectal examination. The prostate gland can be felt through the wall of the rectum and a manual examination will help reveal its size. Urine would also be sent off for tests, and a blood test taken to look for the prostatic specific antigen (PSA) which is raised if there is a cancerous growth in the prostate. Examination of the bladder itself (using a specialized form of X-ray) will suggest whether there is any retention of urine because of blockage. Most prostatic enlargements are now treated by a surgical operation called a transurethral resection (TUR). If cancer is present, then further treatment (radiotherapy or hormone treatment) may be necessary. Following the operation impotence is not uncommon and this will need to be discussed fully.

CERVICAL CANCER

DESCRIPTION

This is an increasingly common cancer of the neck of the womb mainly affecting women over the age of 35, but now found in younger women as well. It can cause bleeding between periods or after intercourse. It is thought to be more common the more sexual partners a woman has, and the earlier sexual activity starts. The cancer will eventually spread if left untreated.

PREVENTION AND SELF-HELP

- Always use a condom during sexual intercourse.
- Reduce your number of sexual partners.
- Have regular cervical smear tests.
- Treat genital warts early (see entry below).
- Seek gynaecological advice if you have irregular periods.
- Reduce or eliminate smoking. Smokers run a greater risk of developing cervical cancer.

ALTERNATIVE THERAPIES

General treatment and alternative therapies for cancer are covered on pages 194-199.

ORTHODOX TREATMENT

Routine cervical smears will identify the "pre-cancerous" stage of the uterus, which can be treated with laser or minor surgery. Advanced disease may require hysterectomy (surgical removal of the uterus), radiotherapy and chemotherapy. Infection with the human papilloma virus (HPV), which is sexually transmitted, predisposes to cervical cancer.

FIBROIDS

DESCRIPTION

These are benign "tumours" in the muscle of the uterus which can be present and cause no symptoms. These are quite common in women over the age of 35 especially if there have been no pregnancies. Symptoms consist of heavy periods, back pain and occasionally anaemia and infertility.

PREVENTION AND SELF-HELP

Little can be done to prevent these growths as it is not known why they occur. Regular gynaecological checks with cervical smears will ensure they are detected early.

ALTERNATIVE THERAPIES

Both **acupuncture** and **homeopathy** may help with heavy bleeding and there have been some reports indicating that

Below: *A nurse is seen preparing a specimen on a glass slide as part of a routine cervical smear test.*

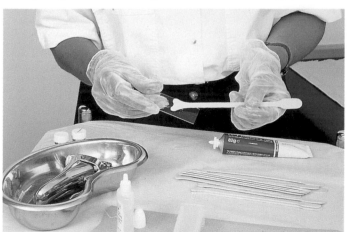

the fibroids have shrunk by such treatments.
Naturopathy would suggest an iron-rich diet (green vegetables, meat and fresh juices).

ORTHODOX TREATMENT

Fibroids can be very small but those causing symptoms can be felt on pelvic examination. Ultrasound scanning will reveal their size and number. No treatment is necessary unless symptoms are severe or anaemia cannot be controlled. They can be removed individually but usually a hysterectomy is performed.

GENITAL WARTS

DESCRIPTION

These are small, multiple, fleshy, cauliflower-like growths around the penis, vagina and anus, often contracted through sexual intercourse. They can be symptomless, or cause pain, irritation and vaginal discharge. Warts are caused by a virus (human papilloma virus, HPV) and predispose to the occurrence of cervical cancer, so should be treated promptly.

PREVENTION AND SELF-HELP

Because of the association with cervical cancer, warts should be treated at a gynaecological clinic, but all the preventative measures for cervical cancer (see above) should also apply.

ALTERNATIVE THERAPIES

Herbal medicine Herbalists use fresh garlic or lemon juice – dab on to the warts daily.
Naturopathy A general wholefood diet with plenty of fresh juices and extra Vitamin A, Vitamin C and Vitamin B is recommended.

ORTHODOX TREATMENT

It is possible to be infected with HPV without having visible warts, so regular gynaecological checks are important. Treatment is with podophyllin paint or laser treatment. Occasionally medication is given to improve the immune system.

HOT FLUSHES

DESCRIPTION

The symptoms are associated with the menopause and come about because of the changes in hormone levels in a woman's body. They cause sweating, changes in skin colour and temperature. They may last anything from a couple of minutes up to a few hours at a time, and usually persist for up to a year after the periods stop.

PREVENTION AND SELF-HELP

- Follow a wholefood diet – stop consuming coffee, tea and alcohol.
- Drink juices and herb teas, and plenty of mineral water.
- Practice meditation and relaxation exercises.
- Take Vitamin C, 1g twice a day.
- Drink a cup of honey and hot water with three drops of essential oil of sage added to it before sleeping to relieve night sweats.

ALTERNATIVE THERAPIES

Many alternative therapies are helpful in the menopause, see pages 172-173. Specifically for hot flushes you can try:
Homeopathy *Lachesis* 30x and *Glonoinum* 30x – take one tablet four times a day for three days.
Herbal medicine Ginseng and sarsparilla taken as teas can be helpful – drink two cups a day.

ORTHODOX TREATMENT

Symptoms if mild are ignored – at least by the doctor! Hormone replacement therapy (HRT) is now quite commonly advised and examination will exclude reasons for not taking HRT. Blood tests are done to check hormone levels (see also the Menopause, Orthodox Treatment, on page 173).

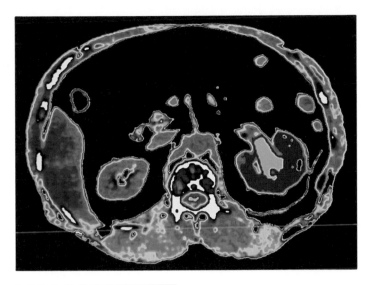

KIDNEY STONES

DESCRIPTION

They are formed by an excess of salts in the urine which crystallize out to form tiny stones. They can be caused by inadequate fluid intake, an inappropriate diet or gout (see page 106).

PREVENTION AND SELF-HELP

Stones are common in dry, hot countries and where the mineral content of water is conducive to stone formation. Plenty of fluid intake is advised.
- If you are bed-bound for a long time, make sure you avoid dehydration.
- Use a water filter to remove calcium in hard-water areas.
- Avoid oxalic acid-containing foods, such as spinach, rhubarb, and chocolate.

ALTERNATIVE THERAPIES

Acupuncture can help with the pain and infection but if the stone is large, orthodox treatment is required.
Herbal medicine Herbs can be given to prevent stone formation, such as gravel root, parsley and chamomile. Seek professional advice.
Naturopathy will recommend that you reduce your intake of calcium-rich foods (milk, cheese) and suggest taking a little cider vinegar daily.

Above: *This CT scan reveals the two kidneys on either side of the spine. The right kidney is enlarged due to the presence of a stone (yellow).*

ORTHODOX TREATMENT

They are usually detected because of the pain they cause as they pass from the kidney to the bladder (renal colic), or they may be seen on a special X-ray of the kidney. They may cause blood in the urine. They are either passed "naturally" or removed surgically, or more recently, broken up with ultrasound treatment.

NEPHRITIS

DESCRIPTION

Inflammation of the kidney often following a throat infection caused by streptococcus bacteria. It can also be caused by poisoning with heavy metals and can be a complication of other diseases.

PREVENTION AND SELF-HELP

General care of our kidneys should encompass the following measures:
- Drink plenty of fluid daily – at least 1¾ litres (3 pints) a day, more in hot weather.
- Use a water filter if you live in a hard-water area.
- Empty your bladder as soon as you feel the need to.

- Get early treatment for an infection (see pages 166-167).

ALTERNATIVE THERAPIES

Although some therapies may help, this is a serious condition and should be seen by an orthodox doctor. Diet, herbs, acupuncture and homeopathy will be recommended, but only if undertaken in conjunction with orthodox treatment.

ORTHODOX TREATMENT

Nephritis will cause cloudy urine with blood, and occasional kidney failure. Chronic nephritis may lead to high blood pressure. Treatment will depend on the cause; antibiotics are often prescribed. However, in serious cases, a kidney transplant may be required.

PROLAPSE OF THE UTERUS

DESCRIPTION

Weakening of the muscles of the "pelvic floor" following childbirth, especially if forceps have been used during delivery, can lead to a "dropped womb" (when the cervix drops down into the vagina and may even protrude beyond the vulva). Incontinence, infection and difficulty with periods and intercourse may occur.

PREVENTION AND SELF-HELP

- Pelvic floor exercises should be practised before and after childbirth. They strengthen the muscles of the vagina.
- Avoid being overweight.
- Exercise regularly for at least ten minutes at a time.

ALTERNATIVE THERAPIES

Acupressure Find the acupoint situated two fingers' width above the pubic bone, and four fingers' width from the centre line of the abdomen. Press firmly with a thumb for two minutes. This can

help a prolapsed womb return to its normal position.

ORTHODOX TREATMENT

This condition will be detected on physical examination. A ring pessary can be placed in the vagina to support the womb. In serious cases, a hysterectomy is performed.

VULVITIS

DESCRIPTION

An infection or inflammation of the female external genitalia which can occur as a result of poor hygiene, through sexual intercourse or as a reaction to soap or deodorant. It causes pain, discomfort and itchiness.

PREVENTION AND SELF-HELP

- Good hygiene and cleanliness are essential (see pages 174-175).
- Avoid vaginal deodorants and powerful sprays and soaps that may irritate the vulva.
- Use tampons rather than sanitary pads.
- Regular bathing of the genitalia with dilute cider vinegar helps.
- Seek medical advice early to exclude serious diseases.

ALTERNATIVE THERAPIES

Herbal medicine Garlic capsules, one twice a day, or propolis (3g daily for three days then 2g daily for eight days) is recommended. Local application of aloe vera gel, twice a day, is another option, but treatment must depend on expert diagnosis.

ORTHODOX TREATMENT

The type of treatment will depend on the cause. Swabs will be taken. The most common infection is candida (see pages 174-175). Occasionally vulvitis is caused by problems with skin or cancer. Local treatment may involve a small biopsy whereby tissue cells are removed for microscopic examination.

ADDICTIVE DISORDERS

Addiction does not, as is commonly thought, relate only to drugs (heroin, crack, LSD, marijuana). For instance, in Great Britain alcohol probably causes over 40,000 deaths a year and tobacco up to 100,000 deaths. Other forms of addiction include reliance on coffee, sweets, tranquillizers and sleeping tablets. The nature of the addiction is often linked to cultural factors, e.g. cannabis is considered "normal" among Rastafarians, while alcohol is prohibited among the Muslim community. It is clear that whatever the form of addiction, be it coffee or heroin, there appears to be a general increase in the problem in society and that many school and health authorities are increasingly disturbed by the younger age groups that appear to be using hard drugs.

Recently, the term "addictive personality" has been introduced to describe the characteristic groupings of behaviour that appear to be present, no matter what the addiction is. It is important to realize that human beings are creatures of *habit* and addiction may be an exaggeration of a normal habit pattern. Often people will become addicted without having a wish to become so. They may be prescribed addictive drugs and then find it difficult to stop taking them. Addiction may be *chemical*, i.e. the body requires a drug such as caffeine, alcohol, heroin, valium, to function and so ceasing taking the drug will produce *withdrawal symptoms*. Often the body develops a level of tolerance to the drug and a higher dose may be necessary to produce the same effect.

CAUSES

Social and cultural influences are clearly important but the addictive personality is described as one who cannot tolerate being frustrated and has to gratify his or her need quickly. He or she can be of any age and from any social background. Often addicts may lead unstimulating, boring lives and feel inadequate and lack self-confidence. On the other hand, some will resort to an addictive drug (alcohol, crack) to help them cope with a demanding and difficult lifestyle, e.g. the social drinker who becomes a heavy drinker under increased stress, or the executive who uses valium to reduce the anxiety associated with a busy work schedule. Ease of access to addictive drugs is clearly a factor in the increase in addiction, but experience suggests that out-and-out prohibition does not work.

Below: *Smoking is addictive, anti-social and bad for your health. Once you are hooked, breaking the habit can be very hard to manage.*

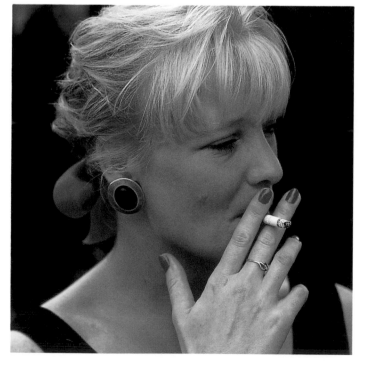

SYMPTOMS

Physical signs and symptoms will depend on the nature and type of addiction and the stage which the addict has reached. General symptoms may include mood swings, behaving out of character, irritability, lack of sleep, unreliability, poor performance at work or frequent illness, neglecting food, change in appearance.

Alcohol will produce gastric symptoms, early morning vomiting, the shakes, loss of memory, loss of sexual interest and potency.

Coffee addicts are often in a terrible hurry, breathe rapidly, suffer from palpitations, frequency of micturation, and gastric disturbance.

Drug addicts may develop pinpoint pupils (from using heroin), red eyes and drowsiness (cannabis), disorientation and giggly behaviour (LSD), sniffing, a dry cough and skin peeling around the lips (cocaine).

Tobacco addicts may smell, cough, have yellow-stained fingers and teeth.

PREVENTION AND SELF-HELP

Probably the most important step for any addict is to acknowledge the problem, because without doing so, treatment is of little value. This is where friends, or a doctor, may be of help. A useful

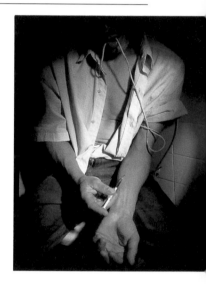

Above: *This heroin user fits the popular image of an addict. But quite "ordinary" people are also addicts.*

test for alcohol abusers is the following questionnaire (**CAGE**):
- Have you ever felt you should **C**ut down on your drinking?
- Have you ever been **A**nnoyed about and critical of your drinking?
- Have you ever felt **G**uilty about your drinking?
- Do you ever drink in the morning (**E**ye opener)?

An answer "Yes" to two or more questions almost certainly suggests a serious problem. A modified form of these four simple questions can be used for other addictions. The first three questions are applicable to all addictions.

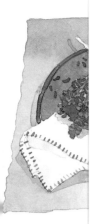

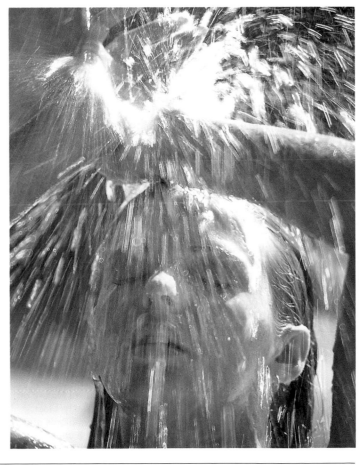

Above: *Most Western cultures accept social drinking, but a simple pleasure can turn into a destructive habit.*

Above: *Pani... mind. Massag... clary sage, lav... help to calm m...*

■ **Organize ...** anticipate ar... demand in y... month.

■ **Develop ... anti-anxiety ...** could includ... breathing ar... meditation, ... achieving y... positively, s... challenges: ... yourself as ... you are in c...

■ **Surround ... calming, re...** Quiet music... calm friends... help to rest... balance.

■ **Speak to ...** Sometimes... trouble half... sulk for lon... repressed a... only by kick... punching th...

■ **Check y...** does not c... stimulants ...

Self-help tips for alcohol abusers
■ Dilute alcoholic drinks.
■ Take smaller sips.
■ Change your normal choice of drink.
■ Drink more slowly.
■ Avoid getting into buying "rounds" in bars and pubs.
■ Start later in the day.
■ Eat before you drink.
■ Abstain for at least one day a week.
■ Join Alcoholics Anonymous if you cannot get your drinking under control.

Self-help tips for smokers
■ Cut each cigarette in two before smoking.
■ Stop for one day a week.
■ Create no-smoking zones in your house and workplace.
■ Try to stop abruptly – plan ahead when you will do that, and make it a definite date in your diary.
■ Use nicotine chewing gum or take up healthy habits to cope with feelings of craving.
■ Take up a relaxation exercise.

The problem for most addicts is that because of their addictive nature (from which you do not "recover"), they will need to replace the old bad habit with a new good habit, such as exercise or meditation, or changing from coffee to herbal teas. Self-help classes, such as those run by Alcoholics Anonymous, Narcotics Anonymous and Tranx Anonymous, are very helpful in ensuring there is adequate support and understanding during the withdrawal phase. Withdrawal symptoms may need to be addressed specifically and with the harder drugs (heroin, cocaine and even valium), it will be necessary for the sufferer to be under some medical supervision. Coffee withdrawal often causes headaches, and tobacco withdrawal may, paradoxically, cause a dry cough. Any aid or support during withdrawal is important and having a co-addict to 'phone up if the person is tempted is a useful addition to the overall treatment plan. The natural therapies described below may also be helpful.

BACH REMEDIES

Agrimony - For alcohol abuse, especially if there is denial.
Larch - Lack of confidence.
Clematis - Wish to escape reality.
Rescue Remedy - Withdrawal symptoms.
Take three drops of the appropriate remedy in a cup of water daily for one week. More than one remedy can be taken at the same time, if necessary.

HOMEOPATHY

An extensive history will be undertaken by a trained homeopath to unravel the "constitutional" remedy (a term relating to a remedy appropriate to the "whole person"), but the following may be helpful on a self-help basis:
Tranquillizer addicts *Nux vomica* 6x, one three times a day for one month.
Alcohol withdrawal *Aconite* 6x, one every half-hour, up to eight tablets.

NATUROPATHY

Treatment will often involve entering a "clinic" or retreat where a regime of fasting, hydrotherapy, vitamin supplements, exercise and massage may be prescribed. Regular hot baths followed by cold showers may be used during the withdrawal period. A regular wholefood diet can overcome some of the withdrawal symptoms associated with alcohol and coffee addiction. High doses of Vitamin B complex (two tablets three times a day) together with Vitamin C (1g twice a day) are often prescribed.

ACUPUNCTURE

Acupuncture, especially auricular acupuncture in the ear, has been used with moderate success in both tobacco addiction and drug addiction.

Below: *Overcoming an addiction often involves enduring a period of withdrawal. Hydrotherapy can help sufferers get through the anguish.*

ORTHODOX TREATMENT

All forms of addiction have increased and as yet treatment packages do not seem to offer more than a 15-18 percent cure rate. A combination of approaches has produced the best results, especially where there is a self-help group to which the client can go for moral support.

DEPRESSION

Depression is both a normal human feeling as well as a serious medical condition, and it is for this reason that it can be difficult to know when to seek help and when to accept your condition as the "natural" response to a disaster – a loss of job, or someone you love. Feeling sad following a disappointment or tragedy is normal and healthy. If this persists for longer than is acceptable to yourself or your family and friends, you may then find the label "depression" being used. For doctors, the two most common forms of depression are *exogenous*, as described above, or *endogenous*, where there is no obvious cause. This can sometimes be associated with other medical conditions such as anaemia or thyroid disorders. Endogenous depression is associated with biochemical changes in the brain and some doctors will compare it to diabetes, i.e. your brain metabolism is not working, in the same way as in diabetes your sugar metabolism is faulty and you may need to take insulin to regulate it. Another form of depression is associated with periods of hyperactivity or mania and is known as *manic-depressive* illness. This can often be an hereditary condition and can be characterized as a tendency to have exaggerated mood swings. *Postpartum or postnatal depression*, also known as the "seven-day blues", is linked to the hormone changes following delivery of a child and can be particularly intense and worrying.

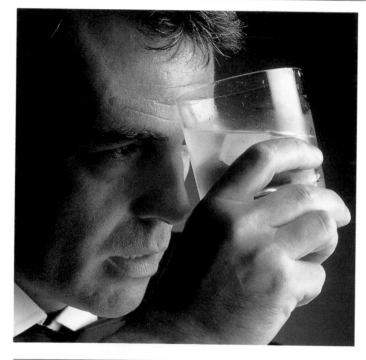

CAUSES

Genetic disposition, early childhood events, hormonal and chemical imbalances, current life events, lack of social support, isolation and cultural factors are all thought to play a part in making depression one of the most common conditions. Some 15 out of every 1,000 patients will present with depressive symptoms to their doctor, while many more try to "soldier on" alone. General surveys, however, suggest that up to 75 percent of people will admit to "loss of energy" and loss of sparkle and feeling sad.

Above: *Alcohol abuse can result from depression as the victim turns to drink to mask out the symptoms.*

SYMPTOMS

Most observers acknowledge that depression is often under-diagnosed and missed both by the person who is depressed as well as the doctor or therapist to whom that person may present. This is often because the presentation may be in the form of a physical symptom or a repeated type of behaviour, e.g. compulsive shop-lifting is often the first sign of someone presenting with depression.

The classic symptoms include flat affect (loss of *joie de vivre*), loss of self-confidence and self-worth, feelings of misery and despair, lack of concentration, chronic tiredness or fatigue, suicidal thoughts. Physical symptoms will include a slowing down of movement (stooped posture, hunched shoulders, expressionless face, slow speech, and a slowing down of the alimentary tract, loss of appetite, constipation). Sleep disturbance is common; early morning wakening is often experienced as is hypersomnia – sleeping through the alarm clock and waking up tired. Depression will affect sexual drive; impotence or loss of libido is common and in some women periods may stop altogether. Minor aches and pains, with constant headaches, are not unusual. Many people who are depressed will present to their doctors with mild hypochondriasis: each cough will be potential cancer, and each headache will be a possible brain tumour. Depression can be masked even further and can present as alcohol or drug-addiction; repeated car accidents or promiscuous sexual behaviour are sometimes a "cover" for underlying serious depression. Depression is both very common but also very serious, as suicide can be the final and, at times, only presentation. It is important, therefore, to be able to pick up clues of depression at an early stage to enable appropriate treatment to commence.

PREVENTION AND SELF-HELP

It is important to separate sadness and "healthy" depression from the more serious kind, because one of the ways to get through times of difficulty, be they the loss of a job, the breaking up of a relationship, or the death of a loved one, is to **accept the change** and **experience the loss,** i.e. do not try to "fight" the low feelings. Allow yourself to cry, **express your feelings** – sometimes there may be anger under the depression – "Why did he leave me?" "Why did this happen to me?".

■ **Keep a diary** – this can be a very good way of allowing yourself to understand what is affecting you.

■ **Talking to a friend** is of course what we all would like to do – it is a "natural" response, a bit like a mother rubbing the bruised arm or leg of her child. It is those who are isolated and have no friends who find that the normal disappointments of life can turn into depression.

■ **Taking exercise** is an excellent way of lifting your mood and increasing your energy levels. Indeed it is now a commonly "prescribed" method for dealing with mild depression (jogging, swimming, cycling, skipping). 10-15 minutes exercise a day will allow you to avoid the physical symptoms of depression.

■ **Correct breathing and relaxation** may also be helpful but exercises need to be carefully

Are you sad or are you depressed?

Since sadness and depression are often confused, the following table contrasts their characteristics, and may help you to determine whether you are sad or depressed.

Sad	Depressed
Periods of expression of feeling (crying, sobbing), which bring relief.	Crying is not "deep" and brings little relief. Sufferers often lose the ability to cry at all.
Feelings (especially emotional pain) are acute. Heartache.	Feelings are numbed. Pain is numbed. Feeling of dull lingering emptiness rather than acute pain.
The ability to laugh and experience other emotions is not lost. After feeling sadness, the ability to experience other feelings may even be heightened.	Loss of sense of humour. Loss of ability to experience any other feeling.
Sense of "movement" – feelings are experienced, "moved through", so that by the end you are ready for a new experience of life.	Sense of stagnant heaviness, of being stuck in a groove and unavailable to new experience.
No loss of self respect.	Loss of self-respect.
No feeling of distance from self and others; in fact the expression of sadness may bring you closer.	Feeling of distance from self or others.
No loss of energy or motivation.	Loss of energy and motivation.
Usually short-lived when fully expressed.	Apart from moments of the blues, it tends to last a long time and is self-perpetuating – the more your energy drops, the worse you feel about yourself, and so the more you give up, and the more your energy drops.

From *Overcoming Depression*, Gillett, R., BHMA, London/Dorling Kindersley.

BACH FLOWER REMEDIES

Tired and exhausted: olive.
Resentful and bitter: willow.
Despair and hopelessness: gorse.
Extreme despair: sweet chestnut.
Major life change: walnut.
Dilute stock remedies – put two drops of essence into a cup of spring water. Take four drops of the dilute remedy four times a day.

NATUROPATHY

Recommendations will include advice on diet, exercise and hydrotherapy. Early morning cold baths have been used with very good results in cases of moderate to severe depression, especially those associated with M.E. or post-viral fatigue.

AROMATHERAPY

Aromatherapy will relieve the feelings of mild depression and sadness through massage, and you can use the oils (basil, clary sage, Roman chamomile, rose and thyme) in your bath (six to eight drops of one of the above). You can also inhale the oils through an impregnated tissue or handkerchief (three drops on a tissue, then inhale through the nose for about one minute). Repeat three times a day.

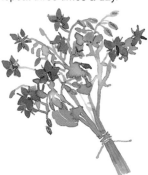

Above: *For centuries borage has been praised as an anti-depressant.*

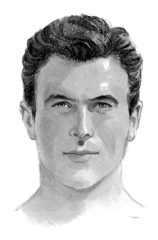

Above: *Governing Vessel 26 may be stimulated to alleviate depression, but use it for short spells only.*

HOMEOPATHY

Homeopathic remedies include the following:
Weeping and sad: *Nat.mur.* 6x.
Feeling under a black cloud: *Aurum met.* 6x.
Melancholic and talkative: *Lycopodium* 6x.
Depressed and hopeless: *Sulphur* 6x.
Fearful and lack of self-confidence: *Calc. carb.* 6x.
In each case take one tablet three times a day for six days.

ACUPRESSURE

■ Acupoint Governing Vessel 26, in the groove of the upper lip below the nose just above the lip, is helpful. Apply *light* pressure with the edge of the nail of the index finger. Do not press hard (it may raise the blood pressure) and for no more than one minute.

HERBAL MEDICINE

Taking a tisane – herbal tea – is a common method of treating depression (try borage or vervain). A hot cup of rosemary tea or ginger will help to raise the spirits.

introduced to someone who is moderately depressed.
■ **Rewards and distractions** are a common way we all deal with mild or even severe depression. These can be harmful in the long run (tobacco, alcohol, promiscuous sex, drugs, comfort eating, compulsive shopping) or beneficial (listening to music, reading a book, having a massage, having your hair done, finding a new hobby).
■ **Diet and nutrition** play a large part in both causing mood changes, as well as relieving depression. Much of Ayurvedic medicine concentrates on how to affect mood states and energy levels by changes in the diet. Cut down on coffee, tea, cola drinks (stimulants) and introduce a wholefood diet with plenty of Vitamin B_1 (thiamine), Vitamin B_6 (pyridoxine) and Vitamin C (ascorbic acid). Take one tablet twice a day of each for up to a month. Specially constructed diets for depression can be worked out with the help of a trained therapist.

ORTHODOX TREATMENT

Early diagnosis is felt to be important and most doctors will now prescribe an approach to include counselling, exercises and anti-depressants. Anti-depressants need to be taken for a long time (months) to allow for the chemical change that is thought to be causing the depression to be countered. On some occasions, the medication may need to be taken for life. Severe cases of depression with suicidal risks will be *hospitalized and in cases that do not respond to medication, electro-convulsive therapy (ECT) may be required. There are several different classes of anti-depressant drugs and the treatment will depend on the type of depression. Long-term counselling and psychotherapy are often offered in exogenous depression, especially when a major loss or death is involved (bereavement counselling).*

INSOMNIA

Sleep disorders are by far the most common disorder known to man. It is calculated that in Great Britain between 7-10 million people suffer from one sort of sleep disorder or another. Up to 50 percent of women over the age of 60 in Scotland are taking sleeping tablets at night. It is surprising, therefore, that we know so little about sleep and that it is only in the last few years that special units (sleep disorder clinics) have been established to study in depth the variety of sleep disturbance. With the aid of video cameras and EEGs (electroencephalograms – recordings of brainwave activity), we now have a far more accurate understanding of the nature of sleep, and it is possible to study with some precision what seems to go wrong. First, sleep appears to be a necessary restorative state, both physically and mentally. There are at least six to eight cycles of sleep during one night when the brain appears to change patterns and alternates between deep sleep and light sleep. During light sleep, dreaming occurs although not everyone will remember their dreams. Disturbed and altered sleep patterns are both a symptom of and a cause of physical illness. The different types of sleep disturbance include: difficulty getting off to sleep; waking up during sleep; waking up tired; over-sleeping; disturbed dreams and nightmares; sleep talking and sleep walking; snoring and sleep apnoea (a brief cessation of breathing).

CAUSES

▪ Illness: pain, high temperature.
▪ Change in climate: extremes of temperature, storms.
▪ Change in environment: new bed, noise from outside, unfamiliar surroundings.
▪ Excess food and drink: over-eating, consumption of stimulants and liquids.
▪ Difficult life situations: bereavement, anxiety, depression, going to bed tense, marital difficulties, sexual frustration, unresolved conflicts, over-excitement.
It is important to appreciate that sleeping patterns vary from person to person and from age to age. Generally, as we get older we need less sleep. Some people

Below: *Scientific research into sleep patterns has shown that brain activity passes through distinct cycles in the course of a night's sleep.*

Age	Average total sleep time (hours)	Average time taken to get to sleep (minutes)	Average no. of wakenings per night
3–6	9.89	14.3	Less than 1
6–9	9.68	12.24	More than 1
10–12	9.33	17.39	Less than 1
13–15	8.08	15.78	More than 2
16–19	7.53	17.75	More than 2
20–29	7.08	17.73	More than 2
30–39	7.06	7.80	More than 1
40–49	6.79	8.91	More than 3
50–59	6.84	11.06	More than 5
60–69	6.77	12.38	More than 5
70–79	6.55	23.0	More than 7

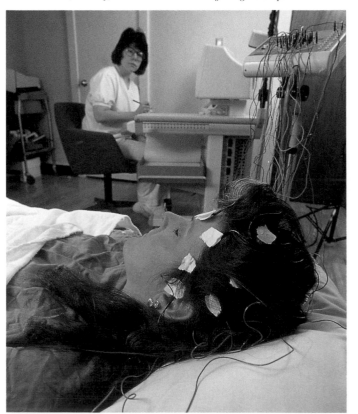

can manage on only four hours' sleep a night, while others need at least eight.

The relationship between sleep disturbance, snoring and sleep apnoea has recently been established, and it is felt to be an important factor in the development of heart disease. Sleep apnoea is the "breath holding" that occurs prior to the act of snoring, and is present when the body is in a state of muscle tension and its breathing pattern is disturbed as in hyperventilation.

SYMPTOMS

These are usually self-evident in that the individual is unable to sleep, has disturbed sleep or wakes up unrefreshed and tired. Sleep apnoea may be apparent only to the wife or husband, and hypersomnia (over-sleeping) is often overlooked as a symptom of disturbed sleep.

PREVENTION AND SELF-HELP

Often a vicious circle is established: sleep disturbance will produce anxiety which will in itself cause sleep disturbance.

Things to do before going to sleep
▪ Listen to a favourite piece of music.
▪ Avoid stimulant drinks before sleep – coffee, tea, cocoa.
▪ Avoid too many liquids, especially if bladder capacity is low.
▪ Practise a breathing and relaxation routine.
▪ Practise a tension-releasing routine.
▪ Go for a brisk walk.
▪ Avoid starting an argument or important discussion which will set your mind racing.
▪ Write down any immediate worries or anxieties on a piece of paper.

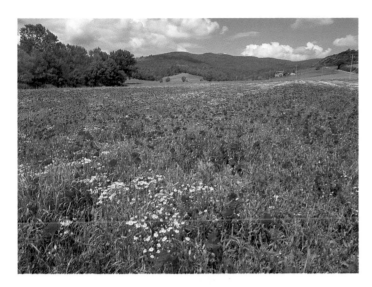

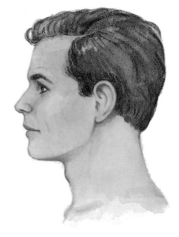

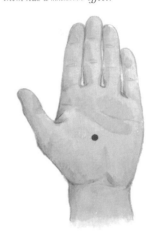

chamomile, lavender or rose to a warm bath will have a sedative effect on the body.

HERBAL MEDICINE

An infusion or tisane (tea) of lavender, lime blossom, lemon balm, chamomile or valerian, will reduce anxiety levels. Take one cup shortly before bedtime.

HOMEOPATHY

The following remedies may all be helpful:

Aconite 6x – if there is a shock or bereavement. One tablet taken every half-an-hour (up to eight in total) will usually help.

Arnica 6x – one or two tablets will help relax the body, especially if overtired.

Coffea 6x – if you wake up in the middle of the night. One tablet, repeated three times if necessary.

Nux vomica 6x – one before sleeping will help if you wake up feeling tired.

Take each of these remedies half-an-hour before going to bed. Try this regime for up to two weeks to give it time to work.

Below: *To Macbeth, sleep is "Balm of hurt minds... chief nourisher in Life's feast". Massage can help you enjoy it.*

Above: *The Gall Bladder 12 points are found behind each ear. Pressure on them has a sedative effect.*

Above: *Acupressure on this acupoint, Heart Governor 8, is also recommended for sufferers from insomnia.*

ACUPRESSURE

Acupressure is also helpful in reducing anxiety and helping to induce a state of peaceful sleep. Use:

▪ Gall Bladder 12: Two fingers' width behind the ear in the small cavity under the bone. Apply pressure with the thumbs on both sides for a minute. Press upwards.

▪ Heart Governor 8: Bend the middle finger until it touches the palm. Press on this point towards the middle finger for up to two minutes.

▪ Read a book that is absorbing, but not overstimulating or frightening.
▪ Do not panic.

Things to do if you wake up
▪ Get up and go to the toilet.
▪ Practise a diaphragmatic breathing routine.
▪ Write down any thoughts or worries on a piece of paper.
▪ Choose a mental image – your last holiday, a favourite film, a pleasing scene – and focus your mind on the details.
▪ If this is frequent, have a cassette tape recorder by you and play a relaxing piece of music or relaxation tape over a pair of earphones.
▪ If you are very tense, get up and expel some of the energy through some form of physical activity.

Things to do during the daytime
▪ Recognize you have a difficulty and decide to deal with it during the day as well as at night.
▪ Check your exercise routine.
▪ Check your diet.
▪ Examine the reasons why you may not be sleeping:
- unresolved psychological problem.
- marital conflict.
- loss of a loved one.

Above: *Calling a restful scene to mind is one way of calming yourself if you wake unexpectedly in the night.*

▪ Be honest with yourself, but also be kind.
▪ Seek the help of a doctor, counsellor, friend, psychologist.

MASSAGE AND AROMATHERAPY

Especially before sleeping a body massage will help to relax the body and restore a rhythmical sleeping pattern. Adding three drops of any of the oils of

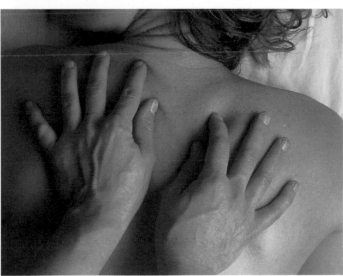

ORTHODOX TREATMENT

General advice as outlined above may be given, but unfortunately the easiest method for doctors to cope with sleep disturbance in their patients is to prescribe sleeping tablets. The latter, although very effective initially, may produce both side-effects and long-term addiction. They should only be taken in short courses. Behavioural therapy (relaxation, biofeedback) is occasionally suggested, as is counselling and hypnotherapy.

OBSESSIVE/COMPULSIVE BEHAVIOUR

Obsessive/compulsive disorders are a form of exaggerated "normal" behaviour which can take over someone's life and dominate them to the extent of requiring hospital admissions. *Obsessions* involve repetitive thoughts that cannot be ignored or dismissed. They can flood someone's mental processes and disable them completely. They may be associated with normal concerns – "Have I switched the light off?", or "Have I remembered my keys?". Sometimes the thoughts are irrational and fearful that something awful will happen – "the cake is poisoned". These thoughts are associated with anxiety symptoms and then may be linked to *compulsions* or repetitive actions which can involve superstitious habits – touching wood, or not stepping on the line of a pavement. When serious, these compulsions may include washing a glass repeatedly, checking the lights are switched off twelve times or more, or warding off the poison coming from the toilet by locking it up. If these habits are not performed, the person may become anxious and experience panic attacks. Some people develop compulsions to collect newspapers or paper bags and their whole house may be filled with these objects.

CAUSES

Not very much is known as to why people develop these disorders. Hereditary factors are occasionally found. Some psychiatrists believe there may be some dysfunctional chemical messages in the brain, while others believe the symptoms to be a sign of underlying deep anxiety and depression. Obsessional personality characteristics are commonly identified among "normal" people, and it is important to differentiate between the disorder as described above and what may only be a character trait.

SYMPTOMS

These may include the keeping of lists and the repetition of daily tasks. Asking someone whether they are plagued by constant thoughts that go round and round will usually reveal how troubled they are.

PREVENTION AND SELF-HELP

This illness may often require professional help, but a general understanding of the problem and an avoidance of punishing or rejecting behaviour on the part of family and friends is essential. Practising techniques which help to induce a state of physical and mental relaxation (breathing, meditation, exercise routines) can be particularly helpful. Sometimes using one of the creative arts (painting, sculpting, sand play or music therapy), will allow some of the "locked-in" tension to be released through the production of a "work of art". Some of these paintings will illustrate the irrational fears that seem to drive the person to commit the repetitive rituals.

The most effective treatments have included a combination of relaxation (autogenic training) together with a behavioural approach. Simple step-by-step behavioural programmes are worked out, much as in the treatment of phobias, so that the client is encouraged not to repeat the thought or action. Each successful step is followed by a reward or positive reassurance from the therapist. Other therapies have involved the use of colour to break through the repetition. An experienced therapist will choose a colour to reflect the client's personality and then gradually introduce shades of the colour to "enlarge" and expand their ability both to "see" and to respond to different colours. It is unlikely that any of the self-help measures available in complementary therapy will alter this distressing disorder, but a general approach of encouraging regular exercise, a wholefood diet, and supplemental vitamins (B_6 and C) will certainly not harm the client.

Below: *Hypnotherapy has been used with some success to treat obsessive behaviour, but the results are patchy.*

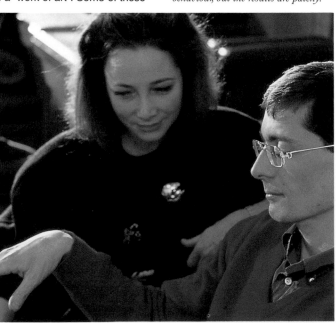

HELPFUL THERAPIES

Hypnotherapy can be of benefit but the effects are unfortunately only short-lived.
Bach Flower Remedies (Rescue Remedy) or **homeopathy** (*Aconite* 6x) will relieve some of the acute symptoms associated with this condition.

ORTHODOX TREATMENT

Counselling and psychotherapy do not seem to have a very good record in dealing with this condition, and so medication will be tried including anti-depressants and mild tranquillizers. In very severe cases, brain surgery is employed, although this is much less frequently undertaken today than in the past.

PHOBIAS

Phobias, from the Greek word meaning "fear", are irrational and persistent fears which are out of all proportion to the actual risk or danger involved. Having fears is a normal and necessary part of growing up – a way of avoiding unnecessary danger. Being afraid of heights is a normal and appropriate response. Being afraid of spiders to the extent that you will not enter a house in case there is a spider there is abnormal. The most common phobias include agoraphobia (fear of leaving home or a safe base), claustrophobia (fear of being shut in), social phobias (fear of social situations), animal phobias (terror of insects, mice, animals etc.), fear of flying or storms or illness. One of the common phobias is the fear of contracting cancer or AIDS and seeking constant reassurance from doctors (with demands for regular blood tests) that you have not got the disease in question. Phobias are relatively common in both men and women, but the degree of severity can vary enormously.

CAUSES

Although there may be hereditary predisposition, it is felt that the majority of phobias are "learned" from our parents or are the result of a particular psychological problem or event in early childhood. The subjects of phobias are commonly avoided by people who suffer from them, but this avoidance may escalate into dysfunction and people can be trapped in their own homes, or be unable to travel or visit a particular part of the country, for fear of encountering the cause of their phobia.

SYMPTOMS

Anxiety symptoms, from mild palpitations through to panic

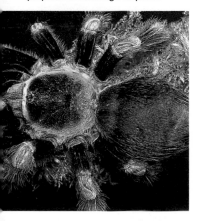

Above: *Someone with arachnophobia may find it hard to look at this picture. Fear has tipped over into phobia.*

attacks, hysterical symptoms and death, have been known to occur if the person is confronted with the phobic cause.

PREVENTION AND SELF-HELP

Sometimes people are ashamed to admit their problem and will cover up to avoid the shame and guilt they feel, thus avoiding the possibility of help. The major successful approach to managing phobic symptoms is a form of desensitization that can be undertaken at home, as well as by a clinically trained psychologist. The desensitization programme involves increasing the awareness of the phobia – i.e. by writing down when, where, how and why you feel phobic. Describe the symptoms you feel and grade each symptom: 0 (none) to 5 (very bad). The cause of the phobia is then introduced in a minimal way. It could be a picture of a storm, or a spider, or it may be in the form of someone who simply repeats the feared word. You are then asked to record all the symptoms you feel in relation to the stimulus. The next stage involves you learning how to modify the symptoms through some form of relaxation or breathing exercise.
You are also given a number of other possible strategies to adopt once you have encountered your phobia. These can include a muscle-relaxing exercise, a

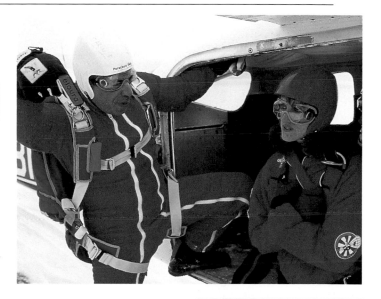

Above: *This woman used hypnosis to overcome her fear of a parachute jump. Similarly, phobias can be relieved through desensitization programmes.*

visualization exercise, or a "cognitive reframing" sentence, e.g. "I am terrified but I will get over it in time". "I think I'll never get over this, but this is just a feeling. In time I will get over this". (Cognitive reframing is the technical term for retraining the mind – the popular term "positive thinking" is sometimes used instead.)
This step-by-step exercise is repeated two or three times a day and gradually the stimulus is increased in intensity until the actual object of the phobia is confronted.

HOMEOPATHY

Certain self-help homeopathic measures can be tried.
Agoraphobia: *Aconite* 30x, one tablet three times a day for ten days.
Claustrophobia: *Argentum nitricum* 30x, one tablet three times a day for ten days, or *Pulsatilla* 30x, one tablet three times a day for ten days.

ART THERAPY

This has been used successfully as a way of expressing the irrational fears on paper, which reduces their intensity. Once the phobia has been confronted, its hold over the imagination can start to be relaxed.

ORTHODOX TREATMENT

Tranquillizers may be prescribed as a way of dealing with short-term anxiety, but their long-term use should be avoided as they are addictive. A desensitization programme, as described in the Prevention and Self-Help section, is a general recommendation.

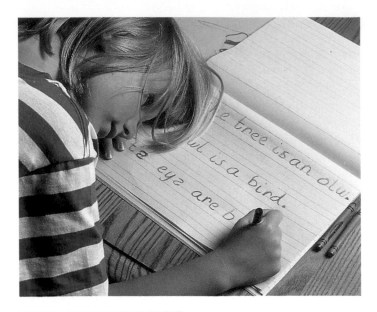

DYSLEXIA

DESCRIPTION

A form of learning disorder in which children have difficulty in reading and writing, affecting one in 25 of the population. It can involve secondary behavioural and emotional problems leading to school refusal.

PREVENTION AND SELF-HELP

Parents can be of great help to children by
- Encouraging the child's efforts.
- Reading to the child.
- Using video and tape recorders to help study set texts at school.
- Getting to know the teachers.
- Avoid punishment for reading and writing mistakes and making unflattering comparison with other children.

ALTERNATIVE THERAPIES

Relaxation and breathing exercises are helpful as is **Yoga**. **Hypnotherapy** has been used and **osteopaths** claim to have helped some children by realignment of the cervical vertebrae.

ORTHODOX TREATMENT

Dyslexia is now thought to be the result of nerve cell

Above: *A dyslexic child working on a writing exercise. Dyslexia appears to be a disorder of the nerve cells and has nothing to do with intelligence.*

disorganization and special psychological and neurological tests are undertaken. Vision disturbances need to be excluded. Educational psychologists and special teachers are of great help to children and parents alike.

SCHIZOPHRENIA

DESCRIPTION

A serious mental disorder which results in loss of contact with reality and may be associated with paranoia and violence. Conversation may be bizarre and the individual may have hallucinations and believe he is a famous historical figure, such as Jesus Christ or Napoleon. Single attacks, often in young adults, may be precipitated by taking drugs.

PREVENTION AND SELF-HELP

- Avoid taking hallucinogenic drugs and other stimulants.
- Obtain expert advice if you do suffer an attack.
- Join a self-help support group.
- Do no try to reason with some-one who has hallucinations. Keep calm. Ensure that they cannot harm themselves, and call a doctor.

- Attention to the effect that this illness has on the whole family will reduce stress. This is a difficult situation for family members to cope with.

ALTERNATIVE THERAPIES

Orthodox advice should always be sought in the first instance, but the following therapies can be both helpful and supportive.
Art therapy Communicating through painting, especially with colour, can help reduce feelings of isolation that a schizophrenic may experience.
Music therapy will also help reconnect the individual with the outside world.
Homeopathy can be tried but only with guidance from a skilled practitioner.

ORTHODOX TREATMENT

Referral for psychiatric assessment is essential and hospitalization may be necessary. The condition may be familial and relapses and remissions are common. Medication with anti-psychotic drugs and long-lasting injections, together with skilled counselling and supervision in the community, are the usual treatments for this condition.

Below: *This image was produced by a technique called positron emission tomography: PET scanning. It shows abnormal activity in the brain of a patient suffering from schizophrenia.*

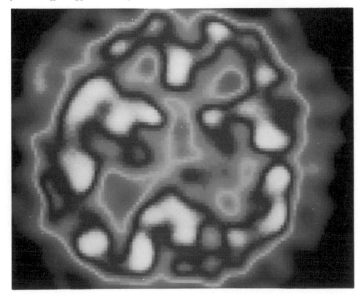

SLEEPWALKING

DESCRIPTION

A distressing occurrence affecting children, often associated with anxiety and emotional trauma. The child rises from his or her bed while still asleep, and may walk to other parts of the house.

PREVENTION AND SELF-HELP

- Gently lead the child back to bed, preferably while still asleep. No harm is done if the child wakes, however.
- Relaxation exercises before bedtime help to ensure an untroubled night's sleep. Sleepwalking may be related to anxiety.
- Block off steep stairs to prevent inadvertent injury during a bout of sleepwalking.

ALTERNATIVE THERAPIES

Massage before sleeping or a hot bath with a few drops of essential oil of lavender added promote relaxation.
Homeopathy Homeopaths will suggest *Coffea* 6x, one tablet to be taken before sleeping.

ORTHODOX TREATMENT

Referral to a psychologist or sleep disorder clinic may be necessary.

Reassurance that the condition is harmless will usually suffice, however.

STUTTER OR STAMMERING

DESCRIPTION

A repetitive and hesitant speech difficulty found in around four percent of the population. It is more common in men than women. Repetition is a normal phase in speech development and repetitive stammering may be a result of delayed maturation or an abnormality of palate and speech muscles. Usually it has a large emotional and psychological component.

PREVENTION AND SELF-HELP

▪ Reducing the emotional atmosphere surrounding a stammering child is important.
▪ Avoid punishment or causing embarrassment which will increase a child's self-consciousness about the speech impediment.
▪ Creative therapies such as singing or voice therapy help improve confidence.

ALTERNATIVE THERAPIES

Bach flower remedies These are often used, especially cherry plum, holly, chestnut bud and vervain.
Acupressure on the outside corner of the thumbnail on the Lung 11 acupoint is said to help with speech problems.
Yoga Breathing with the diaphragm and "bellow breath" is advised to develop breathing control before speaking.
Hypnotherapy is often successful.

ORTHODOX TREATMENT

Treatment will involve appropriate developmental examination and referral to a speech clinic. The use of recorded speech and headphones, together with behavioural modification using rewards, are often successful.

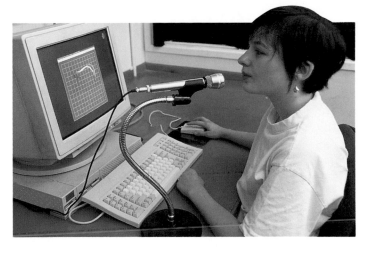

Above: *People who suffer particularly severely from stammering may be referred to a speech clinic which will help them to overcome the problem.*

TEETH GRINDING

DESCRIPTION

This is a common and painful condition, which usually occurs during sleep, often caused by tension in the masseter muscles of the jaw resulting in problems with the teeth, temporomandibular joint dysfunction, pain, malalignment of teeth and occasionally dislocation of the jaw.

PREVENTION AND SELF-HELP

▪ Note the frequency of the condition, and become aware of tension in the jaw muscles.
▪ Learn a new relaxation or breathing technique, and practise it, particularly when you feel tension in the jaw.
▪ Autogenic training is very helpful in making you relax.
▪ Check there is no malalignment by visiting your dentist.

ALTERNATIVE THERAPIES

Alternative therapies can be very effective and several approaches can be offered.
Osteopathy can release the tension by careful manipulation of the neck.
Acupressure Press gently upwards in the hollow under the cheekbone, two fingers' width in front of the ear for two minutes.

Massage and **relaxation** techniques can both contribute to a lessening of muscular tension in the face.
Homeopathy *Rhus tox.* 6x, one tablet twice a day for a week, is a general recommendation.

ORTHODOX TREATMENT

Usually a referral to the dentist reveals the malalignment, which is secondary to the tense muscles, pain or clicking of the joint together with X-ray evidence of mild arthritis. General pain-killers and anti-inflammatory drugs do not address the primary problem of underlying muscle tension. Tranquillizers can sometimes help. Jaw dislocation is treated by manual manipulation of the jaw to ease it back into position.

TEMPER TANTRUM

DESCRIPTION

Children commonly have these around the age of two ("the terrible twos") as the child learns to exercise his or her own authority, often by refusing to eat, sleep or go to the toilet. A tantrum is often associated with breath-holding attacks when the cessation of breathing may cause the child to faint.

PREVENTION AND SELF-HELP

▪ Avoid giving the child stimulant sweets or drinks with added dye and preservatives – check the E-numbers on the packaging carefully.

▪ Stay calm, and ensure the child can come to no harm. Be firm, and avoid "bribing" the child with rewards to overcome the immediate problem.
▪ Seek professional advice if simple measures do not work.

ALTERNATIVE THERAPIES

Homeopathy *Aconite* 6x, one tablet a day, may help to calm the child, but it will be impossible to administer it during a tantrum.
Hydrotherapy A warm bath with three drops of lavender or lemon balm oil can calm an excitable child.
Massage and **aromatherapy** Rosemary oil will help to calm the child. Add three drops of oil to a warm bath.

ORTHODOX TREATMENT

Firm and loving responses are required to help protect the child from harm. Avoid physical punishment and reward *positive* behaviour. Reassurance that the child is not having a "fit" or going mad helps to calm worried parents. Occasionally referral to a child guidance clinic is appropriate.

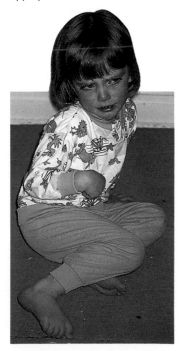

Above: *The body language of this child says it all: "I'm having a tantrum so don't try and stop me."*

CANCER

Every year nearly 250,000 new cases of cancer are diagnosed in the UK alone, and it is estimated that worldwide one in three persons will suffer from some form of cancer before they die. The difficulty with discussing cancer generally is that, like the word "fever", it can both be a sign of a very mild disease or a very serious condition leading to death. The word "cancer" covers a whole range of different conditions which do not necessarily have anything in common. Someone with skin cancer can look forward to a 98 percent likelihood of recovery; some leukaemia (blood cancers) are now curable by modern drugs. Other cancers, such as breast or bowel cancer, do not respond so well to orthodox treatments (i.e. surgery, radiotherapy and chemotherapy). So generalizations about cancer are unwise.

WHAT IS CANCER?

The essential nature of cancer is that the cells of a particular tissue grow beyond their normal life span and can spread both locally and to other organs (secondaries). Of course, cells are always growing, dividing and dying; a cancer cell (often called a "mutant" cell) is one that is no longer under the normal control of the body's own processes. Its growth is uncontrolled. Much greater understanding as to why this happens now exists and many doctors believe that up to 60-70 percent of all cancers are preventable by avoiding those factors that are known to trigger the cells into abnormal growth. Causes such as smoking and pollution have been known for many years; the effect of ultra-violet light on skin is now known to have increased the chance of

Below: *These Australian children are well covered as they play by the sea. Their parents know overexposure to the Sun can lead to skin cancer.*

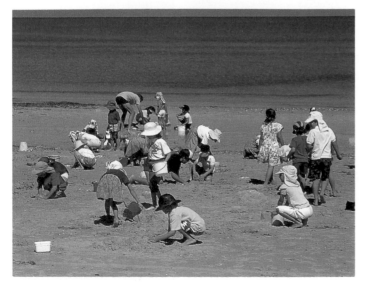

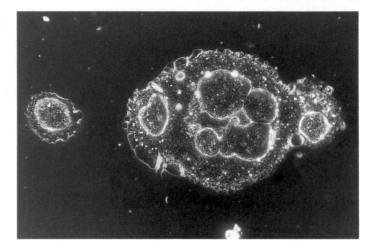

Above: *This is a lymphoma cell, a type of cancer that multiplies in the lymph system producing tumours.*

skin cancer.
The human diet contains many mutagens and carcinogens – cancer-producing substances – and recently a correlation between a high-fat diet and breast and prostatic cancer has been identified. It is known that a high-fibre diet protects against the incidence of bowel cancer. This is almost certainly because it increases the bulk of the stool and aids evacuation of the faeces, thus reducing the amount of time that the carcinogens come into contact with the bowel wall. Some cancers are hereditary, and recent research has begun to identify the gene that may predispose to the development of cancer later on in life.
Because cancer has become such a "fearful" word, it is not surprising that many people have turned to alternative therapies for help, especially when the orthodox approaches – surgery, radiotherapy and chemotherapy – are themselves not always successful and carry with them a degree of unpleasant side-effects that cause many people to question their effectiveness.
It is important before embarking on alternative therapy for cancer that you discuss the issues with your doctor. You may find that the type of cancer you have will respond well to orthodox treatment. Several centres now offer some of the alternative therapies as an additional option to conventional treatment.

ALTERNATIVE THERAPIES

The main therapies that are used in cases of cancer fall into two broad categories: they are sometimes referred to as the Big Six and the Little Six.
The Big Six are:
- Diet therapy
- Megavitamin therapy
- Metabolic and immuno-augmentative therapy
- Counselling
- Relaxation and visualization
- Faith healing
The Little Six are:
- Massage
- Aromatherapy
- Acupuncture
- Homeopathy
- Art therapy
- Reflexology
Of course, many other therapies have been employed to treat cancer, but these are by far the most popular and widely available in the Western world. In the course of this section, I shall outline what they involve.

DIET THERAPY

The diet therapies share a common philosophy: poor diet can help cause cancer, and so a good diet can help to cure it. Some aim to rid the body of toxins that accumulate from the food we tend to eat in the Western world, by such means as fasting or eating only fruit. Common principles found among the dietary therapies are strict vegan or vegetarian adherence, eating large amounts of raw foods, the consumption of foods that are sugar-free and low in salt, the use of vegetable/fruit/liver juices and taking high doses of vitamins, minerals and enzymes.

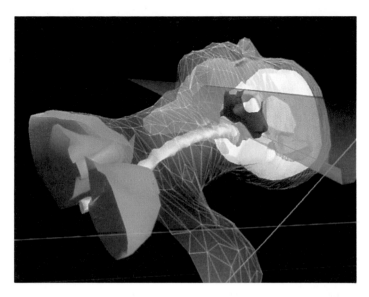

Above: *This picture shows radio-therapy for cancer. The brown area is the tumour, the green cone the radiation.*

There is no doubt that these therapies can be of benefit to some patients. As a population in the West, we generally eat an unhealthy diet and taking an interest in one's diet is a very constructive way of helping oneself when ill.However, it has been argued that the diets generally used in diet therapies are exactly the opposite of the needs of most cancer patients.They are high in bulk and low in calories, often unpalatable, difficult to prepare and costly to follow. The usual outcome is weight loss, weakness, depression (if the diet is not enjoyable), guilt (if the patient has to stop the diet), and anger (if the diet produces no result).
There are also many supporters of the benefit of special diets in both the treatment and prevention of cancer.

The Gerson Diet
This is perhaps the best known. Max Gerson, a German physician, developed the diet originally to treat his recurrent attacks of migraine. He then suggested that this diet could be of use in the treatment of tuberculosis and cancer. He treated his first patient in 1928, and claimed a complete remission. He believed that our normal diet is too far removed from a "natural" diet. Over-use of artificial fertilizers, other chemicals in the soil, poor food

preparation, and a poor environment generally are all parts of this process. Gerson believed that these dietary insufficiencies reduce our natural defences to the point where one trigger-event can produce cancer. Time and commitment are needed to follow the Gerson diet – most practitioners would recommend that it is maintained for at least three months. The dieter cannot lead a normal life while on the diet. It is based on four principles.

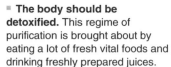

▪ **The body should be detoxified.** This regime of purification is brought about by eating a lot of fresh vital foods and drinking freshly prepared juices.
▪ **Vitamin and mineral imbalances should be corrected.** On the Gerson diet, the daily intake of vitamins and minerals is very high because of the large amounts of fresh fruit and vegetables that are eaten.

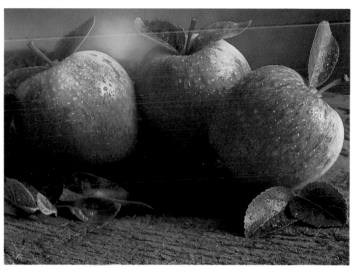

Below: *Pulses are an integral part of the Bristol diet. It is felt that they help the body rid itself of toxins.*

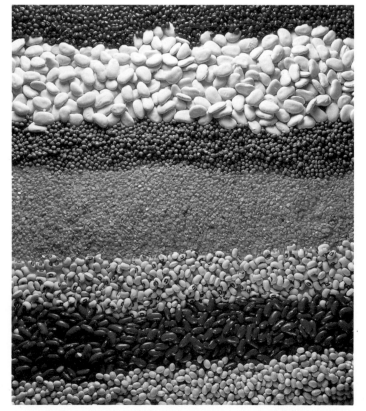

Gerson also advocated the use of supplemental potassium, iodine and Vitamin B$_3$.
▪ **Restore digestion.** Gerson advocated the use of supplemental gastric acid and pancreatic enzymes for this purpose.
▪ **Restore and maintain a positive attitude.** This was thought to be of help both in general and specifically in relation to diet.

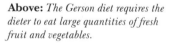

Above: *The Gerson diet requires the dieter to eat large quantities of fresh fruit and vegetables.*

The Gerson diet was widely dismissed by the medical profession at the time, yet there are similarities between the Gerson diet and that now recommended by The American Cancer Society to minimize the risk of developing cancer.

The Bristol Diet
Another such diet is the Bristol diet, developed at the Cancer Help Centre in Bristol in the UK. In many ways this is similar to the Gerson diet. They recommend a slow start to the diet, and emphasize that it is not to be viewed as a punishment or a penance. If patients feel depressed or guilty while on the diet, they are helped to think again about their suitability for it. The diet itself is in two parts:
▪ **The Get Well Diet** The aim of this diet, like the Gerson diet, is detoxification. It is a fruit juice diet, vegan, with 90 percent raw foods, and is 100 percent salt-free. No sugar is eaten, and no salt is added.

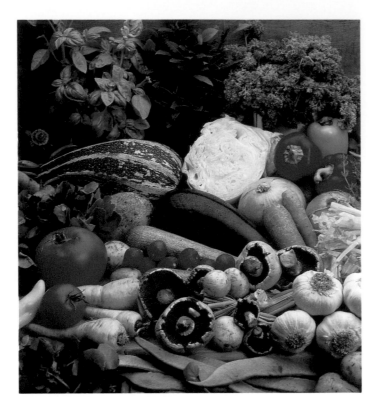

Above: *The daily consumption of fresh, unprocessed foods is a common recommendation in dietary therapy.*

Emphasis is placed upon seeds, grains and cereals, pulses, and nuts. Unlike the Gerson diet, caffeine or coffee enemas are not recommended, but herbs may be used to stimulate the liver. Patients with cancer are advised to stay on the Get Well Diet for at least six months.

■ **The Stay Well Diet** This is the same as the Get Well Diet , with a few additions. Eggs are allowed, up to 50 percent of vegetables may now be cooked, an occasional treat is allowed every fortnight, and honey may be used to sweeten drinks. While on the Stay Well Diet, patients are encouraged to eat lots of carrots or drink carrot juice, to avoid flesh and milk products (which usually contain growth factors fed to the animals) and to take supplemental doses of Vitamin C, selenium and zinc.

Other dietary advice

There are many alternative practitioners who do not use diet in such an aggressive way, but are convinced that a good diet can be of help to the patient suffering from cancer. Such a good diet might include the following:

■ Limitation of sugar intake. This means reading labels carefully – canned foods, bottled sauces, dressings and cereals, even if described as "natural", often contain high quantities of sugar.
■ Avoid highly-processed foods with preservatives and colouring added.
■ Eat natural, wholegrain breads, cereals, pasta and rice, rather than highly-processed varieties.
■ Eat plenty of fresh fruits and vegetables, rather than those which are frozen or canned.
■ Eat high-quality protein sources (low-fat dairy products, whole grains, beans, fish, eggs, fowl) and avoid high-fat meat, high-fat cheese, red meat and processed meats.
■ Find suitable beverages to replace coffee, tea and fizzy canned drinks. Try a variety of juices and drink plenty of spring water.
■ Reduce salt intake by avoiding added salt and snack foods.
■ Keep tobacco and alcohol consumption to a minimum and avoid unnecessary medication.
■ Keep fast-food and canteen eating to the minimum.
■ Reduce fried foods both at home and in restaurants. Cook vegetables in a steamer rather than in a saucepan.
■ Try to eat your largest meal in the earlier part of the day to ensure the body is able to rest more at night.
■ Give yourself time to eat slowly, peacefully, and with concentration. This way you will be aware when you have eaten enough and will be less likely to overeat. Digestion is aided by a peaceful body and mind.

Should I change my diet if I have cancer?

The answer to this question is, I am afraid, not simple. Some cancers, e.g. skin or lung cancer, have never been shown to have any correlation with diet. If you are changing your diet because you think it will affect the rate of cancer growth, you will be disappointed. If you are changing your diet because you want to eat a "healthy" diet, then following the basic guidelines may be all you need to do. However, remember that your morale may be lifted by eating an unhealthy diet that comforts you, e.g. chocolate mousse or fried egg and bacon. The decision on whether you change your diet or not should also be determined by your family's views. Meal times have always been a battleground for families to sort out who is in charge.

Below: *Natural unprocessed pasta is an attractive and healthy source of complex carbohydrates.*

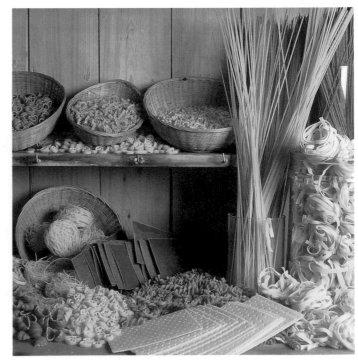

The vitamins most often used in this form of treatment are Vitamins A, C and E. Dosages of these vitamins are dependant on the type of cancer involved and will be modified by the practitioner looking after the patient. "Self-help" doses can be safely taken, both as a form of treatment and as a preventative measure – one tablet twice a day.

■ **Vitamin A** There is some evidence to suggest that Vitamin A may have a protective action in some forms of cancer.
■ **Vitamin E** This is thought to act as an anti-oxidant and to decrease the amount of "faecal mutagens" (substances in the faeces which may promote tumour growth) present in the gut. Like all vitamins in cancer therapy, it has enjoyed a fashionable phase but as yet there has been no reliable evidence to suggest it works.
■ **Vitamin C** In practice, Vitamin C is the most popular of the vitamin supplements used to treat cancer. Vitamin C (ascorbic acid) is an essential constituent of the "ground substance" in which the cells of the body are embedded. Spread of malignant cells is enhanced if this ground substance is defective in any way. In addition, Vitamin C is also

required for the efficient functioning of the immune system. Unlike the other vitamins, Vitamin C has well-known and Nobel prize-winning medical scientists supporting the case for its inclusion in cancer treatment. It is also the one vitamin which has been subjected to good clinical trials. Unfortunately, the results have proved inconclusive although they mostly showed that the Vitamin C has not proved of specific benefit.

Below: *Patients on the Stay Well Bristol Diet are encouraged to drink large quantities of carrot juice.*

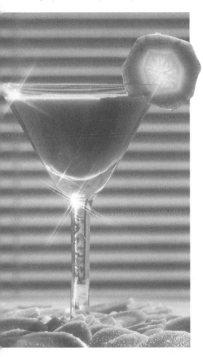

METABOLIC AND IMMUNO-AUGMENTATIVE THERAPY

Vitamin therapy although largely useless in the treatment of cancer is also largely harmless. This cannot be said of many approaches using "metabolic therapy" which claim to boost the immune system. This treatment is often given in the form of injections, and therefore is not suitable as a self-help measure. They are often prepared locally in the clinic in which they are administered and their precise constituents are not always clear. What many of these treatments have in common is a popular belief in their effectiveness and a

hostile response from the medical profession. The two most commonly used therapies are Laetrile and Iscador:

■ **Laetrile:** amygdalin or Vitamin B_{17} is a derivative of bitter almonds and has been used since the birth of Christ. Ancient pharmocopœias (books listing the use and characteristics of drugs) suggest that it was used in the treatment of cancer. The belief in its efficacy was so great that recently a prospective, randomized, controlled trial was carried out. It has been banned in the United States of America at the insistence of the Federal Drug Administration. There are, nevertheless, many anecdotal cases of patients with cancer who claim to have been cured by it.

■ **Iscador** is the extract of mistletoe that is used in anthroposophical medicine ("whole person" medicine based on the work of Austrian Rudolf Steiner) and has been used extensively by homeopathic doctors in the treatment of cancer. It can be taken by mouth as well as injections and a course is prescribed together with enzymes to enhance the digestive processes. Iscador is thought to work by enhancing the body's immunological response and studies have shown a rise in lymphocytes (white blood cells that attack invading organisms) following injections of this substance. No studies have shown that it has had any long-term beneficial effect, however.

PSYCHOSOCIAL FACTORS AND CANCER

The interest in the relationship between cancer, emotion, stress and psychological factors has greatly increased in the last ten years. Many of the psychological therapies that have been popularized by alternative therapists have operated on the principle that changing one's attitude to having cancer can affect the prognosis. Many popular books, such as *A Gentle Way with Cancer – Love Yourself Well Again* and *Fight for Your Life,* have attracted a lot of attention and form part of most alternative approaches to cancer.

Can changing my attitude and level of stress affect the prognosis of cancer?

This is a complex and difficult area and it is important to separate out the cure of the cancer itself from the care of the patient with cancer. We shall examine several approaches that have been used and discuss each in turn. It is important to remember that not all these approaches are either necessary or suitable for all cancers, let alone all patients. They should never be a substitute for good honest communication between the individual who has cancer,

Below: *Capsules of Vitamin E oil. Vitamin E has its advocates as a cancer treatment.*

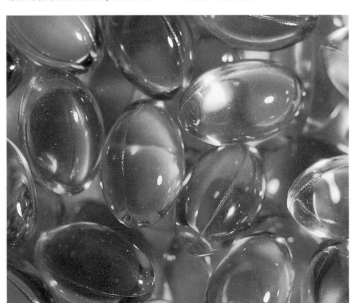

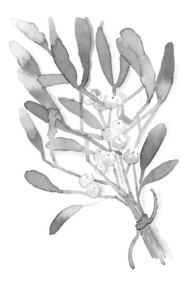

Above: *Iscador, which is extracted from mistletoe, has been used by therapists to treat cancer.*

his/her family and the doctor and nurses who have prime responsibility for looking after the patient. Because there may be a counsellor attached to the radiotherapy or surgical unit, this should not absolve the surgeon from discussing with the patient all that is necessary to ensure that he/she is fully informed.

PSYCHOLOGICAL AND SELF-HELP METHODS

■ Counselling
■ Breathing and relaxation
■ Meditation
■ Visualization
■ Self-help Groups
■ Hypnotherapy
■ Group psychotherapy
■ Spiritual healing
■ Cognitive therapy

COUNSELLING

If there is one thing that unites most people who are involved in the treatment of cancer, it is that the development of a counselling service for patients, families and, at times, practitioners, is long overdue and has been one of the real advances in cancer treatment in the last ten years. Counselling, although not elevated to a profession in its own right, is something that goes on between friends, parents and children, husbands and wives, and it is important to recognize that you

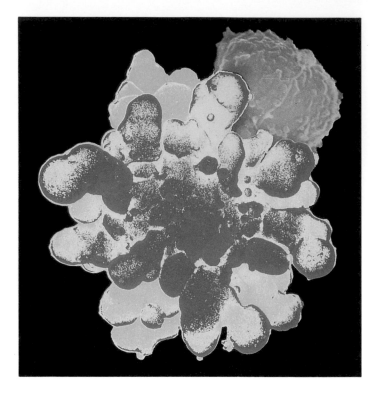

Above: *A cancer cell is here attacked by one of the body's own defenders: a T-lymphocyte cell (green).*

see it as a mental exercise which can help to calm the mind, and so reduce the element of fear, pain, anxiety and depression. All these symptoms are not very far away in people with cancer. In addition, it is very easy to feel "out of control" and become passively dependent on the medical and nursing staff.

People who meditate regularly describe feeling in greater control of their lives. Recently much interest has occurred because regular meditation has been found to increase the efficiency of "T-helper cells", a group of cells in the immune system thought to be required to prevent the spread of cancer cells. So far, however, all studies have shown that although regular meditation decreases the depression associated with cancer, it has not had a long-term effect on survival time.

CREATIVE VISUALIZATION

This is a technique that involves the use of imagination to create positive mental images, e.g. imagine you are lying on a beach with a warm Sun heating your body, or imagine your white cells are destroying all your cancer cells. This imagined scene or mental image occurs during a state of relaxation or meditation. The theory is that by imagining a peaceful scene you will encourage yourself to feel "at

peace". A simple exercise to illustrate how imagination can produce physical changes is to imagine or "picture" a lemon being cut in front of you. Most, if not everyone, who does this will notice how their salivary juices are activated by the thought. It is believed by those who introduced creative visualization into the treatment of cancer that change in the immune system can occur which could affect the growth of the cancer. The therapy which has received the most public interest is that made popular by Carl and Stephanie Simonton, a husband and wife team who ran a cancer treatment centre in Texas. The patient is encouraged to imagine his white blood cells eating/destroying the cancer cells in the body. The Simontons have now modified this approach and suggest that focusing on the cancer in this way may make it difficult for some people to get on with their normal life. They now suggest focusing on feeling better and stronger and reducing the symptoms of cancer and the side effects of treatment, rather than focusing on the cancer itself. Another model describes the cancer cells as "weak" and "confused" while the body's immune cells are described as strong and powerful like sharks attacking meat.

Below: *Group psychotherapy can be very helpful in providing an arena for cancer sufferers to express mutual support for one another.*

do not have to be a counsellor to counsel. The most important ability is *to listen attentively.* Other activities that come under the term counselling include *giving information, providing support, allowing feelings to be expressed, helping with decisions* and occasionally *offering insight.*

BREATHING AND RELAXATION

One of the most useful introductions to modern clinical practice for a variety of conditions from migraine to high blood pressure and cancer is the introduction of a simple breathing and relaxation self-help exercise. Many people with cancer and, indeed, many of the relatives of patients can be helped to relax and experience a sense of calmness if taught these simple methods. Many cancer self-help centres will hold weekly classes. For some, learning with others under the guidance of an instructor has ensured they continue the exercise at home, because one of the disadvantages of many of the self-help exercises is that they require motivation and constant practice if the person is going to benefit. Follow the exercises in Part One if you would like to learn a relaxation routine at home.

MEDITATION

Whereas most people might accept the values of a stress-reduction exercise as described above, for many the word meditation implies a "religious" pursuit which may inhibit its acceptance. One way of understanding meditation is to

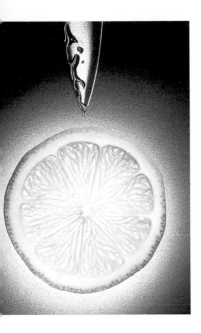

Above: *Does this picture make you salivate? If so, you appreciate the power of creative visualization.*

SELF-HELP GROUPS AND GROUP PSYCHOTHERAPY

One of the by-products of the interest in alternative approaches to cancer has been the emergence of support groups for patients and their families. Often this can be the first opportunity for families to discuss the disease with other cancer patients or cancer "survivors" as they like to be called. These groups can be of great benefit for they not only provide a source of information but they give support and an opportunity for emotional release to many who participate. Similar to the groups set up for alcoholics or people with diabetes, they are not intended to supersede conventional treatment or advice, but will offer much that the professionals cannot. Many such groups are themselves run by cancer survivors. A study recently showed that people attending such groups lived on the average eighteen months longer than those who did not.

SPIRITUAL HEALING

The laying-on of hands, absent healing or spiritual healing has always formed part of the healing ministry of the Christian church and it is therefore not surprising, or indeed inappropriate, that many patients with cancer who are approaching death seek this form of intervention. It can provide an important and very necessary support for the patient as well as his or her family. Those spiritual healers who operate outside a formal religious setting do so in the belief that they may possess a special gift of healing and that the laying-on of hands allows them to act as a channel through which "healing energy" flows into the patient. Such claims have meant that many in the medical profession dismiss spiritual healing as a superstitious remnant from the medieval days, and regard these activities, at best, as quackery and, at worst, as a dangerous deception. Nevertheless, the practice of spiritual healing continues to grow and organizations, such as the Confederation of Spiritual Healers, have attempted to develop a code of ethics and registration for all those who claim to work in this way.

OTHER THERAPIES

Massage/Aromatherapy/ Reflexology Massage can be used systematically to relieve muscle pain and tension, to bring about a sense of relaxation, and, for those isolated and lonely, to reaffirm their humanness by contact with another human being. In the care of the hospitalized or bedridden patient, it can be most powerfully used to help with the sense of hopelessness and despair that can at times occur. Many relatives who sit helplessly round the hospital bed can be taught to massage the foot or hand of their wife, husband, father, mother or

child, which will reduce the levels of anxiety and bring pleasure to both the giver and the recipient. In addition to massage, aromatherapy oils can be used. Cedarwood, because of its sedative effect, will be used in cases of anxiety and troublesome cough, while rosemary, which has an invigorating and refreshing effect, will be used for someone who is depressed, tired and suffers from loss of memory. **Acupuncture** has been shown to be effective as an additional therapy in the treatment of cancer, and in the treatment of the side-effects of contemporary medical anti-cancer therapy. It is used to manage pain, and reduce the side-effects associated with radiotherapy.

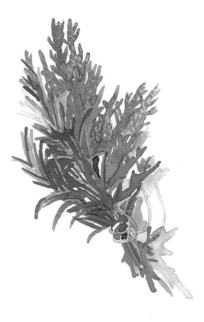

Above: *Cedarwood oil calms anxiety, while oil of rosemary can lift the spirits of the depressed.*

Below: *A simple foot massage can help family members and friends show their love for a terminally ill patient.*

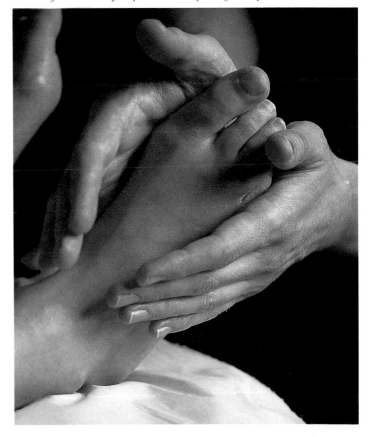

ORTHODOX TREATMENT

The orthodox treatment of cancer will depend on the type of cancer diagnosed. One, or a combination, of the following treatments are normally used: surgery, radiotherapy or chemotherapy. Surgery removes a cancerous tumour or an affected organ. Radiotherapy involves directing controlled doses of radiation at a specific part of the body to kill cancer cells. Chemotherapy relies on drugs to kill cancer cells in the body or to prevent them from multiplying further.

AIDS

HIV (Human Immunodeficiency Virus) and AIDS (Acquired Immune Deficiency Syndrome) have, in the last 20 years, aroused international concern as the "plague" of the later 20th century. The original condition was first detected and described in America among the gay population in the early 1980s. The presumed virus was identified by scientists at the Pasteur Institute in France in 1984 and the connection between the infectious agent (HIV) and the subsequent disease (AIDS) seemed firmly established. The virus itself is part of the retrovirus group: viruses that are so named because they are able to transfer genetic material from one virus to another and multiply within the "host" cells. The cells it invades are those of the immune system itself – the body's normal means of protection from infection. Thus people with AIDS are susceptible to a wide variety of infections bacause their immune system has been largely rendered non-functioning by the HIV. Since its first discovery, several other retroviruses have been identified (HIV II and HIV III) that cause AIDS or AIDS-related illness.

MODES OF TRANSMISSION

Although initially there appeared to be some confusion about the way the virus spread, there is now general agreement that it is transferred from one individual to another when there is prolonged exchange of body fluids. Thus **unprotected sexual intercourse** (vaginal and anal) remains the most common cause of spreading. **Contaminated needles** are another source of infection. People at risk include intravenous drug abusers, and people receiving unsafe injections or needlestick injuries (medical or nursing professionals accidently injuring themselves on a needle used for injection). **Blood transfusion and organ donation** (heart, kidney transplant etc.)

Below: *This computer-enhanced image shows the Human Immunodeficiency Virus magnifed x1,400,000. The virus invades the body's own immune system.*

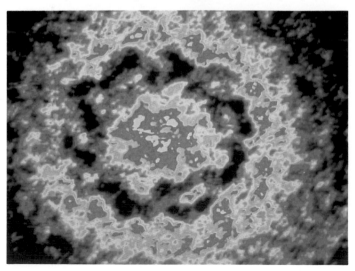

have all caused HIV transmission. Happily current precautions in hospitals and surgeries make this cause of transmission highly unlikely. **Mother-child transmission**, where the mother infects the baby either in the womb or at birth, are some of the saddest cases witnessed. The virus dies rapidly outside the body, so hand-shaking, kissing, hugging, massaging are not modes of transmission. Although the virus has been isolated from saliva, urine and breastmilk, none of these forms of body fluids has been implicated in the transfer of the virus. Nevertheless, current advice about safe sex recommends avoiding deep French kissing.

HIV AND AIDS

The initial infection with HIV rarely produces any noticeable condition, although in some people a minor viral infection may be noted with glandular fever-like symptoms (temperature, enlarged lymph glands, diarrhoea and occasionally meningitis). This minor illness affects susceptible groups only and is usually of a few weeks' duration. The majority of people with HIV infection notice nothing until either they are found when tested to be HIV positive (see below) or when they have developed AIDS itself. The proportion of people who are HIV positive who go on to develop AIDS varies, and figures from 30-55 percent are often quoted. The variation depends on the virulence of the virus itself and the capacity of "host-resistance", i.e. a malnourished African male is more likely to develop AIDS than a well nourished heterosexual white European. The length of time of "conversion" may also vary from anything up to ten years after the original infection.

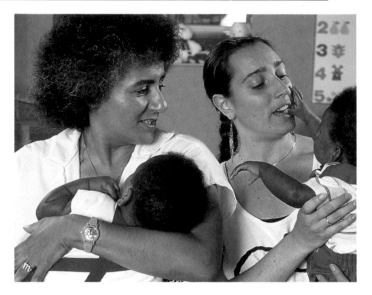

Above: *Volunteers caring for babies who have unhappily contracted HIV from their mothers during pregnancy.*

The nature of AIDS
Once the individual has "converted" from HIV positive to developing AIDS, the course of the disease also varies. Although it is generally understood that no cure for AIDS has as yet been discovered and the majority of people who develop the condition will die within five years, several have survived and some have shown no subsequent evidence of infection. The AIDS-related "complex" (a combination of symptoms that affect people who are HIV positive but have not actually developed AIDS) and AIDS disease manifests itself in a number of opportunistic infections which invade the body as a result of the destruction of the immune system. These infections include viral, bacterial and fungal conditions. They can affect any part of the body, but usually start with the skin, the intestine, the lungs and the brain. Kaposi's sarcoma (a slow-growing skin

tumour) and pneumocystis carinii (a form of destructive pneumonia) are the two most common manifestations of AIDS and, together with "wasting" diarrhoea disease (Slim's disease), characterize the progression of the disease which will eventually, but not in all cases, affect the brain and cause encephalitis.

HIV TEST

Blood tests can identify whether someone has been infected by the virus but do not detect whether he/she has developed AIDS or not. The test usually becomes positive from anything up to three weeks to three months after the infection and will remain positive whether or not AIDS develops later. There is some evidence that some people who have been HIV positive can convert to normal again, and there is an increasing group of people who develop AIDS but who are and remain HIV negative (see below).

It is important for those contemplating HIV testing to discuss the consequences of having a positive test with a counsellor or their doctor. The test is simple to perform – home test kits like pregnancy testing may soon be available – but because of the psychological consequences of a positive result, as well as the practical problems (ineligibility for life insurance and some mortgages; possible difficulties with medical and dental treatment), it is best to seek advice first.

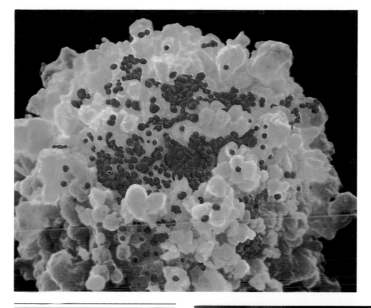

PREVENTION AND SELF-HELP

Much of the campaigning directed against AIDS has been in increasing public knowledge about the condition and ensuring everyone who is potentially at risk has access to information. The safe sex guidelines include the following commonsense policy. Reduce your number of sex partners; know about your partners' previous drug and sex history; practise safe sex and always use a condom.

Safe sex guidelines
- *No risk*
Solo masturbation
Massage away from genital areas

Below: *Blood tests provide a simple way to determine whether someone is HIV positive or not.*

- *Low risk*
Mutual masturbation
Dry kissing
- *Medium risk*
Wet kissing
Fellatio and cunnilingus
- *High risk*
Vaginal and anal sex (may be safe if condom used)
Sharing sex toys and needles
All condoms should be used with a water-based lubricant and should be worn before intercourse. Couples who are monogamous and HIV negative have nothing to fear, but only one "extramural" sexual contact is sufficient for transmission of HIV.
Drug usage is the second most common form of transmission and all users should be warned of the risk and advised to stop taking all forms of injectable drugs. If this is not possible, then they should be

advised to use disposable needles and syringes, which are now available at drug-abuse clinics. They should also be advised regarding sexual transmission of HIV, as well as the high risk of women passing on the infection to their baby.
Vaccine Much research has been undertaken to develop a vaccine that will protect against HIV infection. As yet this is at least ten years away from production and the only reliable way to prevent yourself catching AIDS is by practising safe sex and avoiding drug use.

Left: *A T-lymphocyte cell (green) invaded by HIV (red). The T cell will now produce more viral particles.*

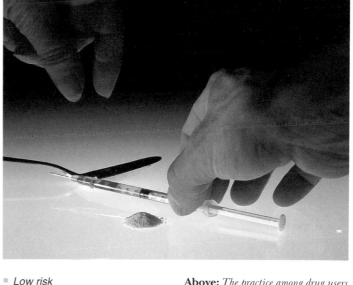

Above: *The practice among drug users of sharing needles is one of the ways in which HIV has been transmitted.*

THE ALTERNATIVE VIEW OF AIDS

Because this condition is so serious and often fatal, many alternative practitioners have rightly felt it inappropriate and dangerous to involve themselves seriously in treating it. But as it has become apparent that orthodox medicine seems unable to identify a worthwhile treatment, and that many patients with AIDS are dying unhelped, several different alternative approaches have been tried, mostly on the basis that "at least they won't harm and they might do some good". In addition, many of the alternative therapies claim to

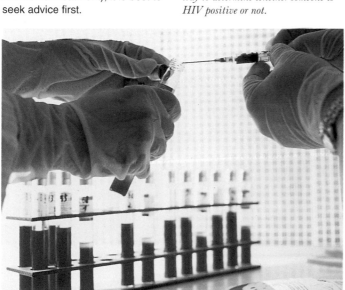

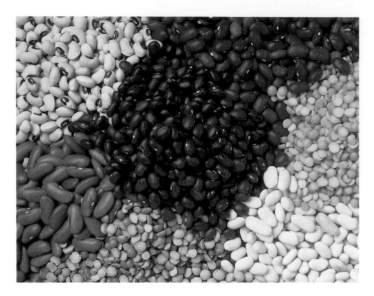

Above: *A balanced diet has its part to play in the care of AIDS patients. Fresh vegetables are essential.*

work by boosting the immune system and AIDS is a condition that essentially arises because the immune system is not working.

Initially several alternative approaches were tried as "supportive therapies", but recently some alternative practitioners have been more outspoken, some claiming to "halt" or "cure" AIDS, others claiming that the orthodox understanding of AIDS is at fault. In any serious and fatal condition it is essential that claims for a cure are exposed when obviously fraudulent, and several orthodox and alternative practitioners have been prosecuted for making such claims. However, like the treatment for cancer, the management of AIDS may have much to learn from some of these approaches. The following advice for treatment regimes should be followed with caution and some scepticism as none has been subjected to controlled trials.

HIV MAY NOT CAUSE AIDS

Several alternative practitioners believe that the fundamental cause of AIDS is not the HIV virus but a disturbed immune system that arises from lifestyle abuse – poor nutrition, over-frequent use of antibiotics, stimulants and drug abuse, sexual permissiveness, and stressful life events. They believe that the presence of the HIV is a coincidential finding and not the causative agent. It is true that not all people who develop

AIDS are HIV positive and not all people who are HIV positive develop AIDS. This minority view is now supported by some scientists in the field of AIDS research, but is still seen as totally false by the majority of AIDS researchers.

If AIDS is a condition that results from a failed immune system, then any intervention that can boost the immune system may help. The following approaches have been tried in people who are HIV positive and those who have AIDS. Like all new treatments there are anecdotal stories of long remissions and cures but it must be stated again that no proper trials have been conducted to indicate that the following regimes work.

DIET AND NUTRITIONAL SUPPLEMENTS

A good diet has always been the cornerstone of any preventative approach to illness and it is equally true for AIDS. A research project called H.A.R.P. (Healing Aids Research Project) suggests a two-pronged approach. Follow this ten-point guideline:

- Eat whole foods with as many essential nutrients and as few additives as possible.
- Fresh, organic vegetables, fruits and proteins (fish and meat) are suggested whenever possible.

- Avoid processed foods.
- Reduce or eliminate refined carbohydrates (sugars, white flour, etc.) and replace with complex carbohydrates such as vegetables, whole grains, and beans, which are rich in nutrients.
- Reduce polyunsaturated and saturated fats and oils. Use monounsaturated oils (olive oil, peanut oil) with special emphasis on omega-3 oils (fish and certain plant oils).
- Eat smaller portions more frequently throughout the day to

Below: *Aloe vera is one of the many herbs that are used to counter specific symptoms. Aloe has powerful antifungal properties.*

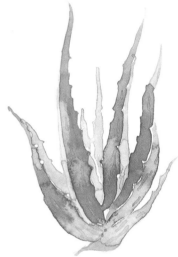

optimize absorption of nutrients from food.
- Try to keep a balanced intake which ensures that 65 percent is complex carbohydrates (vegetables, fruits, legumes and grains), 15 percent protein (fish, yoghurt, eggs and meat) and 20 percent fat.
- Make sure fruits and vegetables are thoroughly clean and free of parasites and bacteria by steaming lightly before eating.
- Eat a wide variety of foods to help avoid becoming sensitized to specific food families through repeated exposure.
- Eliminate chocolate, caffeine and alcohol.

Nutritional supplement guidelines
Supplements of these substances, which are commonly found to be deficient in AIDS sufferers, should be taken under expert guidance.
- Vitamin B$_6$
- Folic acid
- Vitamin B$_{12}$
- Selenium
- Zinc

Other supplements may include:
- Vitamin A
- Vitamin E
- Vitamin C

Below: *This combination of foods provides a healthy balanced diet. AIDS sufferers are advised to avoid eating processed and highly refined foods.*

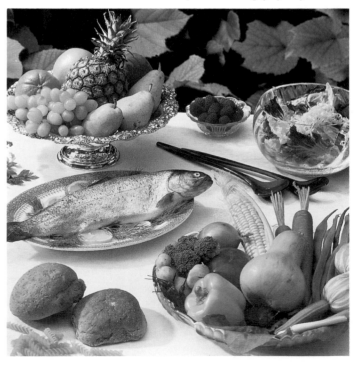

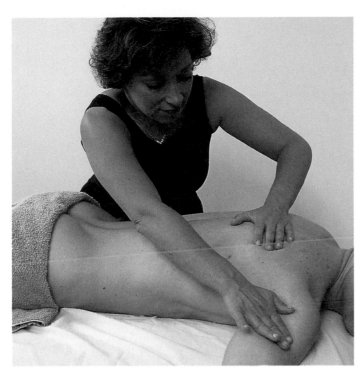

Above: *Massage helps to alleviate the sense of rejection and despair that AIDS patients can experience.*

HERBAL MEDICINE

Various herbs have been used to treat specific AIDS-related symptoms as well as to boost the body's immune system. They can be toxic to the body and self-help is not advised, so no dosages are given here. Consult an expert. Aloe vera, garlic, echinacea and citrus bitter lemon are used to treat viral, bacterial and fungal infections. Carnivora, goldenseal, astragalus and liquorice boost immune response.

HOMEOPATHY

This has been used to help with AIDS-related symptoms and some initial trials suggest that homeopathic remedies may help to delay the point at which HIV positive patients develop AIDS. The following remedies may help with the symptoms noted.
Medorrhinum: sleep problems.
Natrum mur.: grief
Tabacum: nausea, loss of appetite.
Cinchona (or *China*): night sweats.
Pulsatilla: mood swings.

MIND-BODY MEDICINE

Boosting the immune system by reducing stress, and practising a breathing and relaxation routine and learning meditation are all measures that can help sufferers come to terms better with the fact of having AIDS.

MASSAGE AND TOUCH THERAPIES

The sensation of being touched and stroked will reduce tension and pain, induce relaxation, help with depression and boost the patient's self-confidence and sense of self-worth.

ACUPUNCTURE

This form of therapy has been used with AIDS patients but because of the high risk of transmission via infected blood, great care must be taken and disposable needles always used.

COUNSELLING

This form of psychological support has assumed great importance in the management both of people who are HIV positive as well as those who have developed full-blown AIDS. Counselling will involve talking through both the consequences of having an HIV test as well as the significance of being found positive. Allowing for the shock of learning one is HIV positive, as well as being given accurate information as to what this means, are all-important aspects of humane care. Discussion regarding infectivity is important and it may well be helpful to see and talk to the partner, or partners, of HIV positive patients. Responding with anger, fear, depression and denial are all not uncommon reactions and appropriate time and support will have to be given to ensure that the individual can work through what is appropriate to him or her. Sometimes the counselling will need to include "health-boosting" advice and lifestyle changes may be suggested, e.g. relaxation, meditation. Many people with AIDS find help from self-help support groups where they can share their concerns with like-minded people.

Below: *Psychological support of the terminally ill is a mainstay of the treatment of AIDS. Here a male patient is counselled by a social worker.*

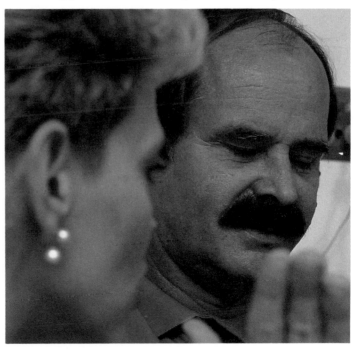

ORTHODOX TREATMENT

As yet, no specific cure for AIDS has been indentified and treatment of the condition has focused on eliminating the opportunistic infections with antibiotic, antifungal and antiviral agents. All of these treatments, especially the latter, carry side effects and the benefits in terms of longevity have not been proven. The only agent that appears to reduce infection and prolong life is an antiviral drug called AZT (azidothymidine). Although there is some evidence that it is helpful, this help appears to be temporary only and the side effects – bone marrow suppressions – can often cause more problems than it cures. In addition AZT causes a host of symptoms from fatigue to hair loss that has made many people with AIDS who are symptomless cautious of taking it. The focus on the treatment of AIDS has been towards counselling and humane care as the therapies so far used have had little effect on the disease itself.

COMPLEMENTARY FIRST AID

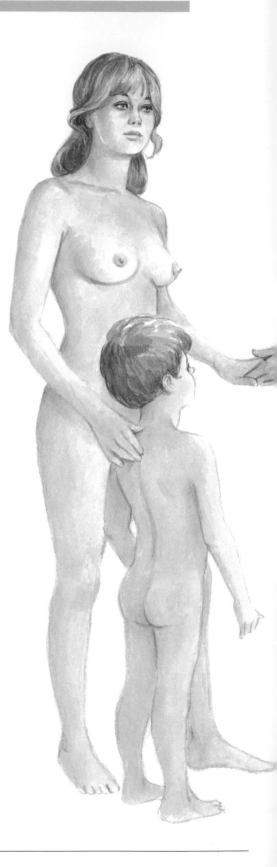

CHILDREN'S FIRST AID

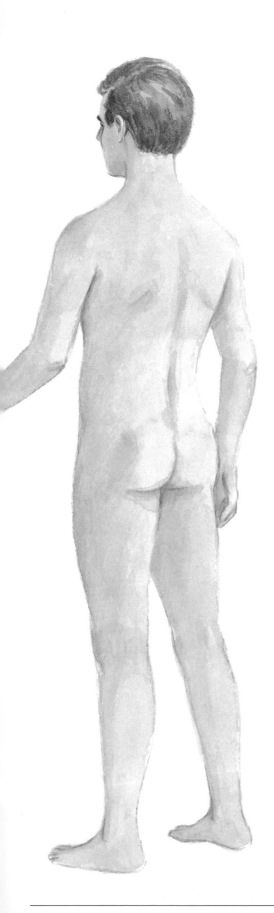

COMPLEMENTARY FIRST AID

The advice given in this section provides a selection of the best of the many possible first aid measures which derive from complementary health care. The topics covered include the most common emergencies that you may encounter. The advice given is not meant to replace emergency medical care, which is often the most appropriate to the situation, but to complement this.

Because our focus is complementary health care, it was decided that it would not be appropriate to include detailed descriptions of standard orthodox medical first aid methods, such as cardiopulmonary resuscitation ("the kiss of life") or the Heimlich manoeuvre (to assist in dislodging something stuck in the throat), or even how to deal with broken bones in an emergency, since there are no complementary methods which can add much to orthodox medical approaches in such a crisis. Details of these standard first aid measures are readily available and well described in a number of reference books, which we highly recommend that you purchase and keep alongside this book in your home.

ALLERGY

Whatever the cause of the allergy taking three to four grams of Vitamin C and/or bicarbonate of soda as a drink will modify the acuteness of the symptoms of an allergic reaction. Vitamin C can be taken either as a powder or in capsule/tablet form. For bicarbonate of soda, add between a half and a full teaspoon to a tumbler of water.

BURNS AND SCALDS

Remove whatever caused the burn and any jewellery and clothing around the area of the burn. If the burn was caused electrically, call for emergency attention.
If the area of a scald or burn is no bigger than 2.5cm (one inch) square, self-treatment is in order – if it is larger call for help.
Do not apply butter, oil or grease, or burst blisters, or cover the burn

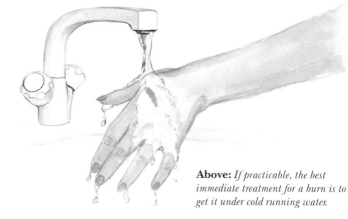

Above: *If practicable, the best immediate treatment for a burn is to get it under cold running water.*

with cloth which could stick to the surface. Only use light gauze bandaging until expert help comes.

IMMEDIATE FIRST AID

Get the affected area under *cold running water* and keep it there for as long as possible – certainly for at least ten minutes. If medical help has been summoned, keep the area under running water until

it arrives. If the cause of the burn was *chemical,* wearing gloves when handling the patient is a sensible precaution. For sunburn apply cold wet packs until irritation subsides and then use calendula ointment.

HOMEOPATHY

For pain take *Cantharis* 3x every hour until relief is noted, or *Aconitum* 12x (one dose only) for severe pain from burn or scalds.

HERBAL MEDICINE

Dress minor burns and scalds with gauze soaked in mother tincture of *Urtica urens* (eight drops to half a cup of water). For more serious burns, once healing is underway apply diluted lavender oil (four drops in four tablespoons of almond oil) or apply diluted witch hazel-soaked gauze and gently bandage. This stops infection and promotes

healing. It is safe to use these also on children.
Aloe vera juice or the sap of the leaf or a gel containing it are all soothing and promote healing. Calendula ointment is soothing as healing advances.

HYDROTHERAPY

A neutral bath soothes the discomfort of burn and sunburn conditions. Have a cushion to support the head and keep your feet out of the water to avoid swelling and wrinkling of skin. Water temperature must remain close to 36.1°C/97°F (body heat) throughout. Stay in the water for 20 to 90 minutes.

NUTRITION

Vitamin C, 3 grams daily (or more in severe cases) and zinc, 50mg daily, promote tissue repair.

CHILDREN: Half the adult dosage of Vitamin C and zinc for children under 12.

CHILBLAINS AND FROSTBITE

Frostbite is a serious condition and requires emergency care. While waiting for this to arrive apply:
■ Cold mashed raw potato (to which salt has been added) or
■ Peeled raw cucumber, mashed. These are traditional folk remedies which have not been

---

HOMEOPATHIC DOSES
In all cases in this section, when an homeopathic remedy is suggested, only take the recommended homeopathic potency and, unless otherwise directed, take two tablets, dissolved under the tongue ideally, every 30 to 60 minutes in acute situations or every four waking hours if chronic, until symptoms start to improve, at which time there is no need to continue with the remedy unless the original symptoms return.

CHILDREN: For children too young to accept a tablet under the tongue, it can be dissolved in pure spring water or the remedy may be obtained as a liquid and added to a drink.

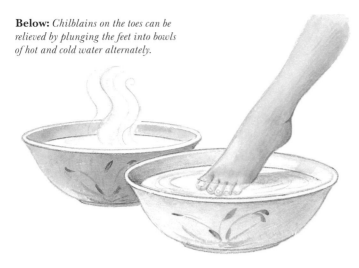

Below: *Chilblains on the toes can be relieved by plunging the feet into bowls of hot and cold water alternately.*

clinically researched but which have stood the test of time and which seem to offer nutrient/herbal substances of value in specific circumstances. The salt encourages the fluids in the mashed plant substance to be released. If the mash is applied as instructed, it will produce a slow warming effect.
▪ Take homeopathy *Agaricus muscarius* 12x.
Never try to warm the area too quickly by placing it near a heat source. Better advice is to place a frostbitten hand under your own arm or, if a companion is available, a frostbitten foot under their arm to warm it gently with body heat. Immersion for a few minutes in warm – not hot – water followed by insulation via a dressing is also helpful.
For chilblains:
Alternating hot and cold therapy is helpful. Place hands or feet in hot water for two minutes and immediately plunge them into cold for one minute. Repeat five more times finishing with cold. Do this twice daily, and/or apply tincture of myrrh while massaging, or rub in Friar's Balsam.

HOMEOPATHY

Take either *Pulsatilla* 6x (if the condition is worse when you are hot) or *Apis mellifica* (if swollen and worse when hot).
For non-bleeding chilblains a compress wrung out in cold water into which *Arnica* tincture has been placed (six drops to 60cl/one pint of water) can be applied to the painful area and left on overnight. If the area is bleeding, then apply calendula cream after the hot and cold alternations described above.

NUTRITION

For chilblains: 3 grams Vitamin C, 1 gram Bioflavonoids, 400 iu (international units) Vitamin E daily and a multimineral tablet.

CUTS AND WOUNDS

Call for help from emergency services if the wound is severe.
▪ Stop the bleeding. If the wound involves arterial bleeding (bright red blood), keep firm pressure over the wound with a pad of lint until bleeding eases or stops. Elevate the area with the bleeding site uppermost. Restrict blood flow from above the wound if bleeding is severe (releasing pressure every minute or so and then introducing it again).
▪ Remove any dirt or foreign bodies (but *not* impaled objects) if they are clearly visible, and gently sponge with clean cotton wool and water.
▪ Draw the edges of the wound together and hold closed with plaster strips before covering with a dressing and a bandage.

HERBAL AND HOMEOPATHIC METHODS

Calendula ointment or tincture offers antiseptic and healing qualities. Alternatively hypericum tincture is antiseptic and eases pain.
Hypericum 6x is the homeopathic remedy for wounds, especially if any dirt has entered the wound (adults and children take one tablet every hour for three to four hours). *Ledum* 6x is the remedy for clean puncture wounds and cuts. Consult a doctor if dirt has entered the wound.

AROMATHERAPY

Dilute essential oils of lavender or cloves, or neat eucalyptus oil are all useful applied directly onto the healing wound several times a day. This is safe for children also.

CRAMP

Cramp occurs when not enough circulation gets to a particular area and the muscle, starved of oxygen, cramps.

IMMEDIATE FIRST AID

Try to stretch the muscle (by standing and leaning forward with your foot flat on floor if the cramp happens to be in the calf, for example) or try to find the "centre" of the pain and press into that point deeply with thumb(s) while at the same time gently trying to stretch the area.
Place a hot, wet towel over the area of the cramp as soon as it has eased, or while it is still easing. Repeat this hot application every five minutes, four or five times in total, and then move the area gently, by walking or stretching.

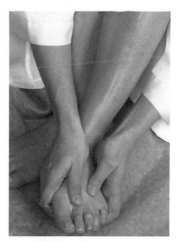

Above: *Cramps are excruciating; massage and gentle stretching of the muscles help to relieve them.*

Try to massage gently over the area, upwards towards the heart, rhythmically squeezing and kneading the muscle.

HOMEOPATHY

Try *Cuprum metallicum* 3x – it can also be given to children.

HERBAL MEDICINE

Cramp bark *(Viburnum opulus)* taken as an infusion or kelp taken as powder (in capsule or tablet form) can both be helpful.

HYDROTHERAPY

Apply hot (one to two minutes) and cold (15 to 30 seconds) applications alternately in the form of wet towels, partially wrung-out, or jets from a hand-held shower to the area where cramp commonly occurs – when cramp is absent. Two or three repetitions each time are recommended. Do this several times daily if possible, but at least after the evening bath or shower if cramps occur at night.

EARACHE

It earache persists for more than a few hours get medical attention. If the earache is due to inflammation of the middle ear, it is more difficult to deal with than when the external ear canal is inflamed. To tell which is which before a doctor is seen, *gently* pull on the lobe of the ear and move the ear in various directions. If the problem is in the outer canal, this will make the pain worse. If it is an inner ear problem (Otitis media), then movement of the ear will not make the pain worse.

FIRST AID MEASURES

In cases of infectious earache soothing heat can be delivered from an oven-heated salt or sand bag applied to the area for half-hour periods with a rest phase of half an hour between applications. Heat one kilogram (two pounds) of salt in a muslin bag in an oven at 220°C (430°F) for an hour, and apply (wrapped in cotton) when the heat is comfortable to the touch. Position the bag so that the affected ear lies on it or it lies on the ear. A *partially* heated (not boiling water), partially filled, well-stoppered and wrapped hot-water bottle can be used instead of the salt or sand.

If the earache is due to atmospheric changes (being at unaccustomed altitude – on a mountain, in a plane) you should chew gum, swallow frequently, suck a sweet or hold the nose closed while *gently* blowing through it to "pop" the eustachian tubes. Do not do this strongly. If the earache arrives soon after swimming (minutes) hold the head at an angle so that the affected ear is facing down towards the ground. Hold two stones close to the ear and bang them together sharply to make a high-pitched sound. The sound waves will often cause a rapid release of the retained water.

COUNTER-IRRITANT MEASURES

Acupressure applied by thumb or finger pressure to a point between the thumb and first finger (in the fleshy mound close to the index finger when these two digits are held together) can ease head and ear pain. Deep, sustained (a minute or so) pressure will hurt but should relieve the ear pain temporarily.

HERBAL MEDICINE

Antiseptic herbals such as liquorice, garlic and myrrh can all be helpful under professional guidance.
To deal with a wax build-up, put a few drops of warm almond oil or castor oil into the ear if the

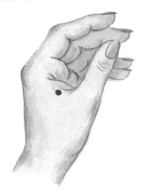

Above: *Press here to relieve earache.*

problem relates to wax compaction which may ultimately need syringing. Do this under expert advice only.
Do not put/push anything solid into the ear – even a cotton bud.

HOMEOPATHY

Depending on symptoms different remedies are indicated for earache:
If the face is red and flushed, *Belladonna* 3x.
If the earache is recurrent and follows exposure to a draught, or in the early stages, *Ferrum phos.* 3x or 6x or *Aconite* 3x.
If earache follows measles or whooping cough, *Pulsatilla* 3x.
If the patient is restless and irritable, *Chamomilla* 3x.

CHILDREN: May take the same dose as adults.

In all instances, if the earache persists, a doctor should be called.

HYDROTHERAPY

A hot foot bath can be soothing whatever the cause of the earache (or headache) because the feet have a reflex connection with the head. 20 to 30 minutes with the feet in a basin of hot water (not scalding) is helpful. Alternatively, try alternating hot and cold applications to the area around the base of the skull and neck. This can help improve local drainage and circulation.

NUTRITION

If the earache is related to infection, fasting for 24 to 36 hours is helpful. Drink water or fruit juice only. The body's immune (defence) functions are enhanced during and after short fasts such as this.

EYE PROBLEMS

In **all** cases professional advice should be sought if eye pain does not go away within a few hours.
Irritation to the cornea This can be caused by a grain of sand or a scratch and is characterized by sharp, stabbing and burning sensations which come on rapidly and which are felt below the

upper lid. The eye will be sensitive to light and will water. *Avoid rubbing it.* Tears will normally wash the irritant away. If this does not happen within a few minutes, wash and irrigate the eye using cool boiled water. If this is difficult put the face into a basin of water and open the eye-lid, holding it open for as long as possible, blinking now and then in order to try to dislodge and/or wash away the irritant object. If this fails to work, cover the eye with a loose bandage and seek medical help.
After removal of a foreign body or if there is a scratch/abrasion, or if irritation is due to chemicals such as chlorine in pool water, use a solution made up of one part in 25 of calendula tincture and pure water to bathe the eye using an eye bath. If the surface of the eye has been scratched, a drop of castor oil can be dropped onto the eyeball and the eye closed and covered with cotton wool and lightly bandaged.
In cases of infection (or allergy) affecting the eyes, such as blepharitis or hay fever, the eyes will be red and irritated. Use a cold compress (see Herbal Medicine below).

COUNTER-IRRITANT MEASURES

Acupressure can help the discomfort of eyestrain caused by reading in poor light etc.
■ Place fingers or thumbs just to the side of the ridge where the bone above the eye meets the nose. Press steadily but not heavily on these points for up to a minute at a time. Repeat every half hour if necessary.

Below: *This acupoint helps tired eyes.*

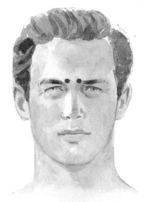

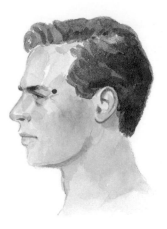

Above: *Pressure here eases eyestrain.*

■ A point will be found in a depression on either side of the head, midway between the outer edge of the eybrow and the outer corner of the eye, just behind the bone. Press here with fingers or thumbs for up to a minute every half hour.

HERBAL MEDICINE

For eyestrain an infusion of the herb euphrasia (also known as eyebright) should be used in an eye bath (eye open) and/or applied by compress soaked in the liquid (eye closed), for 20 minutes every hour until pain and sensitivity eases. An eye compress is best made by placing cotton wool into the bowl of a long-handled wooden spoon, and securing it in place with gauze. This is dipped into either hot or cold plain water or an appropriate herbal infusion or tincture and gently squeezed before being placed gently over the (closed) affected eye. An infusion can be made by adding 15g (half an ounce) of the herb to 30cl (half a pint) of water in a saucepan, bringing the mixture to the boil, turning off the heat, and allowing it to stew for 15 minutes. Strain the liquid and use in an eye bath. For styes bathe the eye every four hours in witch hazel solution – one part witch hazel to four parts cool boiled water.

HOMEOPATHY

Take *Arnica* 6x every four hours for the first 24 hours after injury to the eye. If there has been severe trauma involving the eye itself or surrounding bone or tissue, take the remedy *Symphytum* 6x every four hours after stopping the *Arnica* until healing starts or relief is noted.

CHILDREN: May take the same dose as adults.

FAINTING

If someone feels faint get them seated with their head between their legs. Offer sips of water as they recover. If the faintness is due to emotional upset, encourage deep breathing and slow exhalation. Offer Bach Rescue Remedy (three to four drops in water or directly onto the tongue). If someone has fainted, lie them on their back after raising the legs briefly to allow circulation to the head to be encouraged. Ensure the head is lower than the body; loosen tight clothing and ensure adequate fresh air. Rub the extremities – towards the heart. Offer weak tea, or a warm drink when recovering. Apply firm acupressure to the midpoint of wrist crease (palm uppermost) for a minute. Call for medical help.

HOMEOPATHY

For emotional upset or grief, *Ignatia* 6x.
For an anticipated event (accompanied by trembling and digestive or bladder frequency), *Gelsemium* 6x.
If following fright or shock, *Aconite* 6x.
If from overheating, stuffy environment, *Pulsatilla* 6x.
If accompanied by enormous

Below: *If someone has fainted, raise their legs higher than their head to encourage blood flow to the brain.*

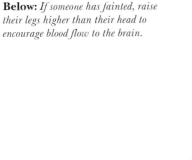

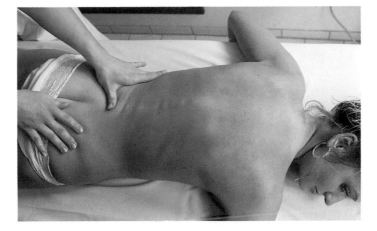

need for fresh air and yet person feels cold, *Carbo veg. 6x.*
Take the recommended dosage every thirty to sixty minutes during the acute phase of any crisis, and less frequently threafter until symptoms ease.

CHILDREN: May take the same dose as adults.

GYNAECOLOGICAL AND MENSTRUAL PAIN

Expert advice should be sought if such problems are persistent or severe.

FIRST AID MEASURES

Menstrual and vaginal cramps can be eased by immersion of the pelvic region (i.e. sit upright in the bath) in hot water (tolerable, not scalding). Stay in the water for up to half an hour.
Note: Do not take hot baths if there is heavy bleeding.

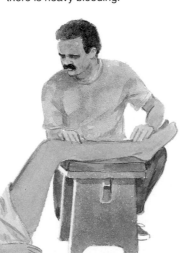

Above: *Massage of the lower back helps to relieve menstrual cramps. Self-massage techniques are also useful.*

AROMATHERAPY

Add ten drops each of essential oils of chamomile and marjoram to a bath for greater relief, while caraway oil (six drops in a bath) is helpful as a treatment for painful menstrual conditions.
For painful vaginal infections use oil of sage (six drops in bath) or for local washing of the vaginal area (three drops into bidet or basin of water).

EXERCISE

A brisk walk and deep breathing both relieve menstrual cramp pains for many people.

ACUPRESSURE

This is often helpful for menstrual pain. Find points which are sensitive about five to eight cm (two to three inches) directly below the umbilicus. Maintain firm pressure on sensitive points as you inhale and lighten up as you exhale. Repeat this ten times.

MASSAGE

Massage of the low back relieves menstrual cramps rapidly if correctly applied. If hand massage is not available, lie on two tennis balls (put into the toe of a pair of socks) so that one ball is on each side of the spine at a level of the low back which gives a "nice" hurt when pressed (usually just below the lower ribs). Move gently, rolling the balls against the tight muscles for several minutes.

HERBAL MEDICINE

Drink well-brewed raspberry leaf tea, or try V*iburnum prunifolium* (black haw): drink 15 to 20 drops of a tincture in water for menstrual cramps, three times a day as needed. *Viburnum opulus* (cramp bark) is effective against uterine cramps: 15 to 20 drops of tincture, three times a day. Ginger root eaten or taken as an infusion or in tablet form is good for general menstrual pain. Garlic relieves heavy painful clotting at period time and up to six capsules of garlic oil can be taken daily at this time.

HOMEOPATHY

Mag. phos. 3x for cramp-like pains which improve with warmth. *Colocynthis* 6x if period pain is extreme but better if pressed. *Chamomilla* 3x if pain is extreme and you feel very irritable.

HEADACHE AND MIGRAINE

First aid for an existing headache is to lie down in a darkened room with either a warm or cold compress on the affected area – whichever helps most.
Eat nothing unless the headache is caused by missing a meal and accompanied by feelings of faintness – in which case low blood sugar could be the cause. In such a case eat a protein food (natural yoghurt for example) and not a sugary one. For all other headaches drink adequately of water or diluted juices and eat little until the headache passes.
If the first signs of a congestion/migraine type headache are recognized, they can sometimes be aborted by a hot foot bath into which several teaspoons of mustard powder have been stirred. At the same time apply a cold compress to the forehead and/or base of the skull area. This is effective because there is a direct reflex connection between the feet (and hands) and the head. Heat applied to the feet will encourage decongestion of the head. Simply placing the hands under a hot running tap (not scalding!) will do the same, but to be effective this needs to continue for 20 to 30 minutes.

HOMEOPATHY

Different remedies exist for different types of headache:
If it is worse for any movement, *Bryonia* 6x.
If pain is like a tight band and is worse when lying, *Gelsemium* 6x.
If it follows over-indulgence (e.g. a hangover), *Nux vomica* 6x.
If accompanied by hot red face, throbbing pain, *Belladonna* 6x.
A blinding head with visual symptoms, worse between mid-morning and mid-afternoon, *Natrum mur.* 6x.

CHILDREN: May take the same dose as adults.

JOINT STRAINS AND INJURIES

The acronym "RICE" should be memorized. This stands for:
- Rest – place the injured area in a position of relative ease and allow only essential movement.
- Ice – Ice or cold compresses should be applied to any sprain, strain, bruised or injured area for at least 20 minutes every hour for the first day or so.
- Compression – to reduce swelling a firm supportive bandage (not too tight) should be placed over the area of injury.
- Elevation – if the area can easily be elevated (ankle, knee, arm) it should be supported in an elevated position to reduce excessive swelling. Just as soon as it is possible to start painless movement the "E" for "elevation" can then refer to "exercise".

HYDROTHERAPY

Tincture of arnica can usefully be added to cold compresses which should be applied to injured joints. A cold compress is made from cotton material wrung out in cold water and applied firmly to the affected area, covered with flannel or woollen material, and firmly pinned in place. The cold material warms up slowly and has a relaxing and decongesting effect on injured areas.
Avoid applying heat directly to joint injuries unless this is followed by a cold application, otherwise tissue congestion will increase. Get expert advice if the strain/injury appears to be severe.

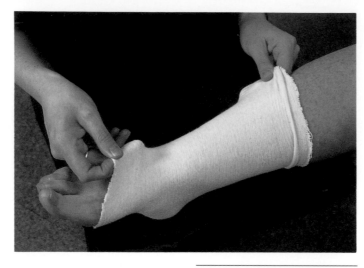

Above: *The application of a firm, supportive bandage is one of the four recommended procedures for dealing with sprains and strains.*

HOMEOPATHY

If there is shock and bruising take *Arnica* 6x for the first day (or *Ledum* 6x if cold applications seem to help). If still painful after a few days take *Rhus tox.* 6x or *Ruta* 6x if the pain eases after use. If there is no improvement of pain with use take *Bryonia* 6x.

CHILDREN: May take the same dose as adults.

MOUTH AND TONGUE PROBLEMS

Specific attention is required to deal with the causes of any mouth or tongue problems which persist.

FIRST AID MEASURES

For rapid relief hold a moistened (Indian) tea bag over a canker sore. The tannin is an astringent and also kills yeast which might be involved.

HERBAL MEDICINE

Plantago mother tincture applied locally by dabbing with soaked cotton wool to sore places in the mouth is helpful. A mouthwash with a solution containing red sage (infuse the leaves as a tea) or tincture of myrrh (diluted five to ten drops in half a tumbler of warm water) may also be tried.

HOMEOPATHY

Plantago 3x or *Kreosotum* 3x. This is suitable for adults and children.

HYDROTHERAPY

An ice chip placed onto a tender canker sore can be helpful, as can sucking an ice cube if the mouth or tongue feels hot and raw.

NUTRITION

Chewing high potency acidophilus tablets helps, as does rinsing the mouth (retaining the rinse for at least a minute) with a solution containing high potency acidophilus dissolved in warm water.
Redness, soreness (and possibly scaling) at the junction of lips and the mucous membrane of the mouth (cheilitis) is often caused by Vitamin B_2 deficiency. Supplement with one B-complex capsule daily (yeast free, taken at a meal time) as well as an individual supplement of 25mg of Vitamin B_2 at a separate meal time daily until symptoms vanish. Cracking and soreness at the corner of the mouth (angular cheilitis) may result from poor denture fitting or hygiene and/or iron, folic acid, Vitamin B_2, B_6 and/or B_{12} deficiency. Supplementation can be attempted but advice from a health care professional is preferable.
Tongue soreness can also result from deficiency, specifically B_2 (tip will be red and sore), B_3 (fissures on tongue) and B_6 (tongue tip red

and sore). If the tongue is sore and bleeding this can mean Vitamin C deficiency. Get expert advice about this.
Aphthous ulcers can be caused by deficiency of iron, B_{12}, B_6 or folic acid. Again get expert advice.
All of the mouth and tongue problems mentioned can be the result of allergies, with wheat/gluten allergy being one of the commonest. This needs professional guidance to assist.

MUSCLE PROBLEMS

When muscles are overused or abused, they become stressed and commonly inflamed as do the tendons which anchor them to bone. Injury, such as a fall, wrench, twist etc., or repetitive minor stress caused by overwork or postural misuse can all be to blame.

SELF-HELP FIRST AID

If you can walk on or use an area which has been injured, try self-treatment for two days, and if it is improving well just continue doing whatever is helping. If it is not a lot better within 48 hours see a professional for advice or help. *If it hurts to use it, rest it.*

HYDROTHERAPY

For strains or bruises try ice massage followed by gentle stretching of the area. For an ice massage, take a cube of ice and rub it gently over the damaged/strained area, avoiding staying in one place so as not to chill or blanch the skin. Keep the ice moving. Anything from a few minutes to 20 minutes every hour is useful. The objective is to reduce fluid stasis and congestion. Alternatively place crushed ice in folded cotton or towelling and apply to the area for ten minutes or so before gently trying to move the muscle by contracting and stretching it within the limits of pain.
Hot and cold alternating applications are recommended. Use hand-towels wrung out in appropriate temperature water and placed over the area – 30 seconds hot/15 seconds cold –

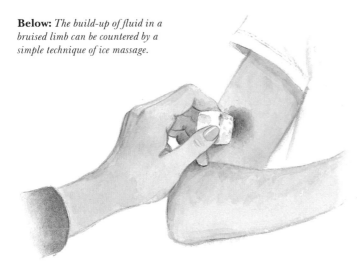

Below: *The build-up of fluid in a bruised limb can be countered by a simple technique of ice massage.*

and repeat up to ten times each, finishing with cold.

Before massage apply a hot wet towel to the area for five minutes. An Epsom salt bath or aromatherapy bath (see list of oils under Aromatherapy below) can also bring relief.

After use of hot moist applications, stretching of stiff or painful muscles to their pain-free limit is useful.

Compression If the area is swollen – a sprained ankle, for example – then as well as resting and icing it, the area should be bandaged for support and compression to reduce swelling. Bandage firmly but not tightly. If swollen, place the area in elevation, higher than the rest of the body.

ACUPRESSURE

This is helpful in relieving pain and tightness. Seek tender/tight areas in muscles and apply pressure to these for 30 seconds at a time to see whether the whole area feels easier afterwards.

HERBAL MEDICINE

Herbs which can ease muscle spasm or irritable muscle conditions include mistletoe, passion flower, skullcap and valerian. Take them as infusions.

AROMATHERAPY

Oils are useful either massaged into the area or used in baths. In particular chamomile, cypress,

eucalyptus and rosemary may be tried. Ten drops of any of these added to a bath or three to four drops to an eggcup of almond oil (for massage) is suggested. Essential oils at this dilution are safe to use on children.

HOMEOPATHY

In case of recent injury take Bach Rescue Remedy.

For bruised muscles, *Arnica* 3x in acute phase (first 24-36 hours). If there is deep bruising or a muscle tear, *Ledum* 3x should then be taken for a few days.

For all muscle aches and pains, *Rhus tox.* 3x.

For damaged tendons or ligaments, *Ruta* 3x every four hours.

If *Ruta* applied locally (mother tincture) and taken internally (3x) does not help tendon pains, using *Symphytum* the same way might.

CHILDREN: May take the same dose as adults.

MANIPULATION AND MASSAGE

Search for localized tender areas in muscles *opposite* those which were stretched or strained or which hurt on movement. The search for "tender points" is in muscles of the region which were not stretched, but which were actually short and relaxed at the time of the strain. So if you turn your foot, twisting it inwards and stretching the outer aspect of the ankle, the tender point would be

on the inner aspect of the lower leg. Hold a firm pressure on the point which hurts, while slowly altering the position of the body or limb so that the pain goes out of the tender point. If you find such a position of ease hold it for a minute before slowly returning to a neutral position, the pain should be very much easier and the muscles more relaxed.

NOSEBLEED

Rest with the head upright or slightly forward of the neck, and place a cold or ice compress on the back of the neck as well as over the nose. For childhood nosebleed, do not tilt the head back at all or blood may trickle down the back of the throat provoking vomiting.

When bleeding stops avoid blowing nose or sniffing strongly or the bleed could start again. Plug the nose with a small roll of lint (soaked in tincture of witch hazel if possible or fresh lemon juice if this is not available), or grasp the soft part of the nose firmly, between index finger and thumb, and hold for up to ten minutes.

If a nosebleed continues for 15 minutes or more despite these measures, seek medical advice.

HOMEOPATHY

Take *Arnica* 3x if nosebleed is due to a blow (in which case also consider getting medical advice as a fracture could exist). Take *Aconitum* 3x if it is due to over-excitement, or *Hamamelis* 3x if due to blood vessel degeneration in an elderly person.

CHILDREN: May take the same dose as adults.

PANIC ATTACK

A first aid measure for an anxiety/panic attack if this is accompanied by hyperventilation – which it usually is – is to re-breathe carbon dioxide by exhaling into a paper bag and re-breathing the stale air until symptoms calm.

Another way of achieving the same effect is to breathe in very deeply and fairly quickly – ideally through the nose – followed by a very slow exhalation through the mouth, taking twice as long to breathe out as was taken to breathe in. If this is repeated about ten times, a calming effect is felt as the biochemical imbalance caused by over-breathing – and the consequent heightened anxiety state – normalizes.

A drink of bicarbonate of soda has a similar effect if this is available.

HYDROTHERAPY

A neutral bath is profoundly relaxing and will reduce anxiety and panic sensations. Place a cushion behind the head and keep feet out of the water to avoid swelling and wrinkling of skin. Water temperature must remain close to 36.1°C/ 97°F (body heat) throughout. Stay in the water for 30 to 90 minutes.

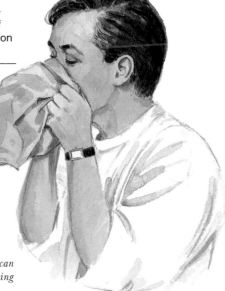

Right: *Hyperventilation often accompanies a panic attack. Calm can be restored by employing a re-breathing technique using a paper bag.*

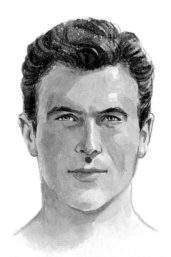

Above: *This acupoint helps with shock.*

SHOCK

An immediate first aid measure is to offer the Bach flower remedy called Rescue Remedy. A few drops in water sipped throughout the day is indicated for severe shock. Advice to rest warmly and not be left alone is also useful.

ACUPRESSURE

For shock acupressure can be applied to two areas:
- The centre of the groove below the nose, on the upper lip. This needs to be located with the thumb nail and firm pressure applied towards the gums under the lip for a minute or so every hour.
- A third of the way down the sole of the foot in line with the middle toe, in a depression below the ball of the foot. Pressure here can allay the effects of shock.

SKIN PROBLEMS

FIRST AID MEASURES

Extract of witch hazel or marigold or chickweed diluted in water and applied to the area as a compress (tepid not hot) soothes most local skin conditions. Make an infusion as explained in the entry on eye problems and apply this diluted 50:50 with pure water by soaking a cotton or lint bandage and applying it to the area. Alternatively use five drops of pure witch hazel extract in 30cl (half a pint) of water and apply in the same way.

For facial herpes or dry eczema add three drops of geranium oil to a little almond oil (an eggcupful) and apply three times daily.
For dry eczema three drops of oil of hyssop in an eggcupful of almond oil can be applied daily.
For wet eczema four drops of juniper oil in an eggcup of almond oil can be applied to the areas affected twice daily.
Aloe vera juice or gel, or in the form of sap directly from the plant, is useful for many conditions, such as burns, shingles, fungal infections, stings, and infected wounds.
For raw, chapped skin use calendula ointment.

CHILDREN: All remedies may be safely used on children.

HOMEOPATHY

For herpes, *Natrum mur.* 3x or 6x. For herpes or eczema, *Rhus tox.* 3x. For urticaria (hives), *Apis mellifica* 3x or *Urtica urens* 3x.

CHILDREN: May take the same dose as adults.

HYDROTHERAPY

To relieve skin irritation from most causes 20 to 30 minutes in an oatmeal bath can be effective. The water should be fairly warm but not hot. Add a few tablespoons of finely ground, uncooked oatmeal to the bath and tie into a cloth half a kilogram (one pound) of coarse uncooked oatmeal. Hang this from the tap so that the water runs through it. When the bath is full, remove the bag and use it as a sponge, gently patting areas of irritation. Stay in the bath for 30 minutes.

NUTRITION

Most acute and chronic skin conditions are helped by controlled fasting – water only (but never for more than 36 hours without supervision).

BOILS

HYDROTHERAPY

Apply towels soaked in hot and cold water. Alternate two minutes hot/one minute cold repeated eight to ten times, two or three times daily.

FOLK REMEDY

Bruise or grate cabbage leaves and apply as a poultice (wrapped in gauze) over the boil whether open or not. Leave in place for at least four hours. Replace daily until healed.

HERBAL MEDICINE

Apply thyme oil (three drops diluted in a cup of warm water) to a boil (once it has opened), using cotton wool, to soothe the skin and promote healing.

POISON IVY STINGS

Wash the skin vigorously with water and simple soap. Apply aloe vera juice or apple cider vinegar. Avoid scratching or the poison will spread!

STINGS AND SPLINTERS

Remove a bee sting or splinter with tweezers, or ease it out using a flat needle pressed against the

Below: *An effective herbal remedy for insect stings is to bandage a sliced onion over the site of the sting.*

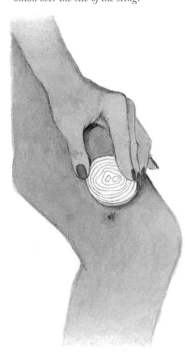

skin. Apply cold running water for up to ten minutes to irrigate the wound. If the splinter cannot be extracted, use a kaolin poultice to draw it out. Kaolin is a clay-based substance that you buy from a pharmacy. Heat it and apply it with a dressing as per the instructions on the packet.
Wasps do not leave stings in the flesh. To deal with a wasp sting apply vinegar or lemon juice or a paste made of bicarbonate of soda mixed with a little water as soon as possible to neutralize the venom.
If the person stung feels unwell or has difficulty in breathing, they may be suffering an acute allergic reaction. Get emergency medical care immediately.

HOMEOPATHY

Ledum 6x can help with both bee and wasp stings – especially if the area feels cold and the symptoms are improved by cold. This is ideal for sharp pricking pains or splinters. (*Hypericum* 6x might help splinters if *Ledum* fails).
If the area is swollen and shiny, take *Apis mellifica* 6x or for heavy itching around sting take *Urtica* 6x.

CHILDREN: May take same dose as adults.

HERBAL MEDICINE

The pulped heads and buds of young marigolds (calendula) make an excellent tincture (preserved in alcohol) which can be applied to stings and splinters. Alternatively a pulped fresh marigold flower can be applied directly to a sting and bandaged in place. A crushed or sliced onion placed over a sting or bite will reduce swelling and ease discomfort.

AROMATHERAPY

Use essential oils of lavender, basil, marjoram or thyme applied directly onto bites and stings. Alternatively, add a total of up to 20 drops (either a single oil or a mixture of oils) to a bath, and bathe the affected area in the water.

CHILDREN: May safely use these remedies as directed above.

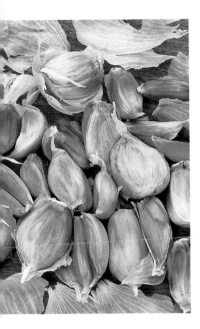

Above: *Garlic is a natural antibiotic and eaten raw, or taken in capsule form, it can help with throat infections.*

THROAT SORENESS

Throat pain can be serious – if it persists or recurs frequently seek medical advice.

FIRST AID MEASURES

Breathe through your nose. If this is impossible, cover your mouth with a thin scarf so that the air is filtered and warm. Ensure humidity is high (steam a kettle periodically or purchase a humidifier). Dry air is extremely irritating to the throat.

HERBAL MEDICINE

Garlic taken in food or as capsules is powerfully antibiotic. Take three to six capsules daily. A teaspoon of red sage extract steeped in a cup of water (sage is available from an herbalist or homeopathic pharmacy) is a useful gargle or mouthwash for sore throats and tonsillitis. Use several times daily.
Or gargle with lemon juice or the following aromatherapy essential oils:
▪ Geranium oil – three drops to a cup of warm water.
▪ Pine oil – two drops to a cup of warm water.
▪ Lemon juice – a small squeeze in warm water.

HOMEOPATHY

If the sore throat is a cold symptom take *Nux vomica* 3x (two tablets every hour until symptoms ease), especially if it started after a chill and there is nasal discharge during the day but not at night and there is restlessness and a feeling of not being able to get warm.
If the cold is worse in the evening and worse in a warm room, then take *Allium cepa* 3x half hourly until symptoms improve.
If the cold is not triggered by a chill, then *Arsenicum* 3x taken half hourly may cut it short.
If accompanied by fever and tonsils are red, *Belladonna* 3x. For other forms of sore throat a professional homeopath would need to advise on appropriate remedies.

CHILDREN: May take the same dose as adults.

HYDROTHERAPY

Irrigation of the back of the throat with very warm (not hot) salt water is useful. Obtain a syringe and fill with warm salt water (a teaspoon of salt dissolved in 60cl/a pint of water is the right dilution). Lean over a basin and squirt this quite strongly onto the back of the throat, washing and irrigating the tender tissues. Use up to 60cl (a pint) of water this way, allowing the "run-off" to sluice out of the mouth (do not swallow it).

NUTRITION

A light (fruit only) diet or a fast (water only) for 36 to 48 hours is the ideal treatment for all sore throats. Consult an expert if you plan on fasting for longer.

THRUSH

If there is severe discomfort around the vagina due to thrush, use one of the following methods for relief.
▪ Live yoghurt applied to the area (ideally to which you have added several teaspoonsful of powdered acidophilus culture). If the burning itch is internal, use a tampon soaked in the yoghurt applied internally for a few hours.
▪ Douche with diluted aloe vera juice (30ml/one fluid ounce to a tumbler of water). Internal use via a tampon is also helpful.
▪ Diluted vinegar can be very soothing for itching and burning. Dilute cider vinegar (ideally) 50:50 with water. For oral thrush, gargle with diluted tea tree oil (two to three drops in a cup of water) or a solution of acidophilus powder (two teaspoons in half a cup of water) several times daily. Avoid sugar and yeasty foods.

TOOTHACHE AND GUM PROBLEMS

Dental attention should be sought as soon as possible. Pain relief from aspirin or other painkillers as well as painkilling mouthwashes can be effective short-term strategies. Do not place such pain killers directly against the gum to ease pain unless they are sold as a mouthwash.

FIRST AID MEASURES

Local application of any of these, several times daily: clove oil (nerve sedative), brandy, peppermint extract, cinnamon oil. Apply any of these directly to gum/tooth margin or into tooth cavity, using soaked cotton wool. Or chew a clove to release its soothing oils.
For pain/swelling of a wisdom tooth, frequent salt water mouthwashes (half a teaspoon of salt in a tumbler of warm water) removes bacteria and is soothing. For any toothache use a solution of tincture of myrrh (five to ten drops in half a tumbler of warm water) as a mouthwash.

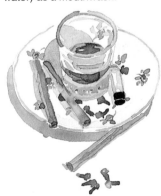

Above: *Applying brandy or the oils of cinnamon or cloves to the gums helps to relieve the pain of toothache.*

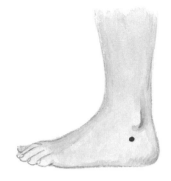

Above: *Pressure here eases toothache.*

COUNTER-IRRITANT MEASURES

Acupressure on two acupoints can be helpful (up to a minute each):
▪ A sensitive point on either index finger on the thumb side of the finger close to the nail-bed.
▪ Just below the ankle bone on either leg, on the outer surface.

HERBAL MEDICINE

Tincture of calendula diluted 50:50 with hot water and applied to painful, swollen gums (after dental surgery for example) rapidly reduces swelling and pain.

HOMEOPATHY

Chamomilla 3x or 6x is good for neuralgia-like pains, especially if accompanied by restlessness and irritability. Take half-hourly until relief is felt.
Pulsatilla 6x, especially if accompanied by feeling weepy.
Calcarea phosphorica 6x, if not helped by either of the above.
Aconitum 3x, ideal if pain is burning/throbbing.

CHILDREN: May take the same dose as adults.

HYDROTHERAPY

Massage the outside of the jaw with ice – either an ice cube or use an ice bag – on the area overlying the sore tooth, for rapid if short-term relief. Keep the ice moving over the skin; do not keep it still.
Apply crushed ice in a plastic bag over painful area (on face not inside mouth!) for ten to fifteen minutes hourly. This is ideal for use after dental surgery or injury.

CHILDREN'S FIRST AID

It is generally acknowledged that emergency attention – dealing with a crisis – is an area of orthodox medical practice which is unsurpassed in excellence. While alternative health care methods certainly have some useful additional methods to offer in first aid settings, it should be recognized that its main benefits are achieved in the treatment and care of more chronic (i.e. long-term) conditions.

In considering first aid for infants and young children, we must stress that the need to involve skilled medical attention at the earliest possible stage is vital, especially for example where dehydration is concerned in cases of fever, diarrhoea and/or vomiting if these do not speedily resolve themselves; or where earache persists; or in cases of heat or sunstroke; or burns; or blows to the head.

See Complementary First Aid section for bites, burns, nosebleeds, ear, eye, throat and mouth problems. General advice on homeopathic dosages for children will be found on page 204.

BUMPS AND BRUISES

Cold compresses and rest are recommended as a first aid measure.

HOMEOPATHY

Arnica 6x every 15 minutes after an injury until pain is reduced is the recommendation.
If bones are bruised, *Ruta* 6x.

HERBAL MEDICINE

Apply distilled witch hazel or comfrey if bones/joints are involved (sprains). A calendula compress (fresh flowers crushed or prepared as an infusion) helps heal bruises rapidly.

Below: *Distilled witch hazel or comfrey ease minor bumps and bruises.*

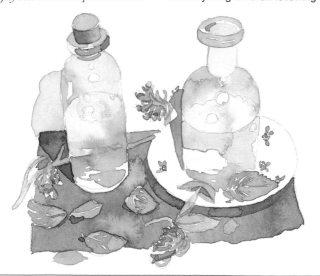

COLIC

Warm or mildly hot compresses to the abdomen help soothe the pain of colic.

HOMEOPATHY

If also very irritable, *Colocynthis* 6c.
If doubled up in pain, *Magnesia phosphorica* 6c.
If combined with nausea (vomiting), *Ipecacuanha* 6c.

DIARRHOEA

Make the child consume a lot of liquid, eat nothing for at least 24 hours and then take puréed apple (no sugar) and live yoghurt in small amounts if the diarrhoea has stopped. If not, call a doctor.

PROBIOTICS

Infant strain "friendly bacteria" (bifidobacteria infantis), which is obtainable from any good healthfood store, is extremely useful in normalizing the intestinal tract of young children following an infection of food poisoning – especially if antibiotics have been used to cure it. In children who have been weaned, standard adult bifidobacteria and acidophilus should be used. A quarter teaspoonful twice daily in water away from mealtimes for a week is suggested.

HOMEOPATHY

The most useful homeopathic remedy is *Arsenicum album* 6x, but others might be needed depending on the individual characteristics of the sufferer – call an expert.

HERBAL MEDICINE

An herbal infusion of agrimony is useful for childhood diarrhoea. Take three cups daily.

FEVER

Treat with a water-only fast for 24 hours, and call a doctor or naturopath.

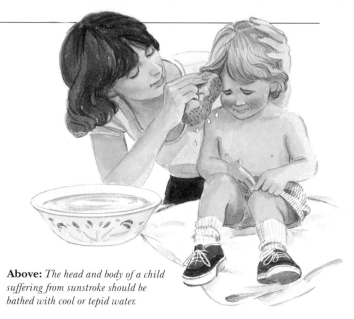

Above: *The head and body of a child suffering from sunstroke should be bathed with cool or tepid water.*

Ensure lots of liquid is consumed at regular intervals.

HOMEOPATHY

For a feverish child before the doctor arrives:
At first sign of fever of sudden onset, very thirsty, restless (perhaps following chill), *Aconite* 6x.
If very red and agitated, use *Belladonna* 6x.
Dry heat – intense thirst worse for movement, *Bryonia* 6x.
Feels chilly and cannot get warm, *Nux vomica* 6x.
Very weepy, cannot be left alone, not thirsty, worse for being hot, *Pulsatilla* 6x.
All remedies should be taken four hourly until symptoms improve.

HEAT OR SUNSTROKE

If symptoms like dizziness, nausea and headache appear along with elevated temperature, and dry or red skin comes on

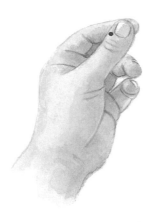

Above: *An acupoint for heatstroke.*

suddenly, and there has been exposure to strong sun and high temperature, the chances are that sunstroke or heatstroke exists. Call for medical help.
Apply cool or tepid water to the head, neck, chest and back using towels or sponging.
If the temperature is very high, elevate the head while the child is in bed and apply a cold compress to the forehead and neck, while sponging the rest of the body with tepid water.
No food should be eaten but water and unsweetened juices should be drunk.
If the child has been exposed to heat and has some of the symptoms listed, but the temperature is only slightly raised and they are feeling exhausted with a cold, clammy skin, then heat exhaustion is a more likely diagnosis. The child should rest, receive cool sponging and have nourishing mineral-rich soups and broths to replenish lost mineral salts.

ACUPRESSURE

A spot just below the thumbnail, on the side nearest the first finger, is a pressure point which helps recovery from heatstroke. Press firmly for half a minute at a time every few minutes.

BACH FLOWER REMEDY

For both heatstroke and heat exhaustion the Bach Rescue Remedy should be taken. Use three to four drops in a glass of water and sip during the course of the day, or apply three or four drops directly on the tongue up to four times a day.

HICCUPS

Place a warm towel (wrung out in hot but not scalding water) over the abdomen/diaphragm area. Re-apply after five minutes or so if hiccup continues. A *warm* water or fruit juice drink may also resolve the problem.

ACUPRESSURE

Apply firm acupressure on either side of the spine (about 2.5cm/one inch distance laterally from the spine itself) at the level of the lower tips of the shoulder blades. The degree of pressure applied should *not* be sufficient to cause pain. Hold for a minute or so and then rest. Reapply pressure if unsuccessful the first time.

Below: *Pressure point for hiccups.*

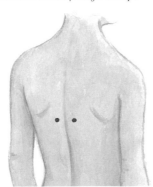

Below: *The Bach Rescue Remedy may help a child suffering from heatstroke. Drops can be added to a glass of water or applied directly on the tongue.*

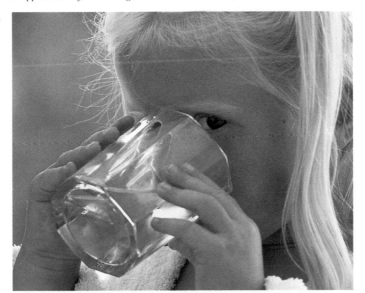

MOTION SICKNESS

ACUPRESSURE

Pressure on the inner forearm two thumb-widths above the centre of the wrist can reduce symptoms of travel sickness and other forms of nausea. "Sea-band" straps which press on the area can be purchased at health stores and pharmacies.

PREVENTATIVE MEASURES

Eat ginger (crystallized) or take ginger capsules. Avoid reading while travelling.

HOMEOPATHY

Cocculus 6x or *Tabacum* 6x taken before the journey can be helpful.

SUNBURN

Apply calamine to affected areas, or calendula ointment, or bathe the skin in black tea infusion, or use a solution containing bicarbonate of soda. A thick liquid consistency is needed for the latter; mix water slowly with the powder to form a paste and then a thick solution which can be applied to the sunburned skin.

HOMEOPATHY

Belladonna 6x if very flushed; if blistered, *Cantharus* 6x.

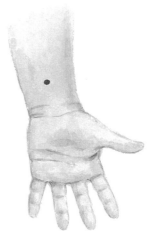

Above: *The anti-nausea acupoint.*

AROMATHERAPY

A few drops of the essential oils of chamomile and lavender used directly onto irritated skin will soothe and promote healing. It is safe to use oils on children's skins provided no allergy to the substance exists.

TEETHING PROBLEMS

HOMEOPATHY

If the child is cross and irritable and wants to be nursed, use *Chamomilla* 6x (also for similar symptoms associated with colds and diarrhoea).
If weepy, clinging, *Pulsatilla* 6x. If not helped by either *Chamomilla* or *Pulsatilla*, *Calcarea phosphorica* 6x.
Infant homeopathic remedies can be purchased as powders, which can be applied directly onto the gums or dissolved in pure water, or in liquid form.

VOMITING

Make sure the child eats nothing and sips liquid frequently. Use pressure points on wrist for relief as described in Motion Sickness.

HOMEOPATHY

Homeopathic treatment would be *Ipecacuanha* 6x or (if there is unproductive retching) *Nux vomica* 6x.

ALTERNATIVE THERAPIES: A SUPPLEMENTARY GLOSSARY

Part Two of this book introduced you to the major therapies, diagnostic techniques and healing disciplines that are the mainstay of complementary medicine as it is practised today. Information about these therapies, which include such well-known systems of healing as acupuncture, homeopathy, herbal medicine, osteopathy etc., will therefore be found between pages 36 and 61. However, as noted in the Introduction, the term "alternative medicine" encompasses a huge range of other activities and therapies, some of which are viewed with some sympathy by the scientific and medical community, others of which are considered of limited therapeutic value by orthodox physicians, and still others which are dismissed as little more than quackery.

This glossary provides a supplementary listing of the best known of these "alternative" alternative therapies, including brief notes about their origins, and, where appropriate, an indication of how their claims are viewed by orthodox medical opinion.

AIKIDO

A form of Japanese martial art where the "contestants" explore their relationship through a form of ritual dance. Developed by Morihei Oyeshiba as a form of "self realization through discipline", Aikido teaches the arts of self defence through the art of non-resistance.

ANTHROPOSOPH-ICAL MEDICINE

A system of medicine based on the work of German philosopher and mystic Rudolf Steiner (1861-1925) who combined a philosophical approach to health with the use of homeopathy, hydrotherapy, and special exercises. Popular in Europe, a few centres also exist in the UK and USA. Steiner believed in "etheric and astral bodies" and several of the approaches used also have a spiritual and religious focus.

ART THERAPY

Developed out of occupational therapy as practised in mental institutions, art therapy enables patients to express their fears, concerns, dreams and fantasies through the medium of paint, charcoal, drawing or clay modelling. The "act" of painting itself is felt to be therapeutic and trained art therapists are able to use the material created to engage with patients in a more traditional counselling format.

AURICULAR THERAPY

A specialized form of acupuncture where the points used (of which there are more than 200) are all located on the ear. It is believed that, as in reflexology, different points on the ear represent different parts of the body. It was developed in the West by Dr. Paul Nogier of Lyons, France and several maps exist indicating how needling parts of the ear will aid migraine, asthma, arthritis, etc.

AVERSION THERAPY

A form of behaviour therapy used to tackle phobias or addictions. Unpleasant electrical shocks or nausea-inducing drugs are applied to the body in association with the addictive substances so that the client associates the substance with pain or discomfort and thus avoids using it. Successful at first, it is no longer used as extensively as it was previously.

BIOENGERGETICS

A form of "postural integration", or Western form of Yoga, using a combination of movements, breathing exercises and psychological commentary to address problems of living – anxiety, depression, lack of confidence,etc. It was developed in the 1960s by Alexander Lowen in the USA after the work of Wilhelm Reich (see Orgone Therapy).

BIORHYTHMS

A way of explaining the ups and downs we all feel during the course of a day or week. Three such cycles are described – physical (23 days), emotional (28 days) and intellectual (33 days). These rhythms can be worked out by charts or computer analysis and are used to predict periods of accident-proneness or intellectual creativity. While agreeing that internal biological clocks exist, orthodox medicine has not supported the precise predictive qualities claimed by practitioners.

CHARISMATIC HEALING

A resurgence of methods of healing first described by St. Paul in his *Letter to the Corinthians* and taken up by both Protestant and Catholic churches, where the power of the spirit is evoked by the priest through prayer or divine guidance, often accompanied by dance, ritual chanting and healing by laying on of hands.

CHRISTIAN SCIENCE

A movement founded in the United States by Mary Baker Eddy (1821-1910), it is linked to devout Christian belief in the healing principle of God. It is not associated with healing disease specifically but with healing sin, which is felt to account for all disease. It is practised by members of the Church of Christian Scientists.

CLINICAL ECOLOGY

An approach to disease based on the belief that environmental factors are often the cause of disease, whether they be food allergies, energies and radiation in the atmosphere or pollution in water and air. Several scientific instruments have now been developed in an attempt to measure whether such environmental causes of illness can be identified.

COLONIC IRRIGATION

A form of hydrotherapy where warm water is passed via a tube into the rectum and excess waste in the bowel – faeces and toxins – are eliminated. Practitioners believe that the build-up of toxins in the large bowel leads to the causation of many health problems. Orthodox practitioners believe this procedure is, at best, useless; at worst, dangerous.

COLOUR THERAPY

Practitioners believe that colours, across the electro-magnetic spectrum affect mood ("having the blues", "seeing red"), and can be used in reverse to address both physical and psychological states. After a diagnosis, clients will be bathed in light of a particular colour, or advised to visualize a colour, or given advice as to what colours to wear. There is some evidence for the benefit of this practice to the extent that colours in an operating theatre have been altered to take their effect into account.

COUÉISM

Established by Frenchman Emile Coué (1857-1926), who is best remembered for his saying "Every day in every way I am getting better and better", this is a form of auto-suggestion and focuses on strengthening the will through the repetition of phrases and cognitive re-framing. Coué believed he was educating the imagination, and much of his work has been taken up by cognitive therapists.

CO-COUNSELLING

A form of counselling in pairs where each individual in turn acts as counsellor, then as client. Guidelines and rules are agreed upon by the pair beforehand, i.e. "just listen" or "give me your advice". Training is offered for those wishing to act as co-counsellors. The major advantage of this therapy is the reciprocity it involves and its cost (nil).

CRANIAL OSTEOPATHY

A specialized form of osteopathy, pioneered in the United States in the 1920s by William Sutherland, where little or no actual physical manipulation need take place. The work is focused on the skull and spinal cord and it is believed that by gentle manipulation of the skull, the cerebro-spinal fluid is permitted to flow freely and balance out energies that can cause disease.

CRYSTAL AND GEM HEALING

Each precious stone is said to emanate certain vibrations which aid healing. Gems are immersed in water which absorbs their energies, and the water is then used to "treat" disease. Other practices involve wearing particular precious stones, e.g. quartz (physical healing), amethyst (spiritual healing). Needless to say, orthodox medicine considers this method as quackery.

CUPPING

A traditional folk-medicine used in France that also forms part of Traditional Chinese Medicine. Glass cups, heated beforehand, are placed, mouth down, on the patient's body and a vacuum is created as the cups cool. This draws the blood and raises the skin under the cup; the theory holds that it removes toxins. Its popularity rests on its dramatic visual effect, rather than any scientific principles.

DANCE MOVEMENT THERAPY

Like other creative arts therapies, dance is used both to release unexpressed emotions, as well as allowing trained therapists to direct clients to particular areas of emotional conflict. Practised widely in tribal healing ceremonies, more sophisticated approaches are used in the West as a form of special education for autistic children or working with the blind.

DO-IN

A self-help routine practised in China and Japan which combines exercise, massage and acupressure as a health-maintenance programme.

DOWSING

A method of diagnosis using a pendulum, which is said to pick up healing energies and "bad" radiation emanating from the body, and guides the therapist to the most appropriate course of action. It is used by practitioners of radionics. This technique is considered to be well beyond the fringe by most orthodox doctors.

DREAM THERAPY

Part of the traditional holistic approach to healing as practised in Greek temples, dreams were seen as portents of the future and no medical or surgical intervention was practised until the individual's dreams were analyzed. More recently, it forms part of traditional psychoanalysis; Freud described dreams as the "royal road to the unconscious".

ENCOUNTER GROUP

A form of group therapy popular in the 1960s and 1970s associated with the human potential movement. Participants are encouraged to encounter their true innermost feelings by direct expression through the use of specific techniques. Many repressed emotions are released and dramatic breakthroughs are described, but vulnerable individuals may be harmed by these techniques, which are not dissimilar to forms of brain-washing.

EXORCISM

A technique associated with religious cults where ceremonial rituals are used to drive out the devil or evil spirits residing in a house or a person. Such practices are not to be recommended as part of a system of health care.

FAITH HEALING

A traditional basis to many spiritual healing practices where "to believe is to be healed". It can be viewed as a very concentrated form of placebo healing, which occasionally has resulted in dramatic cures.

FELDENKRAIS SYSTEM

Developed by an Israeli physicist, Moshe Feldenkrais, this is a combination of Yoga, exercise, stretches and Alexander technique, undertaken to achieve functional integration through "minimum effort and maximum efficiency". Used by sportsmen and women, it has been developed by his followers as a form of body-psychotherapy.

FLOTATION THERAPY

A method of sensory deprivation, achieved by immersion in a dark, warm, soundless water chamber, which can produce both deep relaxation as well as acute panic. This therapy is not for the faint-hearted and should no be tried without careful supervision.

GALVANISM

A form of electro-therapy where direct electric currents (of small charge) are passed through the body as a way of toning the system and unlocking tense muscles or healing sports injuries.

GEOPATHIC STRESS

A system based on the belief that the Earth's electro-magnetic force produces points of concentration of energy (ley lines), which can be both a force for healing as well as a force for producing disease. Instruments are used that can detect abnormal energies and practitioners then suggest ways of countering geopathic stress by moving furniture, or your house!

GESTALT THERAPY

A form of psychotherapy linked to the Human Potential Movement where the focus is on the "here and now", the expression of immediate feelings and the development of experience and living in the moment. Developed by German psychoanalyst Fritz Perls (1893-1970), it is a form of self-awareness programme rather than treatment.

HAY DIET

A form of diet devised by American doctor William Hay (1866-1940) that avoids food combinations – carbohydrates (starches and sugars) with protein being the most common combination that Hay recommended people should avoid. It is felt that this combination decreases the ability of the body to process the food and leads to digestive disturbances.

IONIZATION

Electrically charged particles in the atmosphere can be the cause of both well-being and illness; negative ions are found by the seaside or on top of mountains and positive ions are present in stuffy, over-crowded atmospheres. An excess of positive ions is associated with headaches, tension and irritability. Small ionizers help to change the electric charge in the atmosphere and have been used to effect improvements in offices and for asthma sufferers at home.

IRIDOLOGY

The study of the iris (the coloured part of the eye) is said to be diagnostic of inner disease. Practitioners using a lens, or photographs of the patient's eyes, claim to be able to detect signs of organ damage by identifying abnormal pigments or deposits.

Most doctors do not feel this technique has any scientific validity.

KINESIOLOGY

A form of diagnosis of allergies based on muscle-testing. If the subject is allergic to wheat, then it is believed that holding a piece of bread in an outstretched hand will reduce the power of the muscles in that arm to resist pressure. Muscle testing is the basis of this method but other techniques are also used. Once allergies are detected, then alternative foods are recommended.

MACROBIOTICS

This is a form of diet based on the belief that each food substance has qualities of Yin and Yang, i.e. too much Yin food (milk, cheese, butter) will produce lethargy and depression, and too much Yang food (meat, spices, eggs) will produce aggression, tension, etc. The diet is determined by the right combination of foods, once a diagnosis of the Yin/Yang balance is arrived at by a qualified practitioner.

MCTIMONEY CHIROPRACTIC

A modified form of chiropractic which uses more gentle manipulative movements to address musculo-skeletal problems: it has been used also for treating animals.

METAMORPHIC TECHNIQUE

A modified form of osteopathy, developed by British therapist Robert St. John (1912-), focusing on the hands, feet and head. It attempts to bring the body's energies into balance rather than concentrating on a particular disease.

MUSIC THERAPY

One of the more developed forms of creative art therapies which addresses the issue of

communication problems in autistic children and people with speech difficulties. Its effects can be dramatic and long-lasting, and it is now an accepted form of treatment within orthodox medical practice.

ORGONE THERAPY

This is based on the work of psychiatrist Wilhelm Reich (1897-1957) who believed that blockages in human energy systems (called orgone) were the basis of much human and emotional stress. He constructed an orgone box in which patients sat to balance their energy flows. His ideas are now largely discarded, although some of his work has been developed within Bioenergtics.

POLARITY THERAPY

A combination of Western and Eastern techniques of balancing energy flow in the body devised by American naturopath Dr. Randolph Stone (1890-1983) using manipulation, massage, exercise, diet and relaxation techniques. Through a systematic routine, parts of the body that have polarity relationships are brought into balance with one another.

PRIMAL THERAPY

A form of early regression – usually under hypnotic trance – where clients are encouraged to relive the birth process and, in so doing, explore and express their earliest memories (such as the primal scream). Developed by Dr. Arthur Janov, it is occasionally practised in encounter groups and humanistic psychotherapy meetings.

PSIONIC MEDICINE

A system of diagnosis based on a combination of pendulum power, dowsing and miasm theory (the belief that certain inner disruptive factors inhibit the body's ability to heal itself) combined with treatments, usually homeopathic

or naturopathic in origin. It was developed in the 1960s by a UK general practitioner, Dr. George Laurence.

PSYCHIC SURGERY

A form of shamanistic healing found in primitive tribes, such as in Brazil and the Philippines, which has achieved some notoriety in the West as a result of TV documentaries. Under the influence of a trance, a healer "extracts" poisonous substances from the patient by motions of his hands over the body. It is generally considered to be a particularly clever sleight-of-hand trickery, combined with charismatic influences.

PSYCHOSYNTHESIS

A combination of psychotherapeutic approaches, some analytical, some humanistic, which focus on the transpersonal or spiritual development of the client. Developed by Italian psychiatrist Dr. Roberto Assagioli (1888-1974), it is now more commonly known as Transpersonal Psychology.

PYRAMID POWER

A system of therapy that is based on the belief that pyramids are built in such a way that the energy concentrated underneath them has special healing and preserving powers. Experiments conducted with electro-encephalograms (brain-wave machines) of people sitting inside pyramids purport to show changes in brain activity similar to those found when individuals are in deep meditation.

RADIONICS AND RADIESTHESIA

A system of energy healing developed in the 1920s by a Swiss priest, Abbé Mermet, which purports to analyze the energy flow of patient from a life-history chart, and then corrects any imbalances by sending out natural life-healing energies from a series of electrical machines. It is not accepted as valid by orthodox practitioners.

ROGERIAN THERAPY

A form of psychotherapy developed by Carl Rogers (1902-1987) which is also known as "person-centred-psychotherapy" and encourages the active participation of the client towards positive feelings regarding him/herself/others. The therapist is "non-directive" and allows the client to feel in control.

ROLFING

A form of manipulative therapy through deep massage that can last hours based on the work of American biologist Dr. Ida Rolf (1896-1979), where emphasis is placed on correct body posture and balancing the body's own energy field. The focus is more on encouraging healthy living than on treating specific disease. It is also known as structural integration.

SHAMANISM

The oldest method of healing arising from primitive tribal healers (shamans), which combines a form of ritual dance, prayer and the use of herbal treatments. Shamans tended to focus on groups rather than individuals, and were often used to divine weather-changes and to protect the community from outside attack through their intercession with the spirit world, which came about during trances.

SILVA MIND CONTROL

A form of auto-suggestion, or mind over matter, developed in the 1960s by José Silva, which focuses on integrating body and mind, and uses techniques common in autogenic training and cognitive therapy.

THERAPEUTIC TOUCH

Popular in the United States of America, this form of spiritual healing has developed from the work of Dolores Kruger, a nurse who studied the effects of touch and massage on different states of disease and illness. The healer runs his or her hands lightly over the patient seeking out areas of sickness or energy imbalance, and allowing healing energy to flow into the patient. Several studies have indicated changes in levels of haemoglobin and other objective measures as a result of this technique.

TRANSACTIONAL ANALYSIS

A form of therapy created by American psychiatrist Dr. Eric Berne (1910-1970) based on the belief that three ego states exist within each individual – parent, adult, child – and that we can understand communication problems by analyzing the way we relate to others using these three states of mind. It was further developed and popularized by Eric Berne in his book *Games People Play*.

TRANSCUTANEOUS NERVE STIMULATION

A technique developed for chronic pain sufferers which uses a machine that send minute electrical impulses to the nerves and muscles to block out the pain impulses. Based on a form of electro-acupuncture, these little machines are now widely used in pain clinics.

TURKISH BATHS

Popular in the 19th century, this form of hydrotherapy is returning into use. The combination of steam and heat associated with a Turkish bath means that perspiration does not evaporate, and the treatment is said to relieve the body of toxins and impurities through the copious sweating it encourages.

VOICE THERAPY

A skilled and specific use of the voice accompanied by breathing exercises, which can be used solely for voice training, but which has also found its place as a form of modified psychotherapy through the expressive nature of the technique.

ZEN THERAPY

A systematic series of meditative exercises associated with Buddhist philosophy which aims to bring about integration of body, mind and spirit.

ZONE THERAPY

A specialized and earlier form of reflexology which is based on the belief that different parts of the soles of the feet represent different organ systems in the body. By manipulating these points, correction can be applied and the body's powers of healing encouraged. It was developed by American physician Dr. William H. Fitzgerald in the early years of the 20th century.

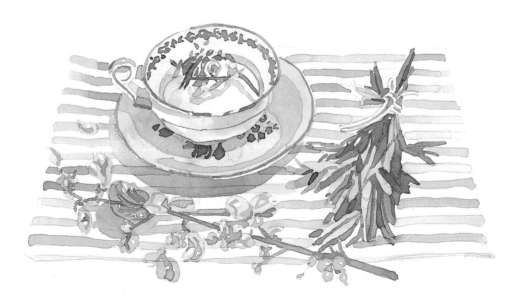

Index

PICTURE CREDITS

The publishers wish to thank the following picture libraries who have supplied photographs for this book. The photographs have been credited by page number and position on the page: (B) Bottom, (T) Top, (C) Centre, (BL) Bottom Left, etc.

The Bach Centre, Mount Vernon: 52, 53T.

Frank Lane Picture Agency: 22 (Silvestris), 34CR (Celtic Picture Library), 37T (Manfred Rutz, Silvestris), 44T (Life Science Images), 57T (E. Coppola), 69B (Life Science Images), 73 (Life Science Images), 87TL (Life Science Images), 88BL (Life Science Images), 89BC (Life Science Images), 93BL (Life Science Images), 96BL (Life Science Images), 97TL (Life Science Images), 99 (Life Science Images), 108T (Life Science Images), 109BL (Life Science Images), 113T (Life Science Images), 155L (Eva Lindenburger, Silvestris), 158BR (Life Science Images), 161BR (Life Science Images), 207 (Silvestris), 209 (Dr. Gerd Wagner, Silvestris).

Images Colour Library: 3, 8TR, 10BL, 11TR, 11BL, 13TR, 19BR, 20BL, 24TL, 24CR, 25, 27, 29, 31TR, 44B, 45T, 45B, 48, 49T, 49B, 55T, 56, 58B, 59, 60, 69T, 76BR, 82, 103B, 105BL, 109TL, 111, 114BL, 115BR, 118BL, 137, 141TR, 141BL, 147TR, 149TR, 154BR, 169, 172BR, 176TC, 183BR, 195CR, 215.

The Image Works: 10 (John Griffin), 12 (Daemmrich), 15TR (M. Siluk), 17BL (M. Greenlar), 18B (R. Lord), 30 (T. Michaels), 32TR (Antman), 33 (W. Hill Jr.), 40B (Bachmann), 58T (M. Schwarz), 61T (Joe Carini), 61B (Bachmann), 80 (Tony Sarino), 91CL (K. Preuss), 108BL (Daemmrich), 116BL (Esbin-Anderson), 118TC (Gontier), 125T (K. Preuss), 136 (W. Hill), 156 (Kolvoord), 203TL (Mulvehill).

The Science Photo Library: 8BL (St. Bartholomew's Hospital), 9TR (Paul Biddle & Tim Malyon), 9BL (Oscar Burriel, Latin Stock), 13TL (Simon Fraser), 13B (Stevie Grand), 14BL (BSIP/Boucharlat), 14TR (BSIP/Zarand), 15BL (BSIP/Barrelle), 16 (Oscar Burriel, Latin Stock), 17TR (Sheila Terry), 18T (Sheila Terry), 19TL (Barrelle/BSIP), 19TR (Sheila Terry), 20TR (Tony Craddock), 20CR (Sheila Terry), 21BL (Tony Craddock), 21TR (E. Nelson/Custom Medical Stock Photo), 23 (Oscar Burriel, Latin Stock), 28 (Jerry Wachter), 31BL (John Mead), 32BL (Oscar Burriel, Latin Stock), 34TC (Martin Bond), 34BL (Simon

Fraser), 35T (Hank Morgan), 35BL (Dr. Morley Read), 35BR (Martin Bond), 36 (Françoise Sauze), 37C (BSIP, Boucharlat), 39T and 39B (Paul Biddle & Tim Malyon), 40T (Andrew McClenaghan), 41 (Hattie Young), 42T (Art Stein), 42B (Françoise Sauze), 43T (Paul Biddle), 43B (Dr. Jeremy Burgess), 46T (David Campione), 46BR (Françoise Sauze), 47T (Hattie Young), 47B (Andrew McClenaghan), 50T (Robert Goldstein), 50B (G. Hadji, CNRI), 51T and 51B (Damien Lovegrove), 53B (BSIP), 54T (Seth Joel), 55B (Paul Biddle & Tim Malyon), 57B (Alexander Tsiaras), 64 (David Scharf), 65 (Hattie Young), 67 (Andrew McClenaghan), 68T (Dr. Gary Settles), 68B (Seth Joel), 70 (Adrienne Hart-Davis), 71T (Dr. Gary Settles), 72 (Alexander Tsiaras), 75 (Oscar Burriel, Latin Stock), 76T (Andrew McClenaghan), 76BL, 77 (Institut Pasteur/CNRI), 78 (Dr. Gopal Murti), 79 (BSIP/Collet), 81 (St. Bartholomew's Hospital), 84 (Western Ophthalmic Hospital), 85 (Jean Perrin/CNRI), 86TR (Westminster Hospital), 86BL (Eric Grave), 87BR (Françoise Sauze), 88TR, 89TL (Seth Joel), 90 (CNRI), 91TC (CNRI), 92TR (Michael Marten), 92BL (Simon Fraser), 93TR (CNRI), 94TR (Dr. P. Marazzi), 94BL (Tony Craddock), 95 (Moredun Animal Health Ltd), 96TR (Damien Lovegrove), 97BR (Françoise Sauze), 98TC (David Scharf), 98BL, 98BR (Astrid and Hanns-Frieder Michler), 100 (Sheila Terry), 101TL (Françoise Sauze), 101BR (Alexander Tsiaras), 102 (BSIP/Boucharlat), 103TR (Françoise Sauze), 104 (St. Bartholomew's Hospital), 105T (Dr. Gopal Murti), 106TR (Clinical Radiology Dept, Salisbury District Hospital), 107 (John Durham), 109BR (Françoise Sauze), 110 (Chris Bjornberg), 112 (Adrienne Hart-Davis), 113B (Damien Lovegrove), 114TR (Sheila Terry), 115TC (John Greim), 116TR, 116BR (Professor P. Motta, University of La Sapienza, Rome), 117 (Seth Joel), 119 (Martin/Custom Medical Stock Photo), 120 (Oscar Burriel, Latin Stock), 121 (Jim Selby), 122TL (Professors P. Motta and F. Magliocca), 122BR, 124, 125BR (Paul Biddle & Tim Malyon), 126 (BSIP/DPA), 127TC (Hattie Young), 127CL (Princess Margaret Rose Orthopaedic Hospital), 127BR (Paul Biddle & Tim Malyon), 128 (Professors P. Motta, P.M. Andrews, K.R. Porter and J. Vial), 129TR (Mike McNamee), 129BL (Françoise Sauze), 130 (Ron Sutherland), 131 (Hattie Young), 132TR (Sheila Terry), 132BL (Professor P. Motta, University of La Sapienza, Rome), 133TR (Sheila Terry), 133BL (Hank Morgan), 134 (St. Bartholomew's Hospital), 135TR (BSIP/Barrelle), 135BL (Custom Medical Stock Photo), 138TL (Dr. H.C. Robinson), 138BR (Dr. P. Marazzi), 139 (Oscar Burriel, Latin

Stock), 140TR (BSIP/MASO), 140BL (Dr. H.C. Robinson), 142TR (BSIP/Collet), 142BL, 143 (Alex Bartel), 144 (Mark Clarke), 145 (Dr. P. Marazzi), 146T (BSIP/Barrelle), 146B (Dr. Jeremy Burgess), 147BL (Dr. P. Marazzi), 148TL (Dr. P. Marazzi), 148TR (St. Bartholomew's Hospital), 148BR, 149BR (BSIP/LECA), 150T (Dr. Jeremy Burgess), 150B (Eamon McNulty), 151TR (Oscar Burriel, Latin Stock), 151BL (Jane Shemilt), 152 (Oscar Burriel, Latin Stock), 153TL (Seth Joel), 153R (Will and Deni McIntyre), 154TL (BSIP/Alexandre), 155BR (Paul Biddle & Tim Malyon), 157 (CNRI), 158C (Paul Biddle), 159CR (Sheila Terry), 159BR (Françoise Sauze), 160TL (Scott Camazine), 160TR (John Greim), 160BR (Damien Lovegrove), 161TC (Paul Biddle & Tim Malyon), 161BL (Simon Fraser, Hexham General Hospital), 162TL (Catherine Pouedras), 162BR (J.C. Revy), 163 (Oscar Burriel, Latin Stock), 164TR (David Parker), 164BL (Dr. Jeremy Burgess), 165 (Chris Priest), 166TR (Adam Hart-Davis), 166BL (CNRI), 167 (Dr. Jeremy Burgess), 168 (Oscar Burriel, Latin Stock), 170 (Mark Clarke), 171 (Paul Biddle), 172TL (Alfred Pasieka), 173 (Sheila Terry), 174TL (Dr. Kari Lounatmaa), 174TR (John Heseltine), 174BR (Alfred Pasieka), 175 (Nicholas de Siose), 176BL (Professor P. Motta, University of La Sapienza, Rome), 177 (Ron Sutherland), 178 (BSIP/MASO), 179 (Astrid and Hanns-Frieder Michler), 180 (Simon Fraser), 181 (Scott Camazine), 182TR (Oscar Burriel, Latin Stock), 182BL (Adam Hart-Davis), 183TL (Peter Menzel), 184 (Sheila Terry), 186 (Oscar Burriel, Latin Stock), 188 (Larry Mulvehill), 189T (John Heseltine), 189B (Doug Plumer), 190 (Philippe Plailly), 191T (Philippe Plailly), 191BL (Vaughan Fleming), 192TL (Will and Deni McIntyre), 192BR (Tim Beddow), 193T (James King-Holmes), 193B (Mark Clarke), 194T (Cecil H. Fox), 194BL (Dr. Jeremy Burgess), 195TL (David Grossman), 195BC (John Heseltine), 196TL and 196BR (John Heseltine), 197CL (Oscar Burriel, Latin Stock), 197BC (Andrew McClenaghan), 198TL (Dr. Andrejs Liepins), 198B (John Greim), 199TL (Phil Jude), 199BR (Andrew McClenaghan), 200TR (Hank Morgan), 200BL (Jon Wilson), 201TC (NIBSC), 201CR (Oscar Burriel, Latin Stock), 201BL (BSIP/LECA), 202TL, 202BR (Sheila Terry), 203BR (Hank Morgan), 210 (Hattie Young), 213 (Astrid and Hanns-Frieder Michler).

Jacket photographs: The Image Works (Daemmrich): left. Images Colour Library: top centre and right. Science Photo Library (David Campione): bottom centre.